Nutrition and Child Health

For Baillière Tindall:

Senior Commissioning Editor: Jacqueline Curthoys
Project Manager: Gail Murray
Project Development Manager: Karen Gilmour
Designer: George Ajayi

Nutrition and Child Health

Chris Holden MSc RGN RSCN
Head of Department, Clinical Nurse Specialist,
Nutritional Care, The Birmingham Children's
Hospital NHS Trust, Diana, Princess of Wales
Children's Hospital, Birmingham, UK

Anita MacDonald BSc PhD SRD
Head of Dietetic Services, Dietetic Department,
The Birmingham Children's Hospital
NHS Trust, Diana, Princess of Wales
Children's Hospital, Birmingham, UK

Foreword by

Brian Wharton MD DSc FRCP FRCPCH
Honorary Professor of University College
London at the Institute of Child Health,
London, UK

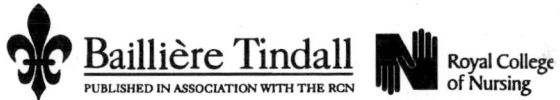

Baillière Tindall
PUBLISHED IN ASSOCIATION WITH THE RCN

Royal College
of Nursing

EDINBURGH LONDON NEW YORK PHILADELPHIA ST LOUIS SYDNEY TORONTO 2000

BAILLIÈRE TINDALL
An imprint of Harcourt Publishers Limited

© Harcourt Publishers Limited 2000

 is a registered trademark of Harcourt Publishers Limited

First published 2000

ISBN 0 7020 2421 X

British Library Cataloguing in Publication Data
A catalogue record for this book is available from the British Library

Library of Congress Cataloging in Publication Data
A catalog record for this book is available from the Library of
Congress

Note
Medical knowledge is constantly changing. As new information
becomes available, changes in treatment, procedures, equipment
and the use of drugs become necessary. The editors, contributors and the
publishers have taken care to ensure that the information given in this text
is accurate and up to date. However, readers are strongly advised to confirm
that the information, especially with regard to drug usage, complies with
the latest legislation and standards of practice.

The
Publisher's
policy is to use
**paper manufactured
from sustainable forests**

Printed in China

Contents

Contributors

Gill Abel BSc(Hons) RSCN
Clinical Nurse Specialist Nutritional Care, The
General Infirmary at Leeds, Leeds, UK

Liz Allott BSc SRD
Senior Community Dietitian (Learning
Disabilities), Ipswich Hospital NHS Trust,
Ipswich, UK

Debra Caney RGN RSCN
Nutritional Care Sister, The Birmingham
Children's Hospital NHS Trust, Diana, Princess of
Wales Children's Hospital, Birmingham, UK

Maureen Chadderton RGN RM RHV
Health Visitor, Broadmeadow Health Centre,
Birmingham, UK

Jane Coad BSc(Hons) RGN RSCN DipNurs
Senior Lecturer, Faculty of Health, University of
Central England, Birmingham, UK

Peter Hodgkinson RGN RSCN ENB 603, 870, 998
Ward Manager, Ward 3, The Birmingham
Children's Hospital NHS Trust, Diana, Princess of
Wales Children's Hospital, Birmingham, UK

Tracey Johnson BSc SRD DipADP
Paediatric Dietitian, The Birmingham Children's
Hospital NHS Trust, Diana, Princess of Wales
Children's Hospital, Birmingham, UK

Jeremy Kirk MD FRCPCH DCH
Consultant Paediatric Endocrinologist, The
Birmingham Children's Hospital NHS Trust,
Diana, Princess of Wales Children's Hospital,
Birmingham, UK

Bob Moloney BSc RGN RSCN DipEd
Senior Lecturer, Faculty of Health, University of
Central England, Birmingham, UK

Carolyn Patchell BSc SRD
Chief Paediatric Dietitian, The Birmingham
Children's Hospital NHS Trust, Diana, Princess
of Wales Children's Hospital, Birmingham, UK

John W L Puntis BM(Hons) DM FRCP FRCPCH
Senior Lecturer in Paediatrics and Child Health
and Consultant Paediatrician, The Children's
Centre, The General Infirmary at Leeds, Leeds,
UK

Elaine Sexton BSc(Hons) RGN RSCN
Nutritional Care Sister, The Birmingham
Children's Hospital NHS Trust, Diana, Princess of
Wales Children's Hospital, Birmingham, UK

Malli Wadge RGN RSCN ENB 603, 870, 970, 998
DipEHCP NLP NNEB
Senior Clinical Sister, Ward 3, The Birmingham
Children's Hospital NHS Trust, Diana, Princess of
Wales Children's Hospital, Birmingham, UK

Foreword

The nutritional health of children has many dimensions. They include the genetic makeup of the individual and the ability to handle each nutrient, the stage of development the child has reached from conception to adolescence, and environmental influences such as infection, socioeconomic circumstances and love. Equally, the practice of paediatric nutrition has many facets: it is a whole body discipline, crossing the presently accepted artificial boundaries between organ specialization, hospital and community, body and mind, and the health care professions.

This book brings together the many dimensions of nutritional health including genetic disorders, the priorities which change with age to ensure successful growth and development, and various environmental stresses. The many facets of nutritional management are presented, calling on a spectrum of experience and discipline. The authors have moulded an attractive amalgam of science and practice.

Brian Wharton

Preface

This is a practical, evidence-based textbook on normal and special paediatric nutrition. It has been written in collaboration with a number of experienced health workers, each of whom has given a foundation of scientific facts and has provided pragmatic, balanced and sensible guidelines, as well as identifying common difficulties and issues relating to their topic.

This book is divided into two sections. Chapters 1 to 6 deal with normal nutrition in pregnancy, infants and children. These chapters cover all aspects of maternal and fetal nutrition, infant feeding, feeding the pre-school child and feeding school-age children and adolescents.

Chapters 7 to 14 deal with feeding sick children, and cover eating disorders, feeding children with special needs, special diets and enteral and parenteral nutrition. There is a chapter on growth and nutritional assessment. Nutritional support for children in the community also features highly as increasing numbers of chronically sick children with nutritional problems are now managed in the primary care setting.

This book has tried sensitively to tackle difficult issues such as ethnicity, culture, poverty and children's rights. Interdisciplinary working is a key theme and, if applied successfully, should help to dispel many of the misleading and conflicting nutritional messages which are widespread.

This book is aimed at providing practical guidance to hospital and community paediatric nurses, health visitors, student nurses, dietitians, medical and dietetic students, and all those in hospital, community and primary care settings who are interested in child nutrition.

In order to make this book easier to read, lists have been used where appropriate, key learning points are identified in many chapters, case histories are used to highlight specific points, and short questions are provided at the end of some chapters to help students assimilate information.

There is a growing awareness among the public that good nutrition is a major determinant of growth, development and long-term health in both the healthy and the sick child. If this book achieves its aims, it should help all health professionals provide accurate, practical and consistent advice to parents and children.

Birmingham 2000

Chris Holden
Anita MacDonald

1

Section One
Normal nutrition and pregnancy

Maternal and fetal nutrition

John W L Puntis

INTRODUCTION

Increasing importance is being attributed to nutritional status during reproductive years. There is evidence that nutritional factors influence fertility, embryogenesis, fetal growth and maternal adaptation to pregnancy. However, the wide variation in dietary recommendations for pregnant women indicates a lack of consensus regarding optimal nutritional intake (Hautvast 1997). Folk wisdom decrees that the mother should 'eat for two', but many studies have shown that energy intake during pregnancy hardly increases. This may be because pregnant women significantly reduce their physical activity and energy expenditure.

Folic acid is one micronutrient of considerable importance, and deficiency is now firmly linked with the risk of neural tube defects. Whether adequate blood concentrations can be achieved by following specific dietary and food recommendations as an alternative to taking tablets or folate fortified products is under investigation. Folic acid regulates the homocysteine status of the body. With increased plasma homocysteine concentrations being implicated as a risk factor for cardiovascular disease, research in the area of folate metabolism is now of much wider general interest.

Iron, another important nutrient, is no longer prescribed for all pregnant women as a routine, but deficiency is still relatively common and should be identified and treated. Maternal and fetal nutrition is now being brought to the forefront of public health and nutrition policy considerations as a result of the increasing scale of epidemiological data linking the risks of adult diseases to nutrition and growth in early life: the Barker hypothesis.

NUTRITIONAL REQUIREMENTS IN PREGNANCY

The pregnant woman must have an adequate supply of nutrients to ensure normal growth and development of the fetus. Evidence related to neural tube defects and other congenital abnormalities (Czeizel 1993) and from studies of low birth weight and prematurity (Scholl et al 1997) also emphasise the importance of nutritional status around the time of conception. In low income women, dietary improvements following one pregnancy can lead to increased mean birth weight in the next (Thomson 1959).

Table 1.1 shows the extra dietary requirements of pregnant women. The reference nutrient intake (RNI) for protein is 45 g/day and women in relatively affluent countries such as the United Kingdom are unlikely to have intakes below this. An increase of 200 kcal/day in energy intake is recommended only for the third trimester of pregnancy. Lower energy expenditure in pregnant women has been shown to be related to a reduction in the amount and pace of physical activity, which in turn is accompanied by a reduction in vitamin

Table 1.2 Percentage of British women with nutrient intakes below the lower references nutrient intake (LRNI) (MAFF 1994. Crown copyright material is reproduced with the permission of the Controller of Her Majesty's Stationery Office.)

	Aged 16–18		Aged 19–50	
	LRNI	%	LRNI	%
magnesium	190 mg	39	150 mg	13
iron	8 mg	33	8 mg	26
calcium	480 mg	27	400 mg	10
zinc	4 mg	6	4 mg	4
vitamin B_2	0.8 mg	9	0.8 mg	8
vitamin A	250 µg	7	250 µg	3
folic acid	100 µg	4	100 µg	4
vitamin B_{12}	1 µg	4	1 µg	1
vitamin C	10 mg	0	10 mg	1

and mineral intake. It is striking that a number of dietary surveys have indicated considerable numbers of women may have an inadequate intake of minerals important in pregnancy (Table 1.2).

Iron

Iron requirements increase during pregnancy and are thought to be met by mobilization of iron stores, increased absorption and cessation of menstrual loss. The prevalence of anaemia (haemoglobin below 110 g/L) during pregnancy may be as high as 10% in industrialized countries, and 50% worldwide. Associated adverse effects are shown in Box 1.1.

However, data on these effects are not conclusive and whether or not iron supplementation during pregnancy should be generally promoted remains controversial (Roodenburg 1995). Iron deficiency in the mother does not seem to increase the risk of the infant being born iron deficient, but

Table 1.1 Reference nutrient intakes for pregnancy – additional daily requirements (DoH 1991. Crown copyright material is reproduced with the permission of the Controller of Her Majesty's Stationery Office.)

	Amount for a pregnant woman	% increase compared with a non-pregnant woman
energy	200 kcal[a]	10
protein	6 g	13
riboflavin	0.3 mg	27
folate	100 µg[b]	50
vitamin C	10 mg	25
vitamin A	100 µg	17
vitamin D	10 µg[c]	c

[a] during last trimester
[b] 400 µg during the first 12 weeks, then 100 µg for the remainder of pregnancy
[c] vitamin D synthesis in skin is sufficient for requirements in an adult with a normal lifestyle including exposure to sunlight. Pregnant women are recommended to take supplementary vitamin D to achieve an intake of 10 µg/day.

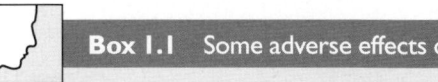

Box 1.1 Some adverse effects of anaemia

◆ Fatigue and decreased work performance.

◆ Increased risk of urinary tract infection and pyelonephritis.

◆ Perinatal death, preterm delivery and low birth weight.

may have a negative impact on iron status in infancy. It would appear reasonable practice to screen high risk groups (e.g. teenagers, low income mothers and vegans) for iron deficiency and treat if confirmed.

Many women increase milk consumption in pregnancy and calcium may inhibit iron absorption. In a recent study of 576 women (Robinson et al 1998) serum ferritin concentrations at the first antenatal visit were typically lower in multiparous, taller, thinner and younger women, and in those who had given blood in the year before pregnancy. Ferritin concentrations fell with increasing calcium intake: the proportion of women with ferritin values below 12 µg/L rose from 14% of those in the lowest quarter of calcium intake to 29% in the highest. This study suggests that dietary effects on iron availability are significant in pregnancy and this may have implications for the definition of dietary iron requirements.

Folic acid and neural tube defects

Neural tube defects (NTDs) include the following:

- ◆ anencephaly – this accounts for about half of all NTDs; most of the brain and skull are absent, resulting in stillbirth or death very soon after birth.
- ◆ encephalocoele – a rare condition in which the brain protrudes through a defect in the skull.
- ◆ spina bifida – the spinal canal in the vertebral column is not closed, although the defect can be covered by skin; spina bifida varies in severity, leading to only minor disability in some cases, but paralysis coupled with incontinence in others.

The prevalence of NTDs fell from about 4 per 1000 births in the 1970s to 0.3 per 1000 in the 1990s, mainly due to screening and selective terminations. A number of studies in the 1980s suggested that taking folic acid from before conception might reduce the risk of NTDs. This was subsequently tested in a large randomized double blind trial (MRC Vitamin Study Group 1991). Women who had previously given birth to a baby with NTD participated, and were allocated to receive 4 mg of folic acid each day, a multivitamin prepara-

Box 1.2 Food sources of folate or folic acid

Rich sources (more than 100 µg per serving)
Fresh, raw or cooked Brussels sprouts, asparagus, spinach, kale, cooked black-eye beans.
Breakfast cereals (fortified with folic acid).
Liver (not recommended during pregnancy because of high vitamin A content).

Good sources (50–100 µg per serving)
Fresh, raw, frozen and cooked broccoli, spring greens, cabbage, green beans, cauliflower, peas, beansprouts, okra, cooked soya beans, iceberg lettuce, parsnips, chick peas.
Kidneys, yeast and beef extracts.

Moderate sources (15–50 µg per serving)
Potatoes, most other fresh and cooked vegetables, most fruits, most nuts, tahini.
Bread, brown rice, wholegrain pasta, oats, bran, Weetaflakes, Weetabix.
Cheese, yoghurt, milk (pint), eggs, salmon, beef, game.

Poor sources (less than 15 µg per serving)
White rice, white pasta, alcoholic drinks, soft drinks, sugar, most pastries, cakes, most other meats and fish.
Most other breakfast cereals not fortified with folic acid.

tion, both, or neither. Folic acid was shown to offer a protective effect of 72%, with multivitamins alone showing no significant protective effect.

It is not known how oral administration of folic acid prevents NTDs, although it may be that folic acid, which is efficiently absorbed and then incompletely converted into metabolically active folates, corrects a folate deficiency. Food sources of folic acid are shown in Box 1.2. The daily dose advised by the Chief Medical Officer for the prevention of recurrence of NTD was 5 mg, continued to the twelfth week of pregnancy (Department of Health 1992). However, 95% of NTDs are in infants born to mothers who have not previously had a baby with this malformation. Evidence suggests that a daily dose of 400 µg of folic acid prior to conception, and during the first 12 weeks of pregnancy is likely to be protective and can be achieved by eating more foods containing natural folate, eating more foods fortified with folic acid, or by taking supplementary folic acid as a medicinal preparation.

Other vitamins

Vitamin A. In pregnancy, extra vitamin A is required for growth and maintenance of the fetus, for providing it with some reserves, and for maternal tissue growth. An increment of 100 µg/day throughout pregnancy (raising the maternal RNI to 700 µg/day) should enhance maternal storage and provide sufficient for the rapidly growing fetus. Most women in the UK have a vitamin A intake in excess of this, and only a small number are likely to need supplementation. High intakes (more than 3300 µg/day) may be associated with craniofacial, cardiac, thymic and central nervous system birth defects. As a precautionary measure women in the UK who are, or might become, pregnant have therefore been advised not to take multivitamin supplements containing vitamin A, and to avoid eating liver and liver products, which are very rich in retinol. In many parts of the world where dietary intake is poor, vitamin A deficiency is common and, through its effects on the integrity of epithelial surfaces, may be an important risk factor in transmission of the human immunodeficiency virus (Mostad et al 1997).

Vitamin D. This is essential for maintaining calcium homeostasis (plasma calcium being kept within narrow limits), in part by varying the proportions of dietary calcium absorbed and excreted. Vitamin D is the precursor of 25-hydroxy vitamin D (25-OH D), which in pregnancy shows a seasonal variation; there is a significant correlation between maternal and cord blood 25-OH D. Women with poor dietary intake and little exposure to sunlight may be deficient in vitamin D. Pregnant women should receive supplementary vitamin D to achieve an intake of 10 µg/day. Vitamin D deficiency is relatively more common in the Asian community.

Vitamin C. This prevents scurvy and aids wound healing; it also assists in the absorption of non-haem iron and is an important antioxidant. During pregnancy there is a moderate extra drain on tissue stores with the fetus concentrating the vitamin at the expense of maternal stores and circulating vitamin levels. The RNI for vitamin C therefore increases by 10 mg/day during the last trimester (to 50 mg), the equivalent of one large orange or 130 ml of orange juice.

Box 1.3 Terms used to describe small infants

Low birth weight (LBW) – below 2500 g

Very low birth weight (VLBW) – below 1500 g

Small for gestational age (SGA) – below 10th centile for gestational age

Large for gestational age (LGA) – above 90th centile for gestational age

Appropriate for gestational age (AGA) – between 10th and 90th centile

Intrauterine growth retardation (IUGR) – a pathophysiologic process resulting in restriction of fetal growth

FETAL GROWTH AND SMALL INFANTS

A number of different terms are commonly used to describe small infants. These are shown in Box 1.3.

It should be noted, therefore, that SGA refers to a statistical grouping of infants (the 10% who fall below this centile) and therefore includes both small normal infants, as well as those who are growth-restricted. In addition, some AGA infants will in fact be growth-restricted, having 'fallen down' the centiles but not actually crossed the 10th centile. Thus, IUGR may more commonly result in a failure to meet growth potential than being SGA, a concept analogous to 'failure to thrive' in infancy (Edwards et al 1990).

Being born small at term may reflect either a reduced growth potential, or growth restriction as a consequence of malnutrition during fetal development. Reduced growth potential results from:

◆ genetic factors
◆ chromosomal abnormalities
◆ major congenital malformations
◆ intrauterine infection (e.g. rubella, cytomegalovirus and toxoplasmosis).

Malnutrition as a consequence of insufficient nutrient supply can be the result of either maternal problems, or impaired placental function due to:

◆ maternal hypertension
◆ smoking
◆ severe maternal cardiac and renal disease
◆ severe maternal nutritional deficiency
◆ placental failure.

Antenatal ultrasound measurements are generally regarded as the most sensitive method for detecting poor growth. Intrauterine growth is an important indicator of fetal health as growth-retarded infants are known to have both greater morbidity and mortality (Heinone et al 1988). However, maternal variables which are known to affect fetal growth include maternal weight and height, ethnic origin and parity. If these factors are

KEY POINTS

◆ Growth retardation is known to be associated with increased risk of morbidity and mortality.
◆ Being small at birth may reflect a reduced growth potential, as with some genetic defects, or failure of nutritional supply: for example, as a result of placental failure.
◆ Ultrasound examinations are used to assess fetal growth during pregnancy.
◆ It is easier to pick out 'small' babies (some of whom will in fact be normal) than the larger group of those who are compromised and failing to meet their full growth potential yet not unduly small.

taken into account, a large proportion of babies are found to be incorrectly classified as growth-retarded when they are normal, and vice versa (Gardosi et al 1992).

THE FETAL AND INFANT ORIGINS OF INEQUALITIES IN HEALTH

The inequalities in health between social classes and geographical regions represent one of the greatest challenges for the makers of health and social policy at the present time. It has been hypothesized that these inequalities are intimately related to maternal and fetal nutrition (Barker 1988). Being small at birth may therefore have very important long-term implications for health. Variation in adult mortality in Britain reflects differences in death rates from a number of chronic diseases, with ischaemic heart disease, stroke and chronic obstructive lung disease being the most important. Evidence now points to the fact that nutritional influences in fetal and infant life can have a permanent effect both on organ structure and metabolism, and hence on the risk of developing these conditions. Such long-lasting effects of transitory influences during a critical period of development is referred to as 'programming' (see below).

Geographical and social class differences in fetal and infant growth which existed when today's generation of middle-aged and elderly people were born, were reflected in the wide range of infant mortality at that time. For instance, towards the beginning of the 20th century infant mortality was almost three times higher in northern industrial towns than in rich southern areas.

Differences in infant mortality were found to be related to differences in maternal physique and health, infant feeding, housing and overcrowding. If mortality statistics for England and Wales are now used to compare today's distribution of adult death rates from specific causes with the past geographical distribution of infant mortality, the results are often striking. Today, for example, the mortality from chronic obstructive lung disease is concentrated in large towns and cities and distributed in a pattern closely matching infant mortality from bronchitis and pneumonia in the early years of the century.

If respiratory infection in early childhood is an important cause of chronic obstructive airway disease, this finding can be easily understood: following exposure to the same pathogens, some children died in infancy and others survived only to develop chronic respiratory disease in adulthood. Further evidence for the role of respiratory infection in chronic respiratory disease has come from follow-up studies of children contracting bronchiolitis, bronchitis or pneumonia which have shown that abnormalities in pulmonary function may persist throughout childhood. Particular adverse influences which are implicated include poor infant nutrition, inadequate housing, overcrowding in the home and large family size.

When it comes to cardiovascular disease, the geographical pattern of death rates today closely resembles that of neonatal mortality (deaths before one month of age) in the past when most deaths were attributed to low birth weight. The geographical distribution of maternal mortality, from causes other than puerperal fever, was very similar to neonatal mortality. Poor physique and health of the mothers was clearly implicated as a cause of high maternal mortality, and was partly a result of poor nutrition and impaired growth of young girls. A follow-up study of men born in Hertfordshire around 1920 has highlighted the importance of nutritional status in infancy as a risk factor for heart disease in adult life (Barker et al 1989). A cohort of men were traced, causes of death established, and records of weight at birth and early life examined. Among men with weight at one year of 18 lb (8.2 kg) or less, death rates were around three times higher than for those who attained 27 lb (12.7 kg) or more. Both prenatal and postnatal growth are important for determining weight at one year. All these findings suggest that processes linked to growth and acting in prenatal or early postnatal life strongly influence the risk of ischaemic heart disease. In addition, there is an inverse relation between adult blood pressure and birth weight pointing to a major effect of intrauterine environment on adult blood pressure. One of the clear implications of such findings is that instead of focusing on environmental causes of cardiovascular disease in adult life, it may be more important to consider the health of babies, for whom mothers are the dominant environmental influence.

Programming

The precise mechanisms linking nutritional factors in early life with adult disease are still being elucidated. The process by which nutritional influences in utero can permanently change the body's structure, physiology and metabolism is referred to as 'programming'. The specific effects of under-nutrition include altered gene expression, reduced numbers of cells, imbalance between cell types, altered organ structure, and changes in the pattern of hormonal release and of tissue sensitivity to hormones. Much supportive data for programming comes from animal studies, which confirm that restriction of nutrients or oxygen in utero leaves permanent marks on the physiology and structure of the body. One example of this is how a low protein diet given to pregnant rats leads to a permanent increase in blood pressure in the offspring (Langley & Jackson 1994).

Animal studies have also shown that under-nutrition at different times has different effects. In early gestation, it leads to proportionate loss of body size as in the small but proportionately grown newborn baby. In late gestation, it leads to disproportionate growth, as in the short or thin human baby. The risk of coronary heart disease in adult life appears to be related more to disproportionate growth as a fetus rather than simply small size.

Inadequate maternal food intake or deficient transport or transfer of nutrients by the placenta may result in programming which manifests in the next generation. For example, girls conceived during the 1944 Dutch famine had normal birth weight, but when they were adults and had babies of their own, these infants were small. This observation would suggest that a mother's ability to transfer nutrients to her fetus is affected by the nutritional experiences to which she herself was exposed as a developing fetus. The placenta may also play an important role in programming the baby. Placental enlargement in animal studies is known to be an adaptation to lack of nutrients including oxygen. In humans, mothers who exercise during pregnancy, anaemic mothers, and those who live at high altitude develop disproportionately large placentas. This has been interpreted as a compensatory response by the fetus to overcome deficiency of nutrient supply by increasing the area of its attachment to the mother. Epidemiological studies have linked a high ratio of placental weight to birth weight with cardiovascular disease, impaired glucose tolerance and raised plasma fibrinogen concentrations in later life as well as to hypertension.

Maternal nutrition and birth weight

A mother's body size before pregnancy is the most important determinant of the size of her baby, with those of low body weight having small babies (Thomson 1959). Chronic under-nutrition influences birth weight through its effect on maternal stature and, in addition, may be associated with specific nutrient deficiencies which influence fetal growth. These include vitamins A, C and D, folate, iron and zinc. In Europe, mothers gain around 12 kg in weight during pregnancy. The maternal component averages 7.7 kg and is made up of fat, extracellular fluid, uterine and breast tissue. Fat stores are laid down in the first half of pregnancy and used as an energy store for the fetus in the second under the influence of placental growth hormone and other hormones. Plasma volume and cardiac output increase and such adaptations which determine placental perfusion may be important for fetal nutrition.

Studies relating birth weight to calorie intake during pregnancy have often shown effects which were less than expected. In one study, the diets of primigravid women were recorded by weighed food intakes and food diaries during the seventh month of pregnancy. There was an association between calorie intake and birth weight in that women who consumed less than 1800 calories per day had babies who weighed 240 g less than those of mothers who ate 3000 or more calories (Naeye et al 1973).

Fetal malnutrition at different times in gestation may lead to newborns with different overall body size, or with similar body size but marked differences in the proportional size of different organs. Variation in growth at birth appears to have different long-term associations:

◆ small size at birth is associated with raised death rates from cardiovascular disease
◆ coronary heart disease is also associated with thinness and stunting at birth, and with small head circumference

---

KEY POINTS

◆ Epidemiological evidence points to strong links between nutritional status during fetal life and early childhood and the risks of adult disorders such as ischaemic heart disease, chronic bronchitis and stroke.
◆ Rather than focusing on changing adult lifestyles, a more sensible strategy for prevention of these diseases may be to concentrate on improving the nutritional status of mothers and their infants.
◆ Intervention strategies will require an understanding of the basic mechanisms involved.
◆ A central concept is that of 'programming', whereby nutritional influences acting at key periods during in utero development can lead to permanent changes in tissue structure, physiology and metabolism.

◆ stroke is associated with low birth weight and placental weight in relation to head size and may originate in restriction of placental growth
◆ cardiovascular disease in men, but not women, is strongly associated with failure of weight gain in infancy.

KEY POINTS

◆ A mother's size before pregnancy is the most important determinant of the size of her baby.
◆ The effects of fetal malnutrition on subsequent body size and proportion as well as risk of adult disease vary according to the time it occurs during fetal development.

The role of the placenta

Much of the work reported in this area is derived from animal studies. Species differences and developmental considerations inevitably complicate understanding of the relation between fetal growth and placental function (Battaglia 1997). One essential role for the placenta is to modify the maternal reproductive tract into a hospitable and nutritive environment for the developing embryo and fetus, a role for which paternal genes appear to be essential. Important signalling systems responsible for determining the surface area available for maternal–fetal exchange have now been identified in the mouse. What has become clear is that fetus and placenta work together as an integrated unit, such that the supply of some amino acids (e.g. branched chain) to the fetus depends not only on placental transport but also on placental metabolism. Similarly, gluconeogenesis in the fetal lamb liver increases only when placental delivery of glucose falls to a low level.

Hormones from the placenta are fundamental to the establishment and maintenance of pregnancy, the trophoblast secreting steroids and trophic peptides which are essential for fetal growth and development. There is a complex regulatory system which involves neuropeptides, growth factors and cytokines. Primate placental lactogens are structurally similar to growth hor-

mone and may serve as an important mediator of the in utero environment. In conjunction with hormones, dietary constituents also play a role in the regulation of gene expression. In the hyperglycaemic diabetic mother, for example, there is a fourfold increase in messenger RNA for the glucose transporter GLUT-3, which probably plays a major role in placental glucose uptake and metabolism. The postnatal development of hepatic long chain fatty acid (LCFA) oxidation and ketogenesis are closely related to the increase in the enzyme system which allows the transfer of LCFA into mitochondria. This is important because postnatal energy needs are met by LCFA. The molecular mechanisms involved are not yet understood, but are key areas of interest.

Physiological and structural changes as gestation progresses increase the placental transfer capacity for oxygen, another essential substrate for the fetus. It is known that chronic oxygen deficiency restricts and modifies the pattern of fetal growth, although this does not seem to operate through a reduction in the availability of carbohydrate substrates. Plasma amino acid profiles in fetal blood are altered, however, while anabolic hormones decrease and catabolic hormones increase. Whether inducing maternal hyperoxia might offer a safe intervention for IUGR is not known, although such an approach has been suggested. To what extent diminished blood flow in human pregnancies may restrict glucose provision to the fetus is unclear. Similarly, there is little information on the role of placental amino acid transporters in relation to fetal growth. It is known, however, that prolonged alcohol consumption, excessive smoking, and use of cocaine can all reduce the transport of specific amino acids.

Fetal demands for lipids are met both by placental transfer and by endogenous synthesis. Arachidonic acid and docosahexaenoic acid concentrations increase in the fetus with gestational age, probably because there is preferential transfer of LCFA across the placenta. LCFAs accrue substantially during the last trimester of development in brain and are essential for cell membranes. The increase in maternal fat deposits during the first two trimesters is mainly a result of increased lipogenesis. Enhanced lipolysis increases free fatty acid production and formation of ketone bodies which rapidly cross the placenta and may be used as fetal fuels or substrate for brain lipid synthesis.

Essential fatty acids

Phospholipids make up about one quarter of the solid matter of the brain and are integral to the vascular system on which the brain depends. Rapid brain growth and phospholipid incorporation occur during fetal life, so that lipid nutrition during pregnancy may be especially important to future development. The essential fatty acids (EFA) linoleic and α-linolenic acid are precursors of polyunsaturated fatty acids (PUFA) and cannot be synthesized by humans but must be supplied in the diet. Fetal development is associated with a high EFA requirement and there is a strong correlation at birth between maternal and fetal EFA status. The PUFA docosahexaenoic acid (DHA) is an important component of cortical neuronal membrane phospholipids. DHA stores appear to be mobilized during pregnancy and DHA status appears significantly higher in primigravida than multigravida,

indicating a possible need to increase maternal EFA intake during pregnancy. A reduction in maternal EFA status during pregnancy appears to be a general phenomenon, and is largely independent of differences in dietary habits and ethnic origin (Otto et al 1997). However, the functional implications of this finding remain uncertain.

PRACTICAL NUTRITIONAL ADVICE DURING PREGNANCY

Box 1.4 shows the groups of women most likely to require nutritional advice during pregnancy.

Animal work shows that suboptimal nutrition before implantation can retard growth and development. Very thin women may have difficulty conceiving, and those who do are at increased risk of having a premature or low birth weight infant. They should be encouraged to eat a nutrient-rich balanced diet. For overweight women, stabilization of weight before pregnancy is recommended by a reduction in fat and sugar content so that micronutrient intake is not jeopardised. Pregnancies that are closely spaced may result in maternal nutrient depletion and are associated with low birth weight and congenital malformation. Optimal spacing between pregnancies is probably 2 to 4 years.

KEY POINTS

- ◆ The fetus and placenta act together as an integrated unit.
- ◆ Hormones and trophic factors from the placenta are essential to fetal growth and development, and dietary constituents may play a role in the regulation of gene expression, with nutritional implications for the fetus.
- ◆ Long chain fatty acids are preferentially transferred across the placenta and are important for brain development and cell membrane structure.
- ◆ The polyunsaturated fatty acid DHA is an important component of neuronal membrane phospholipids, and dietary deficiency may have adverse neurodevelopmental effects.

 Box 1.4 Women most likely to require nutritional advice during pregnancy

- ◆ Women with a past history of low birth weight or spontaneous abortion.
- ◆ Women who are overweight or underweight.
- ◆ Women with dieting or eating disorders.
- ◆ Women who have had a short interval since their last birth (less than 2 years).
- ◆ Women with more than four children.
- ◆ Teenagers.
- ◆ Women with low incomes or living in poor housing.
- ◆ Vegans or vegetarians with inadequate diet.
- ◆ Smokers.
- ◆ Women with chronic medical disorders.

Alcohol consumption should be limited to no more than one unit a day (equivalent to one glass of wine, half a pint of beer or one measure of spirits). Alcohol is recognised as an important teratogenic agent for developmental brain damage and long-lasting central nervous system dysfunction (Brown et al 1997). Together with Down's syndrome and neural tube defects, it is a leading cause of congenital mental retardation and is estimated to affect 0.3 to 1.9 per 1000 live births in western societies. Maternal alcohol abuse can produce a recognised pattern of abnormalities comprising:

◆ prenatal or postnatal growth retardation
◆ learning and memory problems, attention deficits, developmental delay, intellectual impairment
◆ characteristic craniofacial abnormalities including at least two of the following: short palpebral fissures, poorly developed philtrum, thin upper lip and flattening of the maxillary area.

Some foods also represent a potential hazard to the fetus in early pregnancy because of their association with foodborne infection. Soft cheeses such as Camembert and Brie may transmit listeria infection. Raw eggs or any food containing raw egg should be avoided because of the risk of salmonella transmission. Raw meat and poultry may also contain this organism and should always be well cooked. There is no evidence to support the contention that nausea and vomiting in early pregnancy protect the mother from harmful foods which might cause miscarriage or congenital abnormality (Godfrey et al 1996).

Following the birth of the infant, women who breastfeed should be guided by their increased thirst and appetite (an additional 450 to 570 kcal of energy per day is required). Calcium requirements increase to 1250 mg per day, and women not consuming milk or dairy products will need calcium supplementation. Vitamin D supplements are advised to ensure a daily intake of 10 µg. Additional iron is unnecessary as losses are decreased through lactational amenorrhoea, however iron status should be ascertained in the high risk groups listed above, and treated if found. A

Table 1.3 Suggested eating plan for pregnant or breastfeeding women

Food group	Daily servings
Bread and cereals	4 or more to satisfy appetite
Vegetables and fruit	at least 4
Milk and milk products	3[a]
Lean meat, poultry, fish eggs, beans and nuts	2
Spreading and cooking fats	in small amounts
Sugar and confectionary	limit quantities consumed and do not eat instead of nutrient-dense foods (i.e. those in the first four groups)
Alcohol	no more than 1 unit per day

[a] 4 servings for breastfeeding mothers

KEY POINTS

◆ Attention to a well balanced diet should be integral to pregnancy planning and antenatal care.
◆ Some groups of women are more likely to have inadequate diets than others (e.g. teenagers, women with low incomes, smokers).
◆ Surveys suggest that mineral intake during pregnancy is often sub-optimal.
◆ Alcohol is an important cause of fetal brain injury with long-term adverse effects on development.
◆ Some foods represent a potential hazard to the fetus because of their association with foodborne infection (e.g. soft cheeses and listeria; raw egg and salmonella).

suggested eating plan for pregnant or breastfeeding women is given in Table 1.3.

Intervention strategies

The fetal/infant origins of disease hypothesis has been challenged (Kramer & Joseph 1996), but even its detractors accept that the studies done so far have yielded sufficient evidence to justify further work. The possibility that growth in utero and during early life has profound effects on the

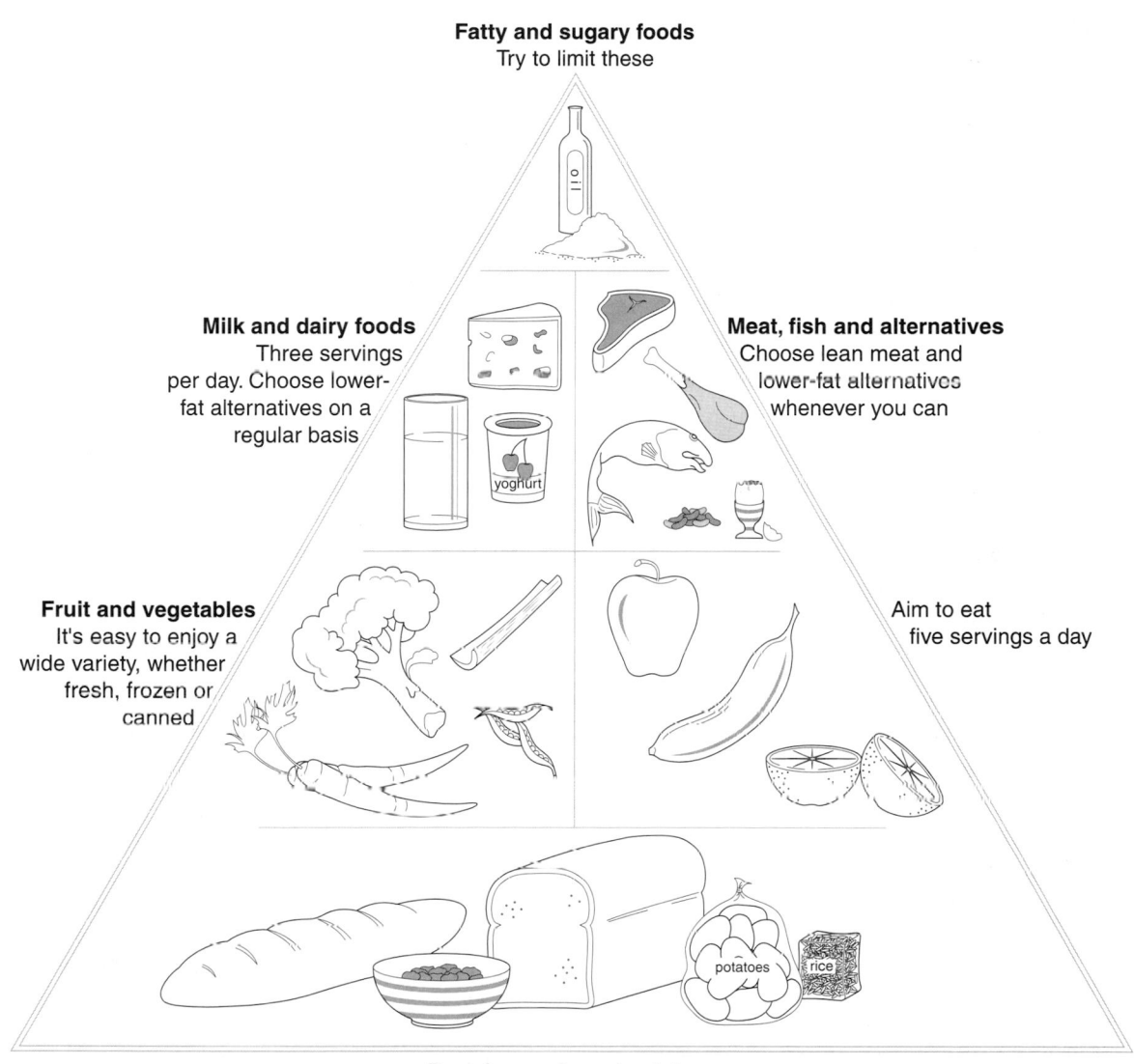

Fatty and sugary foods
Try to limit these

Milk and dairy foods
Three servings
per day. Choose lower-
fat alternatives on a
regular basis

Meat, fish and alternatives
Choose lean meat and
lower-fat alternatives
whenever you can

Fruit and vegetables
It's easy to enjoy a
wide variety, whether
fresh, frozen or
canned

Aim to eat
five servings a day

Bread, cereals and potatoes
Base all meals and snacks on starchy foods from this group and choose high-fibre varieties whenever you can

Figure 1.1   Recommended food choices during pregnancy

risk of disease in adult life has potentially important implications for preventive health policies. Rather than attempting to persuade adults to change their lifestyles and reduce risk factors for coronary heart disease, for example, it may be more important to improve the health and nutritional status of girls and young women, and mothers during pregnancy and lactation. The balance of protein and carbohydrate in the diet during late pregnancy, and the amount of fat and protein in the diet appear to exert considerable influence on placental and fetal growth (Spohr 1997). Although such effects could be important in terms of their influence on long-term health, there is no basis as yet for changing dietary recommendations to pregnant women. Epidemiological data have opened up this fascinating area for further study. In order for preventive strategies to be developed what is now needed is an understanding of the processes involved at a cellular and molecular level. This challenge will undoubtedly continue to stimulate much medical research.

SUMMARY

- Nutritional factors are important in terms of fertility, embryogenesis, fetal growth and maternal adaptation to pregnancy.
- Folic acid deficiency is a major cause of neural tube defects; how to ensure adequate folate status in women of childbearing age before they become pregnant remains an issue of debate.
- There is a modest increase in energy requirements during the third trimester.
- Nutrition surveys suggest inadequate intake of some minerals is common during pregnancy.
- Small infants may be normal, but growth retarded because of factors reducing growth potential, or malnourished as a result of insufficient nutrient supply.
- Epidemiological evidence points to strong links between nutritional status during fetal life and early childhood and subsequent risk of chronic disorders in adult life such as coronary heart disease, hypertension and diabetes.
- Research is focusing on the basic mechanisms underlying this link, but as yet the public health implications in terms of dietary advice and intervention remain unclear.

 FURTHER READING

Barker D J P 1998 Mothers, babies and health in later life, 2nd edn. Churchill Livingstone, Edinburgh

This highly readable book gives a comprehensive overview of the epidemiological research which has firmly established the link between disease in later life and nutritional influences acting in utero and throughout infancy.

Battaglia F C (ed.) 1997 Placental function and fetal nutrition. Nestlé Nutrition Workshop Series, vol. 39. Lippincott-Raven Publishers, Philadelphia, PA

From current scientific research, a more precise description of normal fetal growth and metabolism is emerging, with the possibility of exploring how specific maternal diseases affect fetal and placental nutrition. This book summarizes work presented by experts including basic scientists and clinicians to a workshop held in 1996. Topics discussed include the study of placental transport, the interaction between fetal liver and placenta, the endocrine function of the placenta, and regulation of gene expression by nutrients during the perinatal period.

Ramakrishnan U, Manjrekar R, Rivera J, Gonzales-Cossio T, Martorell R 1999 Micronutrients and pregnancy outcome: a review of the literature. Nutrition Research 19:103–159

The authors of this comprehensive review examine the published evidence in relation to micronutrients and their importance for pregnancy outcomes, concluding with suggestions for the direction of future research.

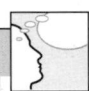 **Questions**

Answers are given in Appendix 2.

1. An unemployed teenage mother of a 9-month-old infant is living in rented accommodation and expecting her second child. What factors make her at nutritional risk and what specific dietary advice might be offered in the antenatal clinic?

2. A woman who has just had confirmation of being pregnant consults you because she has routinely been taking a daily multivitamin supplement for some years. She is worried about the possible damaging effect of vitamin A on her fetus. What advice would you give?

3. A woman of Indian origin who follows a lacto-ovo-vegetarian diet is planning to become pregnant and seeks general dietary guidance. Which aspects of her diet have implications for the fetus?

REFERENCES

Barker D J P 1988 Mothers, babies and health in later life. Churchill Livingstone, Edinburgh

Barker D J P, Winter P D, Osmond C, Margetts B, Simmonds S J 1989 Weight in infancy and death from ischaemic heart disease. Lancet ii:577–580

Battaglia F C (ed.) 1997 Placental function and fetal nutrition. Nestlé UK Ltd, London

Brown J E, Kahn E S, Hartman T J 1997 Profet, profits, and proof: Do nausea and vomiting of early pregnancy protect women from 'harmful' vegetables? American Journal of Obstetrics and Gynecology 176:179–181

Czeizel A E 1993 Prevention of congenital abnormalities by periconceptional multivitamin supplementation. British Medical Journal 306:1645–1648

Department of Health 1991 Dietary reference values for food energy and nutrients for the UK, Report on Health and Social Subjects 41. HMSO, London

Department of Health 1992 Folic acid and the prevention of neural tube defects. Report from an Expert Advisory Group. Department of Health, London

Edwards A G K, Halse P C, Parkin J M, Waterston A J R 1990 Recognising failure to thrive in early childhood. Archives of Disease in Childhood 65:1263–1265

Gardosi J, Chang A, Kalyan B, Sahota S, Symonds E M 1992 Customised antenatal growth charts. Lancet 339:283–287

Godfrey K, Robinson S, Barker D J P, Osmond C, Cox V 1996 Maternal nutrition in early and late pregnancy in relation to placental and fetal growth. British Medical Journal 312:410–414

Hautvast J G A J 1997 Adequate nutrition in pregnancy does matter. European Journal of Obstetrics and Gynecology and Reproductive Biology 75:33–35

Heinone K, Hakulinen A, Jokela V 1988 Time trends and determinants of mortality in a very preterm population during the 1980s. Lancet ii:204–206

Kramer M S, Joseph K S 1996 Enigma of fetal/infant-origins hypothesis. Lancet 348:1254

Langley S C, Jackson A A 1994 Increased systolic blood pressure in adult rats induced by fetal exposure to maternal low protein diets. Clinical Science 86:217–222

Ministry of Agriculture, Fisheries and Food 1994 The dietary and nutritional survey of British adults – further analysis. HMSO, London

Mostad S B, Overbauch J, DeVange D M et al 1997 Hormonal contraception, vitamin A deficiency, and other risk factors for shedding HIV-1 infected cells from the cervix and vagina. Lancet 350:933–937

MRC Vitamin Study Group 1991 Prevention of neural tube defects: results of the Medical Research Council Vitamin Study. Lancet 238:131–137

Naeye R L, Blanc W, Paul C 1973 Effects of maternal nutrition on the human fetus. Pediatrics 52:494–503

Otto S J, Houwelingen A C V, Antal M et al 1997 Maternal and neonatal essential fatty acid status in phospholipids: an international comparative study. European Journal of Clinical Nutrition 51:232–242

Robinson S, Godfrey K, Denne J, Cox V 1998 The determinants of iron status in early pregnancy. British Journal of Nutrition 79:249–255

Roodenburg A J C 1995 Iron supplementation during pregnancy. European Journal of Obstetrics and Gynecology and Reproductive Biology 61:65–71

Scholl T O, Hediger M L, Bendich M L, Schall J L, Smith W K, Krueger P M 1997 Use of multivitamin/mineral prenatal supplements: influence on the outcome of pregnancy. American Journal of Epidemiology 146(2):134–141

Spohr H L 1997 Environmental influences on the embryo and fetus: alcohol. In: Cockburn F (ed), Advances in perinatal medicine. Parthenon Publishing Group, London

Thomson A M 1959 Diet in pregnancy, 3. Diet in relation to the course and outcome of pregnancy. British Journal of Nutrition 13:509–525

Practical breastfeeding

2

Maureen Chadderton

INTRODUCTION

The importance of breast milk to the infant and child has been the focus of much research during the past decade and has left the nutritional, anti-infective, immunological, hormonal and enzyme properties of breast milk undisputed. Some mothers will have decided to breastfeed well before the baby's birth. Others, who had previously thought that they would feed artificially, may have a change of heart when they discover that their baby is sick and has special needs. There will, too, be infants admitted to the ward who are already fully established breastfeeders. Whichever is the case,

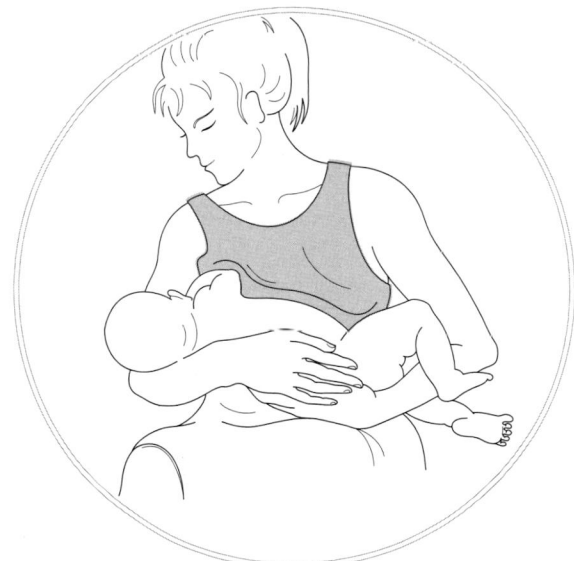

Figure 2.1 Cradle or madonna hold

the support, encouragement and knowledge offered by staff in the paediatric ward to the mother will play a crucial part in the success or failure of breastfeeding.

This chapter is about helping mothers to breastfeed or to supply breast milk during the very difficult time of a child's sickness. The benefits of breast milk and breastfeeding to both mother and baby will be discussed, as will the anatomy and physiology of lactation, some practical aspects of breastfeeding and some alternative methods of feeding breast milk to a baby. Throughout the chapter the term 'breastfeeding' will be used to encompass all methods of giving breast milk to babies. The term 'nursing' will sometimes be used to describe the physical act of breastfeeding. (Figure 2.1 shows a mother breastfeeding her baby using the cradle or madonna hold.)

KEY POINTS

◆ Almost all babies, well or sick, preterm or term, newborn or toddler, will benefit from being breastfed; contraindications to breastfeeding are extremely rare.
◆ It has been estimated that fewer than 10% of women worldwide may not be able to breastfeed.

THE BENEFITS OF BREAST MILK AND COLOSTRUM

Breast milk changes to suit the baby's needs. Not only does it change from colostrum to mature milk, but from the start of the feed to the end. Mature breast milk also changes from day to day and from feed to feed (Lammi-Keefe et al 1990).

At the beginning of a feed, breast milk has a high lactose content but not very much fat, whilst later in the feed the breast milk will be four to five times higher in fat content and therefore provide more calories and be more satisfying.

It is important that babies receive both the high lactose and the high fat parts of breast milk. Mothers should, therefore, be encouraged to allow the baby to empty the first breast before nursing on the second.

Breast milk will always have health benefits for the baby. However, in order to gain greater and longer term benefits, research suggests that exclusive breastfeeding should continue for a minimum of four months.

Babies who are breastfed receive greater protection against disease in both the long and short term. A recent interim report from a longitudinal study shows that children who have been breastfed continue to have better health and greater protection from infection at the age of nine years (Howie et al 1998). Some of these benefits are shown in Box 2.1.

Benefits of breastfeeding to mothers

Mothers also derive health benefits from breastfeeding. These include:

◆ reduced risk of breast cancer (Cumming Klieneburg 1993, UK National Case Control Study Group 1993)
◆ ovarian cancer (Gwinn et al 1990)
◆ osteoporosis (Cumming & Klieneburg 1993)
◆ as well as providing a natural contraception through lactational amenorrhoea (Gross 1991, Lewis et al 1991, Perez et al 1992).

THE COMPOSITION OF HUMAN MILK

Breast milk is a source of carbohydrates, fats, protein and vitamins. Table 2.1 shows the composition of colostrum and of transitional and mature milk.

Carbohydrates

Lactose is the main carbohydrate constituent of breast milk and will provide 37% of the baby's energy needs. Lactose is easily broken down into glucose, which provides energy to the developing brain and into galactose, which is essential for the development of the central nervous system (Akre 1998). Lactose also aids the absorption of calcium and iron, and plays a part in inhibiting the growth of enteropathic organisms.

Breast milk contains the enzyme amylase, which aids the digestion of carbohydrate. Amylase is found in the pancreatic juices and saliva of adults but is almost absent in the young infant.

Box 2.1   Health benefits of breastfeeding for children

◆ A reduced risk of infant mortality associated with necrotizing enterocolitis (Lucas & Cole 1990) and from sudden infant death (Ford et al 1993, Gilbert et al 1995).

◆ Reduced morbidity throughout infancy and childhood from illness including gastro-intestinal, respiratory and urinary tract infections and otitis media (Howie et al 1998).

◆ Lower blood pressure (Howie et al 1998).

◆ A reduced risk of juvenile onset diabetes (Karajalainen et al 1992).

◆ A lower risk of dental caries and possibly malocclusion (Labbok & Hendershot 1987).

Research has also demonstrated that the neurological development of breastfed children is different from those who are artificially fed, and there appears to be a significant advantage in the cognitive function of the breastfed child (Lucas et al 1994), as well as visual acuity (Uuay et al 1990).

Table 2.1 Composition of human milk (Holland et al 1991. Crown copyright material is reproduced with the permission of the Controller of Her Majesty's Stationery Office.)

Nutrient		Colostrum	Transitional	Mature
Energy	kcal	56	67	69
	kJ	236	281	289
Protein	g	2.0	1.5	1.3
Fat	g	2.6	3.7	4.1
Carbohydrate	g	6.6	6.9	7.2
Sodium	mg	47	30	15
Calcium	mg	28	25	34
Iron	mg	0.07	0.07	0.07
Retinol	µg	155	85	58
Vitamin C	mg	7	6	4

Fats

Breast milk fat is abundant in long chain fatty acids of which arachidonic acid (AA) is more concentrated in colostrum and in the breast milk of mothers of preterm babies.

Fat is the most variable constituent of breast milk. Variations arise during each feed with the lowest fat content in the foremilk and the highest levels occurring in the hindmilk. The quantity of fat also varies at different times of day, with the frequency of feeds, and at different stages of lactation.

Protein

Mature breast milk has the lowest protein content of all mammalian milks, with the whey protein being four times greater in quantity than that of casein. This produces a soft curd in the stomach, which is easily digested. A large proportion of the whey protein of transitional and mature breast milk is made up of the same anti-infective properties of immunoglobulins, lactoferrin, lysozymes and active white cells, macrophages, neutrophils and lymphocytes that are present in colostrum. Together, these properties break down and kill susceptible bacteria in the gut (Lawson 1992). Lactoferrin is a whey protein fraction which binds iron in the breast milk, leaving it unavailable for iron-dependent bacteria, such as *Escherichia coli*. Maternal antibodies in the form of secretory immunoglobulin A (IgA) prevent entry of bacteria and viruses into the intestinal mucosa. One study of the anti-infective properties of breastmilk in relation to gastroenteritis demonstrated, after weighting for socioeconomic factors, that the prevalence of gastroenteritis was much less in babies who had been breastfed for at least 3 months (2% compared with 20% of babies who were artificially fed during the first three months; Howie et al 1998).

The child that is breastfed is protected from infections to which his mother has been exposed and has become or is becoming immune. This is because white cells that have spent some time in the maternal gut and lymphatic system are present in colostrum and breast milk. This process is known as enteromammary axis.

The epidermal growth factor (EGF) which is necessary to the stimulation of epidermal and epithelial cell growth is also present in breast milk (Carpenter 1980, Jannson et al 1985).

Vitamins

Both fat-soluble and water-soluble vitamins are likely to vary in quantity. However, with the possible exception of vitamin K, breast milk will almost always meet the needs of the infant of less than 6 months of age who is solely breastfed. Because vitamin K is essential to the blood clotting mechanism, and because the quantity of vitamin K in each mother's breast milk is unknown, almost all babies are given prophylactic vitamin K in order to prevent haemolytic disease of the newborn.

COLOSTRUM

Colostrum is produced for the first 3 to 4 days following the baby's birth. It is a valuable fluid, although its properties are not fully under-stood. What is known of colostrum, however, is that it is a low-volume, highly concentrated nutrition for the newborn in quantities that can be readily taken. The fat and lactose content of colostrum is less than that of breast milk, but it contains a higher concentration of fat-soluble vitamins A and E. Colostrum plays a vital part in protecting the newborn from infection. The anti-infective properties of lactoferrin, immuno-globulins and lyzosomes that occur in transitional and mature breast milk are in colostrum but in much higher concentrations. Some studies have suggested that colostrum not only protects against infection but can also be used as a treatment (Reissland & Burghart 1988). The epidermal growth factor (EGF) which stimulates the proliferation of cells in the gut as well as epidermal and epithelial cells is present in concentrations five times greater than in mature breast milk (Jannson et al 1985). Colostrum also has a mild laxative effect, which helps to clear meconium from the gut and prevents the reabsorption of bilirubin.

The typical yellow colouring of colostrum is caused by the fact that it has a 10 times greater concentration of carotene than breast milk (Lawrence 1989). This colouring may be a significant reason that mothers from some cultures commonly refuse to give colostrum. These mothers will cite a number of reasons for the refusal, but an explanation often given to health workers is that the appearance of yellow and sticky colostrum is thought to indicate that it is 'stale' or 'dirty', having sat in the breast for too long. These mothers prefer to wait for the breast milk to flush it through. Another common misconception is that there is not enough colostrum to satisfy the baby's needs and these mothers will prefer to feed artificially for the first few days. Education and good information is perhaps the long-term solution to these misconceptions. However, confronted by the mother of a sick baby with these beliefs, a knowledgeable member of the paediatric team should do everything possible to persuade the mother of the benefits of giving colostrum. In some cases the services of an interpreter or link worker who is well versed in breastfeeding will be indispensable.

THE ANATOMY OF THE LACTATING BREAST

The development of the female breast

The breast or mammary gland begins its development before birth during the first weeks of pregnancy. Development continues throughout childhood, puberty and sexual maturity. It is during pregnancy, however, that the breast undergoes the final growth.

The size and shape of the breast varies considerably depending on the amount of fatty tissue present. This does not, however, affect the production of milk or the quality of milk produced. Any enlargement of the breast during pregnancy and lactation is brought about by hormonal influences and indicates a functional mammary gland.

The appearance of the breast

The outward appearance of the breasts can be described as being circular at the base, where the breasts lie, one on either lateral margin of the sternum, from the second to the sixth rib and extend to the mid axillary line. The breast is roughly semispherical in shape, covered by skin with a darker pigmented area, the areola, towards the centre and from which the nipple protrudes.

The structure of the breast

The breast tissue is arranged in 15 to 20 lobes rather like the design of the segments of an orange. Each segment or lobe points toward the nipple at the centre of the breast and is divided from the next lobe by a septum of fibrous tissue which extends from the skin to the fascia of the pectoral muscle to which the base of the breast is anchored.

Each lobe is divided into 20 to 40 lobules, which in turn contain clusters of alveoli, tiny sac-like structures, which are lined by the cells of acini, cells that secrete milk in response to the release of prolactin. The alveoli are surrounded by a network of blood vessels and myoepithelial cells (muscle cells). Between 10 and 100 alveoli in each lobule are connected by tiny ductules to a larger duct, the lactiferous or mammary duct. The lactiferous ducts widen out underneath the areola to become lactiferous sinuses. This is where milk collects throughout the feed so that the suckling baby can empty the sinuses, which now narrow to lead to the surface of the nipple. The breast is supplied with blood from the upper intercostal arteries (which branch from the aorta), from the internal mammary artery (which originates in the subclavian artery), and from the external mammary artery (which branches from the lateral thoracic artery). Venous drainage is via the internal mammary veins and the axillary veins. A network of lymphatic vessels drain mainly into the axillary, parasternal, pectoral and liver nodes.

Nipple and areola

Sited within the areola are 18 to 20 montgomery tubercles. These tiny projections are oil-producing glands, which are thought to lubricate the areola and to change the pH of the areola and nipple, thus protecting against harmful bacteria. The nipple is situated in the centre of the areola. In most cases, the erectile muscle fibres that criss-cross the ducts respond to touch, cold or sexual stimulation by projecting the nipple forward. However, a few women have non-projectile, flat or inverted nipples. This does not mean that the mother cannot breastfeed, only that more time, patience and skill may be needed. Sphincter-like muscles also circle the ducts that lie within the nipple tissue.

Both nipple and areola, which are well supplied with nerve endings, are remarkably elastic and flexible and so conform to the baby's mouth and tongue during the breastfeed.

Hormonal influences during pregnancy and lactation

Early in pregnancy, when under the influence of progesterone, the amount of glandular tissue multiplies, increasing the size of the breast. The increase in oestrogen lengthens and broadens the ducts and ductules. The main functions of pro-lactin and oxytocin are described below. However, a secondary function of prolactin is that of conservation of water and salt from the kidneys, and possibly through its effects on the ovary to prolong amenorrhoea. Both these functions reduce the metabolic stress of lactation (Akre 1998). Research into postnatal maternal mood and mother's adjustment to her infant suggests that oxytocin plays a role as a 'bonding' hormone (Newton 1978).

For some days following delivery, the release of oxytocin also causes the uterus to contract. Some mothers, particularly those that have had other babies, will find this a painful experience and require an explanation of what is taking place and may possibly need an analgesic.

THE PHYSIOLOGY OF LACTATION

Following the expulsion of the placenta, oestrogen and progesterone levels in the blood begin to fall, allowing the hormone, prolactin, to begin milk production. This event is completely under endocrine control and will happen whether or not the mother is breastfeeding. However, frequent suckling will increase the prolactin levels in the body and the milk will come in more quickly, possibly within 2 to 3 days. At this time the composition of the milk begins its transition from colostrum to mature breast milk as the amount of lactose that is synthesized rises, resulting in an increase in the volume of breast milk. The production of milk from now on is under autocrine control and dependent upon the regular emptying of the breasts. The baby's suckling is now the driving force of lactation. As the baby suckles, the nerve endings in the nipple and areola are stimulated, sending impulses via the afferent neural-reflex to the hypothalamus. This results in the secretion of prolactin (for the production of milk) from the anterior pituitary gland and oxytocin from the posterior pituitary. Oxytocin causes the myoepithelial cells to contract and expel the milk into ductules; this milk then drains into the ducts and on to the lactiferous sinuses. As the baby's cheek or lips are touched, the 'rooting' reflex is stimulated. This induces the baby to search for the nipple and with wide open mouth to grasp a good mouthful of breast tissue. The suckling reflex then comes into play, and with a rhythmic action of the jaw the infant compresses the area immediately behind the areola between the hard palate and tongue. With the tongue compressing the areola with a peristaltic action the infant strips the milk from the breast.

Initiation of lactation without suckling

Babies admitted to neonatal or paediatric units are often too tiny or too sick to go to the breast. Their mothers therefore will not be able to initiate lactation by breastfeeding. Important though suckling is, fortunately the cycle of oxytocin-release stimulating milk ejection ('let-down') is not only triggered by suckling, but can also be triggered by a mother seeing, touching or smelling her baby or hearing her baby's cry. The let-down reflex is often also found to be a conditioned response, when close proximity to or even thinking about the baby will arouse the reflex and milk will leak, probably fairly vigorously, from the breast. By expressing and emptying the breasts frequently by artificial means, mothers can take advantage of these responses to initiate and maintain lactation until she and the baby can nurse together. The baby may then be given the expressed colostrum or milk. Methods of expressing that may be considered include:

- hand expression
- electrically or battery-operated mechanical breast pump
- hand-operated breast pump.

Delay in lactation

Mothers whose babies or children are admitted to neonatal or paediatric wards may experience a slight delay in initiating lactation, or indeed a temporary halt in established lactation, whether nursing or expressing breast milk. One reason for this is that the reflex can be temporarily inhibited by the effects of increased amounts of adrenaline in the blood, such as when mothers are subjected to stressful situations. Oxytocin secretion is inhibited and the let-down reflex is temporarily suppressed. If the breasts are full and are not being adequately emptied, a second reason for a temporary delay might be that back pressure in the breast is preventing the release of oxytocin. However, if a mother believes and has confidence that she can provide breast milk for her baby, she will quickly overcome this difficulty. It is essential, therefore, that the mother is surrounded by staff who are supportive, encouraging and knowledgeable, as well as by supportive family and friends.

COMMON BREASTFEEDING PROBLEMS

Sore or cracked nipples

Some women can experience nipple tenderness, without any nipple trauma, at the beginning of each feed for the first few weeks of breastfeeding. This situation is resolved in the course of time. However, nipples that are sore throughout the feed and between feeds, or nipples that have become cracked, have almost always been traumatized by friction caused by incorrect attachment and the baby only being allowed to suck the nipple, rather than being able to take in enough of the surrounding breast tissue to form a teat that reaches the back of the mouth (Woolridge 1986a,b).

Successful treatment is achieved by ensuring correct attachment and positioning at the breast. It is important to spend some time helping the mother to get this right and teaching her how to recognize correct attachment when she first begins breastfeeding. (See Figures 2.2 to 2.4.) If the mother complains of sore nipples then the attachment should be checked immediately and corrected in the same way. A mother with sore or

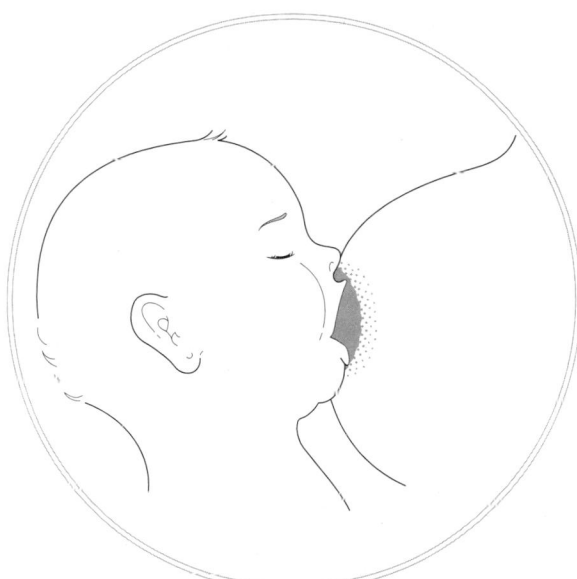

Figure 2.3 An outside view of the breast when attachment is good

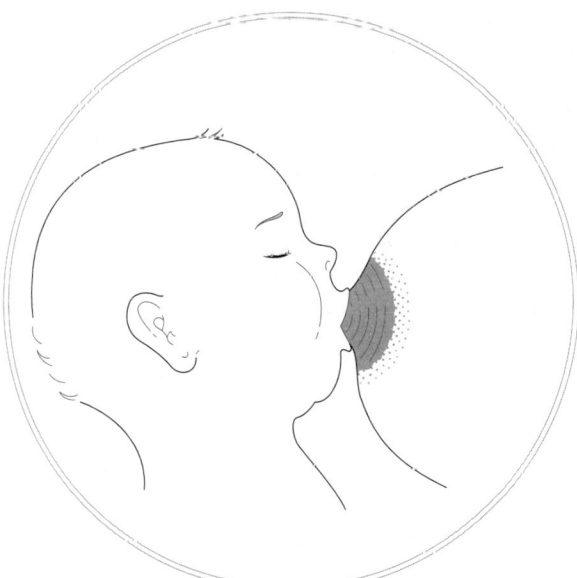

Figure 2.4 An outside view of the breast when attachment is poor

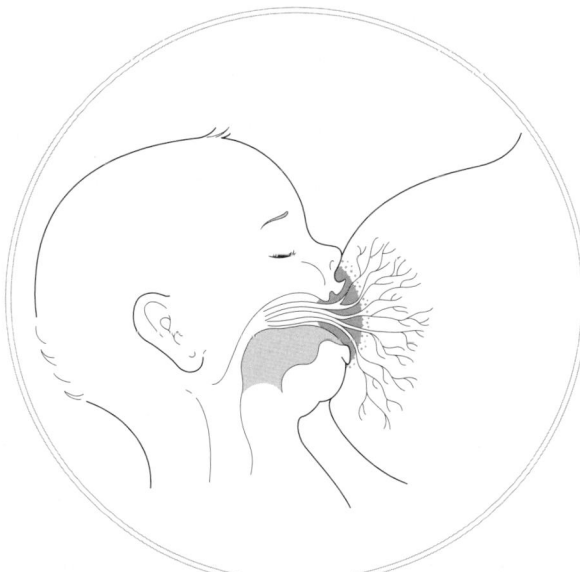

Figure 2.2 An inside view of the breast when attachment is good

cracked nipples will often be reluctant to nurse, but she can be reassured that the condition will be alleviated and recovery will begin as soon as the attachment is corrected.

Other, less common causes of sore nipples include:

◆ short frenulum
◆ thrush.

Short frenulum (tongue-tie)

In some babies the frenulum, the membrane that attaches the tongue to the floor of the mouth, may be so short that it prevents the tongue projecting past the lower lip. This will usually not prevent successful suckling but the mother will need more help to get a good attachment. However a small surgical procedure to nick the frenulum can be performed if it is thought necessary in order to free the tongue and facilitate easier attachment and suckling.

Thrush

Factors that predispose to thrush are maternal antibiotic treatment, maternal vaginal thrush infection, or oral or anal thrush in the baby. Signs and symptoms of a thrush infection are nipples that are painful throughout the feed and possibly accompanied by deep breast pain which lasts for several minutes after the feed has finished. The nipple soreness continues between feeds and can be so severe that even light clothing brushing against the nipple will cause extreme pain. The nipple and surrounding skin will often be raised, red, shiny and itchy. Sometimes, however, these signs are absent and one must rely upon the mother's description of the symptoms. Treatment should be with a prescribed antifungal preparation to both mother and baby.

Engorgement

There are two types of breast engorgement: vascular engorgement and milk engorgement.

Vascular engorgement

Vascular engorgement can occur in the mother, whether breastfeeding or not, 2 to 4 days after delivery, and is caused by the cardiovascular changes that are taking place in the breasts as they prepare for milk secretion. Both breasts are affected equally and become oedematous, painful and tense. The condition resolves naturally within 24 to 48 hours. Treatment to relieve the discomfort includes wearing a well supporting bra and taking mild analgesic. However, women who feed their babies frequently may well find that venous engorgement passes almost unnoticed and the discomfort is minimal.

Milk engorgement

Milk engorgement can occur at any stage of lactation but is most common during the early days of breastfeeding. The condition affects the whole breast and commonly affects both breasts, causing an uncomfortable fullness with the breasts feeling heavy and tense. If the condition is not resolved satisfactorily, a non-infective mastitis may develop. (Mastitis is discussed later in this chapter.)

Clearly, prevention of milk engorgement is preferred but, because engorgement is caused by the breast not being emptied effectively, the course of action for both prevention and treatment is the same. Box 2.2 shows some methods for preventing and treating milk engorgement. Treated correctly, mothers can be reassured that the engorgement will last no longer than 24 hours.

Box 2.2 Preventing and treating milk engorgement

◆ The breasts need to be emptied frequently and without delay after the mother has given birth. As long as the baby is well enough to nurse then unrestricted baby-led feeding should be encouraged, with great care being taken to ensure the baby's correct positioning and attachment at the breast.

◆ If the baby is too small or too sick to nurse, then the mother should be encouraged to keep her breasts comfortable and free from engorgement by expressing the colostrum or breast milk frequently (this can then be given to the baby in the most appropriate way).

- A well supporting bra will help to alleviate the discomfort of heavy breasts.

- Some mothers may benefit from a breast compress of cabbage leaves which is thought to contain a substance that reduces oedema and temporarily increases the milk flow.

- Cool or cold packs applied as a compress may benefit some mothers.

- Warm water compresses. Bathing or showering the breasts with warm water will also stimulate the milk flow and relieve discomfort.

- Expressing a small amount of milk between feeds or between regular expressing may also be helpful.

- A mild analgesic may be necessary.

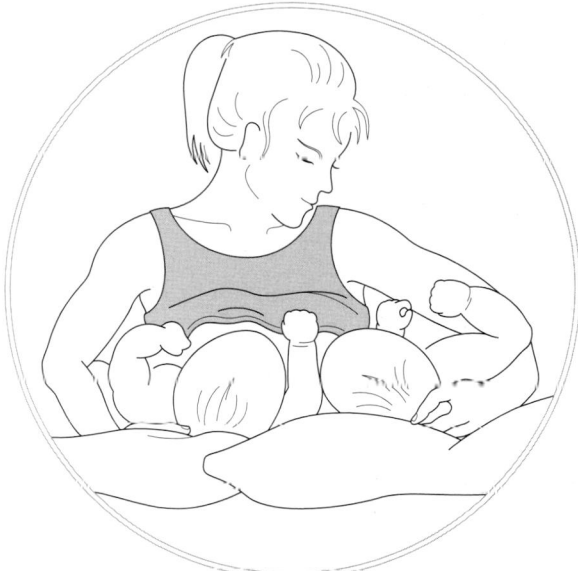

Figure 2.5 Under arm or football hold – here being adapted to feed twins

Blocked duct

A blocked duct will obstruct the flow of milk from one particular lobe and will lead to a hard, tender lump developing over the site of the blockage. If it is unrelieved, the condition may progress to mastitis.

The blockage is often caused by poor positioning of the baby at the breast or by pressure from a tightly fitting or an underwired bra. The condition can also be caused by the presence of a small granule that occurs naturally in the breast milk becoming lodged in the duct. Treatment aimed at improving the flow of milk from the affected area includes:

- ensuring correct positioning (see Figure 2.5 and Figures 2.1 to 2.4)
- changing the feeding position of the baby or of the mother so that all lobes are emptied equally
- ensuring the baby's most vigorous suck at the affected breast by beginning the feed on that side at each feed until the blockage clears (a small amount of milk may need to be expressed from the unaffected side to prevent discomfort)
- gently massaging the area toward the nipple as the baby feeds
- applying warm compresses to the breast

- expressing a little more milk at the end of the feed.

Mastitis

Mastitis can occur at any stage of lactation but is uncommon within the first 2 weeks. The mother will often feel ill with flu-like symptoms and will have a raised temperature. The breast will have a painful site which may be inflamed and hot.

Non-infective mastitis

The causes of non-infective mastitis are often the same as those for a blocked duct or milk engorgement but may also include a recent trauma to the breast. Another cause is an abrupt change in the feeding pattern or the temporary cessation of feeding.

The prevention and treatment is to ensure regular and frequent emptying of the breasts, and so is the same as for preventing and treating milk engorgement with the addition of bed rest while the flu-like symptoms continue. Antibiotic treatment is not necessary.

Infective mastitis

The difference between non-infective and infective mastitis can be difficult to distinguish except by laboratory examination. However, it may be assumed that the mastitis is infective wherever the breast has failed to respond to treatment for a non-infective mastitis and the flu-like symptoms persist. There is the possibility of an ascending infection from a cracked nipple.

Treatment is the same as for non-infective mastitis, with the addition of antibiotic treatment. Breastfeeding from the affected side or expressing and giving the expressed milk to the baby should continue. Delay in treating an infective mastitis can result in a breast abscess, in which case surgical intervention will become necessary.

ALTERNATIVE METHODS OF GIVING BREAST MILK

When babies are being cared for in a neonatal or paediatric unit, circumstances will arise when an alternative or additional method of giving breast milk must be found. Most of these methods will be familiar to paediatric staff. However, methods such as cup feeding, direct expression of breast milk or using a nursing supplementer may not be. Each method is a useful and preferable alternative to giving a bottle as the baby makes the transition to breastfeeding. In fact, studies have shown that preterm babies find breastfeeding easier than bottle-feeding (Meier & Anderson 1987).

Cup feeding

Allowing the baby to lap expressed breast milk from a small cup will help him to develop a suck and swallow reflex and will introduce him to feeding orally at his own pace. A recent study has shown that preterm babies as young as 30 weeks' gestation can be successfully cup-fed (Lang et al 1994).

Nursing supplementer

A nursing supplementer is useful in situations where the baby is suckling at the breast but where he either tends to tire easily or to lose interest after a short time, when the baby has a weak or inefficient suck, or where the mother is establishing relactation.

Direct expression of breast milk

Expressing breast milk directly into the baby's mouth, or expressing a little onto the baby's lips so that it might be licked off, is a useful way of introducing a baby to breastfeeding. It will give the baby the taste of breast milk and will stimulate the suck and swallow reflex.

A fully explained and detailed description of these methods can be found in Sandra Lang's book Breastfeeding special care babies, details of which are given in the recommended reading section at the end of this chapter.

DRUGS AND BREASTFEEDING

Drug exposure to the nursing infant may sometimes be minimized by having the mother take the medication just after completing a feed. The British National Formulary (BNF) provides information on drugs known to be excreted in breast milk.

Prescribed medication

Most prescribed drugs do not pass into the breast milk in quantities that would have a significant effect either on the baby or on lactation, and are therefore usually compatible with breastfeeding.

However, because some prescribed drugs can be harmful to infants and others may inhibit lactation, only essential drugs should be prescribed. Mothers should be encouraged to remind their medical practitioner that they are breastfeeding, and to ask what the possible effects on the baby or on lactation might be.

Over-the-counter medication

Mothers should be advised to be as careful of medication when breastfeeding as they were during pregnancy. Even drugs that may be thought of as harmless in normal dosages may affect the baby or lactation. Mothers should be encouraged to seek the advice of the pharmacist.

A good principle to use is *if the medication is not essential, don't use it.*

Recreational drug use

There are no known safe levels for drugs used recreationally. Therefore, mothers should be strongly advised against their use.

Drug addiction and breastfeeding

The weight of opinion is that it is safer for drug users and addicts not to breastfeed their babies. This especially applies if the method of administration is erratic or intravenous, thereby increasing the risk of human immunodeficiency virus (HIV) and hepatitis infections.

However, 'most drugs of misuse do not pass into the breast milk in quantities which are sufficient to have a major effect on the newborn baby' (Shapiro 1995, p 30).

The benefits of breast milk are so great that, for some women, these benefits should be weighed against the possibility of transmitting small quantities of the drug and, in some cases, against the increased risk of transmitting infection.

Mothers who are drug users or who may test positive for HIV or hepatitis B but who want to breastfeed should be given all the information that they need to make an informed decision, and should be encouraged to discuss this issue with their GP, consultant and key worker.

SUMMARY

This chapter has attempted to give an overview of the help and encouragement that health professionals can give to breastfeeding babies and their mothers. With such a great deal to learn on

	Box 2.3 Training providers

- ◆ The UNICEF UK Baby Friendly Initiative provides training courses for health professionals.
- ◆ The National Childbirth Trust (NCT) provides training to members of the NCT who wish to become breastfeeding counsellors.
- ◆ La Leche League (LLL) provides training to its members.
- ◆ Local trainers may also be available in your area.

this subject, it is recommended that paediatric and neonatal staff receive updated, high-quality training in breastfeeding and its management. Box 2.3 shows some sources of training provision in breastfeeding.

FURTHER READING

Royal College of Midwives 1991 Successful breastfeeding, 2nd edn. Churchill Livingstone, Edinburgh

This is a very readable introduction to the practical aspects of breastfeeding. The clear, down-to-earth manner in which it is written gives practical advice and confidence to all those who are helping mothers to establish breastfeeding. A must for all health workers who have contact with newly delivered mothers and their infants.

Henschel D, Inch S 1996 Breastfeeding: a guide for midwives. Books for Midwives, Hale

A reference book that covers both the theory and practical aspects of initiating and establishing breastfeeding. The authors identify common problems and discuss solutions.

Lang S 1998 Breastfeeding special care babies. Baillière Tindall, London

This book is unique in that it comprehensively addresses the practical aspects of breastfeeding

babies with special care needs. All aspects of breastfeeding are discussed, from anatomy and physiology, fixing and positioning to suggested alternative methods of offering breast milk to a baby who is unable to breastfeed. The book is well illustrated and well referenced and is essential reading for all those involved with preterm, small for dates or sick babies.

La Leche League International 1997 The breast-feeding answer book (revised edition). Schaumburg, Illinois (available from NCT Sales Scotland)

*This is **the** most comprehensive reference book available. It is laid out in a format that is easily accessed by mothers and by those who help them to breastfeed. Breastfeeding situations are thoroughly investigated and discussed and ways of approaching problems always consider the possible emotional state of the mother.*

Akre J (ed) 1998 Infant feeding – the physiological basis. Bulletin of WHO 67 (Suppl.)

This scientific publication is of great value to those health professionals, GPs, paediatricians, nurses, nutritionists, midwives and those working in the field of public health who prepare and implement guidelines on infant feeding. The book covers the nutritional aspects of prenatal and immediate postpartum periods, lactation, the composition of breast milk, its nutritional and immunological qualities. Health factors that may interfere with breastfeeding are also considered, as are low birth-weight infants and infants during periods of acute infection and convalescence.

REFERENCES

Akre J (ed) 1998 Infant feeding – the physiological basis. Bulletin of WHO 67 (Suppl.)

Carpenter G 1980 Epidermal growth factor is a major growth promoting agent in human milk. Science 20 April:198–199

Cumming R G, Klieneburg R J 1993 Breastfeeding and other reproductive factors and the risk of hip fractures in the elderly. International Journal of Epidemiology 22:684–691

Ford R P, Taylor B J, Mitchell E A et al 1993 Breastfeeding and the risk of sudden infant death. International Journal of Epidemiology 22(5):885–890

Gilbert R E, Wigfield R E, Fleming P J, Berry P J, Rudd P T 1995 Bottle feeding and the sudden infant death syndrome. British Medical Journal 310:88–90

Gross B 1991 Is the lactational amenorrhea method a part of natural family planning? American Journal of Obstetrics and Gynecology 166:2014–2019

Gwinn M L, Lee N C, Rhodes P H, Layde P M, Rubin G L 1990 Pregnancy, breast feeding, and oral contraceptives and the risk of epithelial ovarian cancer. Journal of Clinical Epidemiology 43:559–568

Holland B, Welch A A, Unwin I D, Buss D H, Paul A A, Southgate D A T 1991 McCance and Widdowson's 'The composition of foods'. The Royal Society of Chemistry and MAFF, HMSO, London

Howie P W, Forsythe J S, Ogston S A, Clark A, Florey C Du V 1998 Protective effects of breastfeeding. British Medical Journal 300:11–15

Jannson L, Karlson F A, Westermark B 1985 Mitogenic activity and epidermal growth factor content in human milk. Acta Paediatrica Scandinavica 74:250–253

Karajalainen I, Martin J M, Knip M et al 1992 A bovine albumin peptide as a possible trigger of insulin-dependent diabetes mellitus. New England Journal of Medicine 327:302–307

Labbok M H, Hendershot G E 1987 Does breastfeeding protect against dental malocclusion? American Journal of Preventive Medicine 3:227–232

Lammi-Keefe J C, Ferris A M, Jensen R G 1990 Changes in human milk at 0600, 1000, 1400, 1800 and 2200hrs. Journal of Pediatric Gastroenterology and Nutrition 11:83–88

Lang S, Lawrence C J, Orme R 1994 Cup feeding: an alternative method of infant feeding. Archives of Disease in Childhood 71:365–369

Lawrence R A 1989 Breastfeeding: a guide for the medical profession, 5th edn. CV Mosby Company, St Louis

Lawson M 1992 Non nutritional factors in human breast milk. Modern Midwife Nov/Dec:18–21

Lewis P R, Brown J B, Renfrew M B, Short R V 1991 The resumption of ovulation and menstruation in a well-nourished population of women breastfeeding for an extended period of time. Fertility and Sterility 55: 529–536

Lucas A, Cole T J 1990 Breastmilk and neonatal necrotising enterocolitis. Lancet 336: 1519–1523

Lucas A, Morley R, Coles T J, Gore S M 1994 Breastmilk and subsequent intelligent quotient in babies born pre-term. Archives of Disease in Childhood 70:F141–146

Meier P, Anderson G 1987 Response of preterm infants to bottle and breastfeeding. American Journal of Maternal Child Nursing 12:97–105

Newton N 1978 The role of oxytocin reflexes in the three interpersonal reproductive acts, coitus, birth and breastfeeding. In: Carenza, L et al (eds) Clinical psychology – endocrinology in reproduction. Proceedings of the Serono Symposia, vol. 22. Academic Press, New York

Perez A, Labbok M H, Queenan J T 1992 Clinical study of the lactational amenorrhoea method of family planning. Lancet 339:968–970

Reissland N, Burghart R 1988 The quality of a mother's milk and the health of her child: beliefs and practices of the women of Mithila. Social Science and Medicine 27:461–469

Shapiro H 1995 Drugs, pregnancy and childcare. Institute for the Study of Drug Dependence, London

UK National Case Control Study Group 1993 Breastfeeding and risk of breast cancer in younger women. British Medical Journal 307:17–20

Uuay R D, Birch D G, Birch E E, Tyson J E, Hoffman D R 1990 Effect of dietary omega-3 fatty acids on retinal function of very-low-birth-weight neonates. Pediatric Research 28(5):485–492

Woolridge M W 1986a The aetiology of sore nipples. Midwifery 2:172–176

Woolridge M W 1986b The anatomy of infant sucking. Midwifery 2. 164–167

Appendix 2.1 The breastfeed observation chart

The breastfeed observation chart was designed for national 'Invest in Breast Together' training and is intended to be used with nursing mothers.

The BREAST feed observation chart – 'Invest in Breast Together'

Mother's name ....   Date

....

Baby's name ....   Baby's age

....

(Bracketed items refer only to the newborn infant, not to the older baby who sits up.)

Signs that breastfeeding is going well: **Signs of possible difficulty:**

Body position

☐ Mother relaxed and comfortable   ☐ Shoulders tense, leans over body

☐ Baby's body close to mother's   ☐ Baby's body away from mother's

☐ Baby's head and body straight   ☐ Baby must twist neck

☐ Baby's chin touching breast   ☐ Baby's chin does not touch breast

☐ (Baby's bottom supported)   ☐ (Only shoulder or head supported)

Responses

☐ Baby reaches for breast if hungry   ☐ No response to breast

☐ (Baby roots for breast)   ☐ (No rooting observation)

☐ Baby explores breast with tongue   ☐ Baby not interested in breast

☐ Baby calm and alert at breast   ☐ Baby restless or fussy

☐ Baby stays attached to breast   ☐ Baby slips off breast

☐ Signs of milk ejection (leaking, afterpain)   ☐ No sign of milk ejection

Emotional bonding

☐ Secure, confident hold   ☐ Nervous, shaking or limp hold

☐ Face-to-face attention from mother

☐ No mother–baby eye contact

☐ Much touching by mother

☐ Little touching between mother and baby

Anatomy

☐ Breasts soft and full

☐ Breasts engorged and hard

☐ Nipples stick out, protractile

☐ Nipples flat or inverted

☐ Skin appears healthy

☐ Fissures or redness of skin

☐ Breasts look round during feed

☐ Breasts look stretched and pulled

Suckling

☐ Mouth open wide

☐ Mouth closed, points forward

☐ Lower lip turned outward

☐ Lower lip turned in

☐ Tongue cupped around breast

☐ Cannot see baby's tongue

☐ Cheeks round

☐ Cheeks tense or pulled in

☐ Slow, deep sucks, bursts with pauses

☐ Rapid sucks

☐ Can see or hear swallowing

☐ Can hear smacking or clicking

Time spent suckling

☐ Baby releases breast

☐ Mother takes baby off breast

☐ Baby sucked for...minutes

Infant feeding

Anita MacDonald

INTRODUCTION

Appropriate nutrition in infancy is essential for optimal growth and development. It has also been shown to influence adult health. Infants are particularly vulnerable to under- or inappropriate nutrition for five reasons:

1. Low nutritional stores – newborn infants, particularly preterm, have poor stores of fat and protein.
2. Rapid growth and development – energy and nutrient requirements are relatively high per unit body size in infancy.
3. Rapid neuronal development – the brain grows rapidly during the last trimester of pregnancy and throughout the first 2 years of life.
4. Many body systems are still immature – particularly gastrointestinal, renal and immune function. Inadequate feeding can result in problems caused by inadequate digestion, poor absorption, impaired excretion or infection.
5. There is evidence that poorer growth in utero and during infancy are contributory factors to the development of adult diseases such as coronary artery disease, hypertension and diabetes.

Health professionals working with mothers and children are ideally placed to influence the diet of infants. It is therefore essential that any advice offered is consistent and accurate and fully supports the local health trust's own infant feeding policy.

NUTRITIONAL REQUIREMENTS OF FULL-TERM INFANTS

Energy

Energy is needed for growth, metabolism and activity (See Table 3.1).

The neonate is almost immediately dependent on exogenous energy sources. Fat and carbohydrate each provide 40 to 50% of the energy in breast and formula milk. Lactose is the predominant carbohydrate in breast and most normal formula milks.

The estimated average requirements (EAR) for energy (Department of Health 1991) are summarized in Table 3.2. The figures are intended only for formula-fed infants and the EARs for energy for both girls and boys are assumed to be identical when expressed on a body weight basis.

Different infants grow at different rates, and adequate daily weight gain in term newborns has been estimated to be about 10 to 12g/kg per day.

Table 3.1 Utilization of energy in infancy

Energy use	kcal/kg per day
Resting metabolic rate	48–55
Growth	25–40
Activity	10–15
Thermogenic effect of food	5–10
Losses	5
Total	93–120

Table 3.2 Estimated average requirements for energy in infancy. (DoH 1991. Crown copyright material is reproduced with the permission of the Controller of Her Majesty's Stationery Office.)

Age in months	Energy requirement kcal/kg per day
1	115
3	100
6	95
9	95
12	95

Table 3.3 Reference nutrient intake for protein in infancy (DoH 1991. Crown copyright material is reproduced with the permission of the Controller of Her Majesty's Stationery Office.)

Age in months	Protein g/kg per day
0–3	2.2
4–6	1.6
7–9	1.6
10–12	1.5

Protein

Protein is necessary for the synthesis of body proteins, enzymes and hormones, and is crucial for linear growth. The protein dietary reference values for infants, shown in Table 3.3, are calculated from the Committee on Medical Aspects of Food Policy recommendations for infants aged 0 to 3 months, and from the FAO/WHO/UNU expert consultation report (WHO 1995), with additions made for growth for infants aged 4 months and older (Department of Health 1991).

The protein:energy ratio should be within the range 7.5 to 12% for infants. This means they should receive 7.5 to 12% of their energy from protein.

Ninety percent of the protein in breast milk is absorbed by term and some preterm infants. Protein absorption from infant formula is above 80%.

Micronutrients

Dietary reference values for common vitamins and minerals are given in Table 3.4.

Vitamin A and vitamin C deficiency have not been seen in breastfed infants or in infants on normal infant formula. Vitamin B deficiency is rare in breastfed infants. However, infantile beriberi has been reported in a breastfed child of a mother eating polished rice in south-east Asia and vitamin B6 deficiency was reported in a group of Finnish infants exclusively breastfed for over 6 months (Wharton 1997).

Term infants on adequate volumes of normal infant formula do not develop nutritional rickets,

Table 3.4 Reference nutrient intake for vitamins and minerals. (DoH 1991. Crown copyright material is reproduced with the permission of the Controller of Her Majesty's Stationery Office.)

Nutrient	0–3 months	4–6 months	7–12 months
Vitamin A µg	350	350	350
Vitamin D µg	9	9	7
Vitamin C mg	25	25	25
Calcium mg	525	525	525
Iron mg	1.7	4.3	7.8

Table 3.6 Guidelines on the average number and volume of feeds at different ages. (From Wardley et al 1997 with permission of Oxford University Press.)

Approximate age	Approximate volume per feed	Number of feeds per day
1–2 weeks	50–70 ml	7–8
2–6 weeks	75–100 ml	6–7
2 months	110–180 ml	5–6
3 months	170–220 ml	5
6 months	220–240 ml	4

as they receive about 8.5 µg per day of vitamin D from the infant formula. Breastfed infants show a seasonal variation in plasma 25-hydroxyvitamin D, and for babies born in the autumn the concentration can decline to very low levels because winter milk contains little vitamin D.

The dietary reference values for calcium are based on the relatively poor absorption of calcium from infant formula milk. Calcium absorption efficiency from breast milk is 66%, compared with only 40% in infant formula milk.

The term infant is born with adequate iron stores for the first 4 months of life. In addition, total body iron remains at 250 mg between 0 and 4 months, so a dietary source is not important at this stage.

Fluid

Water comprises 70 to 75% of the weight of the newborn term infant. It is required for formation of urine, stool and insensible water losses, as well as for growth. This is summarized in Table 3.5.

Demand feeding with breast or formula milk should ensure that the healthy term infant gets the

Table 3.5 Maintenance water requirements. (Adapted from Moya 1993.)

Use	ml/kg per day
Insensible (lungs and skin)	20
Urine	60–75
Stool	5
Growth	1–3
Total	86–103

right volume of fluid and nutrients. As a guide, in the first 4 months of life most infants ingest 150 to 200 ml/kg per day. After this age, volumes usually fall if other foods have been introduced. Infants should not normally be given more than 1200 ml of feed per 24 hours as this may induce vomiting. Table 3.6 gives guidelines on the average number and volume of feeds at different ages.

FULL-TERM NORMAL INFANT FORMULA

In the UK, the majority of babies are still given an infant formula at some stage. In 1995, although only 34% of mothers gave infant formula from birth, 62% of infants were being given infant formula exclusively at around 6 to 10 weeks, and 77% were using infant formula either exclusively or in combination with breast milk at 2 months (Foster et al 1997). Interestingly, in a survey on infant feeding practices in Asian families in the UK, as few as 10% of Bangladeshi, 24% of Pakistani and 18% of Indian babies had only ever bottle-fed (Avery & Thomas 1997).

In the UK, bottle-feeding is a safe and nutritionally satisfactory alternative to breast-feeding, providing that modified infant formula milk is used. Infant formulae have been designed to match the nutritional composition of breast milk closely, but there are still major differences:

◆ The bioavailability of many nutrients in human milk is superior to that in infant formulae: e.g. calcium and iron.

Table 3.7 Modification of cow's milk to infant formula

Nutrients	Cow's milk	Whey-based infant formula	Casein-based infant formula
Protein			
Quantity	High	Lowered	Lowered
	3.3g/100 ml	1.4–1.9g/100 ml	1.4–1.9g/100 ml
Type	80% casein	40% casein	80% casein
	20% whey	60% whey	60% whey
Carbohydrate			
Quantity	Low	Increased	Increased
	4.9g/100 ml	7.0–8.6g/100 ml	7.0–8.6g/100 ml
Type	Lactose	Usually all lactose	Usually all lactose, but occasionally other carbohydrates added
Fat			
Quantity	3.6g/100 ml	2.6–3.8g/100 ml	2.6–3.8g/100 ml
Type	High in buttermilk	Vegetable oils and other fats replace buttermilk	Vegetable oils and other fats replace buttermilk
		Correct quantity and ratio of essential fatty acids added	Correct quantity and ratio of essential fatty acids added
		Some formulae have very long chain fatty acids added	
Minerals	High in phosphorus, sodium, potassium and calcium	Minerals reduced	Minerals reduced
Quantity			
Sodium	2.3 mmol/100 ml	0.65–1.1 mmol/100 ml	0.65–1.1 mmol/100 ml
Calcium	3.0 mmol/100 ml	0.88–2.1 mmol/100 ml	0.88–2.1 mmol/100 ml
Phosphorus	3.2 mmol/100 ml	0.9–1.8 mmol/100 ml	0.9–1.8 mmol/100 ml
Vitamins and trace minerals	Low in iron, zinc, copper, vitamins C, D, and folic acid	A range of added vitamins and minerals to meet nutritional requirements	A range of added vitamins and minerals to meet nutritional requirements

◆ Breast milk composition varies significantly: e.g. fore and hind milk, time of day, mother's diet and prematurity.
◆ The low levels of vitamins D and K in human milk are considered inappropriate for infant formulae.
◆ The non-nutrient substances – immunological, hormonal and enzymes – in breast milk are not reproduced in infant formulae.

Normal infant formulae, produced from cow's milk, are modified in five main ways to provide a composition more similar to breast milk (see Table 3.7). There are two main types of infant formulae that differ mainly in their protein composition. These are:

◆ whey-based formula (60% whey, 40% casein)
◆ casein-based formula (20% whey, 80% casein).

The practical significance of the two different types of infant formula relates to their digestibility characteristics and to the utilisation of nitrogen:

◆ Whey proteins are quickly eliminated from the stomach.
◆ Casein forms curds which are more slowly digested.

Full-term normal infants readily digest both types of formula. However, infants with poor gastrointestinal function, such as those born preterm, may experience occasional problems with intestinal obstruction with casein-based formulae. In addition, low birth-weight infants have been shown to have better nitrogen and fat absorption with whey-based infant formulae (Brown et al 1989).

Although it is widely believed by mothers that casein-based formulae are more satisfying for hungrier babies, clinical evidence has shown that this is not the case (Taitz & Scholey 1989). The Infant Formula and Follow-on Formula Regulations 1995, which enact EC Regulations 91/321/EC in the UK, regulate minimum and maximum nutrient concentrations for infant

Table 3.8 Guidelines on the composition of infant formulae. (HMSO 1995, reproduced under the terms of Crown Copyright Policy Guidance issued by HMSO.)

Nutrient		Analysis (per 100 kcal)
Energy	(kcal)	60–75 per 100 ml
Protein	(g)	1.8–3.0
Fat	(g)	3.3–6.6
Carbohydrate	(g)	7–14
Vitamin A	(μg)	60–180
Vitamin D	(μg)	1–2.5
Vitamin C	(mg)	8–NS
Calcium	(mg)	50–NS
Phosphorus	(mg)	25–90
Sodium	(mg)	20–60
Iron	(mg)	0.5–1.5
Zinc	(mg)	0.5–1.5
NS = not stated		

formulae. A summary of some of the major nutrients stipulated by these regulations is given in Table 3.8.

Addition of novel nutrients to normal infant formulae

Long chain polyunsaturated fatty acids

There has been debate about the need to add long chain polyunsaturated fatty acids (LCPs), particularly docosahexaenoic acid (DHA) and arachidonic acid (AA), to normal infant formulae. These are components of the phospholipids in the retina and brain, and deficiency may cause impaired visual function and cognitive ability. DHA and AA can be synthesized from their respective parent essential fatty acids (linoleic acid and α-linolenic acid), but the enzymes necessary to do this may not be active until an infant is a few months old.

Term infants fed formulae devoid of LCPs have lower levels of AA and DHA in their red cell membranes, lower levels of DHA in the brain phospholipids, and different visual function to breastfed infants. So far, LCPs are only added to a small range of the formulae available. However, this remains an active area of research, and it may be desirable to add LCPs to all normal infant formulae (Wells 1998).

Nucleotides

Nucleotides are found in human milk. They are compounds of purine or pyrimidine bases, and help make up a substantial proportion of the non-protein nitrogen content of breast milk. Nucleotides are involved in several biological functions:

- cellular immunity
- intestinal microflora
- iron absorption
- synthesis of long chain polyunsaturated derivatives of ω-3 and ω-6 fatty acids
- gastrointestinal development.

Despite their potential benefit, term infants should be able to produce sufficient supplies by endogenous synthesis. For this reason, nucleotides are added to only one manufacturer's normal infant formula in the UK.

β-carotene

β-carotene is an antioxidant and has an important role in the immune response. It is proposed that antioxidants may help the infant's defence against oxygen toxicity by stabilizing free radicals during normal metabolism. However, β-carotene is added to only a few normal infant formulae available in the UK.

Guidelines and legislation on normal infant formulae

The Infant Formula and Follow-on Formula Regulations 1995 gave compositional and labelling requirements for infant formulae intended for use by infants in good health. In addition, it promoted the principles and aims of the WHO/UNICEF International code of marketing of breast-milk substitutes (WHO 1981). This is intended to promote breastfeeding and ensure that infant formulae are used correctly. It includes the following guidelines:

- Milk formulae should not be advertised to the public.
- There must be no free samples given to the public.
- Health professionals must not promote milk formulae.
- Baby milk manufacturers should not use pictures of bottle-feeding babies on labels.
- All information on milk formulae must include reference to the superior nature of breast-feeding.

Preparation of normal infant formulae

Although most babies are given a bottle at some stage, only about one quarter (27%) of mothers of first babies have been shown how to make up a bottle at antenatal classes (Foster et al 1997). Health workers should therefore ensure that parents are instructed on the reconstitution, sterilization and storage of normal infant formulae. (See Boxes 3.1, 3.2 and 3.3.)

Figure 3.1 shows some sterilizing equipment.

Box 3.1   Reconstitution of normal infant formula

- The formula should be mixed exactly according to the manufacturer's instructions.
- In the UK, this is standardized to one level scoop of formula powder to 30 ml (1 fluid ounce) of water.
- Scoops should be level – not heaped.
- Scoops from different infant formula brands hold different amounts of powder and are not interchangeable.
- The water should be brought to the boil – however, prolonged boiling will increase the content of minerals and nitrates by evaporation.
- The water should then be allowed to cool a little – a temperature of about 50 to 60 °C allows easy mixing without clumping of the powder.

Box 3.2   Sterilization of bottles, jugs and teats

◆ Sterilizing tablets or fluid is the most common form of sterilization method by white and Asian mothers (Avery & Thomas 1997).

◆ With all methods, the bottle and teat must be thoroughly cleaned, before the film of milk hardens, by rinsing and then cleaning with detergent, warm water and a bottle brush and further rinsing.

◆ With a chemical agent (usually sodium hypochlorite), a fresh solution should be made every 24 hours.

◆ Bottles and equipment must be completely submerged in the sterilizing fluid for at least the minimum recommended length of time.

Box 3.3   Storage and warming of feeds

◆ If more than one feed is made up at a time, they must be stored in a refrigerator.

◆ The Avery & Thomas (1997) survey found that 22% of Bangladeshi and 16% of Pakistani mothers did not store feeds in a refrigerator, with some leaving made-up bottles in the bedroom at night.

◆ Cold feeds direct from the refrigerator are well accepted by babies.

◆ If feeds are warmed first, this should be for a minimum length of time to avoid incubation of bacteria.

◆ Unfinished infant formula should not be reused.

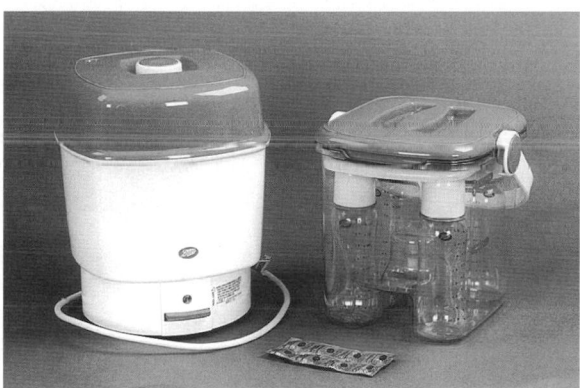

Figure 3.1   Sterilizing equipment

Availability of infant formulae welfare food scheme

Infants in families receiving Income Support, Job Seeker's Allowance or related benefits can receive 900 g per week of a range of specified brands of infant formula by exchanging milk tokens at their local health clinic. Alternatively, they may receive 7 pints or 8 half litres of cow's milk. However, they are not entitled to follow-on formulae or 'ready to feed' formulae. Breastfeeding mothers may take the entitlement in the form of cow's milk to drink themselves.

OTHER MILKS

Follow-on formulae

These are designed for older infants over the age of 6 months. They are based on modified cow's milk and contain less protein, calcium and phosphorous than cow's milk, but more than standard infant formulae. Most follow-on formulae contain almost double the iron and 45% more vitamin C than standard infant formulae.

Follow-on formulae provide a useful drink for older infants if breastfeeding has been stopped, or if the volume of standard infant formulae is less than 400 ml day. However, follow-on formulae should not replace breast milk or standard infant formula milk if the volume is adequate.

Unmodified cow's milk

Cow's milk is low in iron, vitamin C and vitamin D. Although it may be used in small quantities in the preparation of solid foods, it is not recommended as the main drink before 1 year of age.

WEANING

Weaning is defined as the process of expanding the diet to include foods and drinks other than breast milk or infant formula (Department of Health 1994). Weaning is a gradual process, starting with semi-solid foods between the ages of 4 and 6 months, and gradually progressing over a period of months to the age of 1 year, when a child should be managing similar foods to the rest of the family.

Weaning fulfils a number of functions:

◆ to add or replace energy and protein received from milk
◆ to add micronutrients such as iron and vitamin D
◆ to help develop chewing
◆ to introduce a diet similar to the rest of the family.

Box 3.4 identifies the key developmental changes relevant to weaning.

KEY FACT

In 1995, 55% of infants had been given solids by 3 months of age. Asian babies were given solids slightly later than white babies, but 90% still had solids by 4 months of age (Avery & Thomas 1997).

Early weaning is associated with:

◆ increased risk of food intolerance
◆ reduced absorption of nutrients in breast or infant formulae milk
◆ persistent cough
◆ obesity
◆ poor neuromuscular coordination
◆ potential reduction in breast or infant formula milk intake.

What foods and when?

Stage 1: 4 to 5 months

At this stage foods should be thin, smooth and semi-solid.

Box 3.4 Developmental changes relevant to weaning. (Adapted from Wharton 1997.)

4 months:
◆ can maintain posture if supported in a chair.

5 months:
◆ can take soft, puréed food from a spoon, form a bolus and swallow it
◆ can hold objects and put them to mouth to suck.

6 to 8 months:
◆ teeth begin to erupt
◆ sits without support
◆ can chew
◆ can hand-feed items like biscuits
◆ learns to shut mouth, turn head and indicate feed refusal.

9 to 12 months:
◆ can sit easily
◆ attempts to use spoon
◆ indicates and understands 'no'
◆ pincer grasp of small objects.

Suitable food

◆ Puréed fruits, vegetables, mashed potato, custard, natural yoghurt, gluten-free cereal, baby rice.
◆ When an infant has accepted eating from a spoon, different tastes and textures can be introduced, including well-cooked puréed meat, pulses and a wider variety of cereals.
◆ Breast, infant formula milk or cereal can be added to puréed fruit or vegetables to improve the energy and nutrient density.
◆ Salt should not be added.
◆ Sugar should be avoided, or used minimally for palatability only.

Process

◆ Initially offer one or two teaspoons at a midday or teatime feed.
◆ Give milk to ease hunger first.

◆ Gradually increase the quantity and frequency of solids to three times daily according to appetite.
◆ Infants will vary in the time they take to accept solids. It may vary from a short time to several weeks.
◆ Initially the contribution of non-milk foods to total energy and nutrient intake is small. The breast or infant formula should still supply the main source of nutrition.

Stage 2: 6 to 9 months

At this stage foods should be minced or mashed and may include soft finger food.

Suitable food

◆ Coarsely puréed meat.
◆ Soft cooked fish or pulses.
◆ Introduce wholemeal cereals or instant oat cereal.
◆ Introduce well-cooked egg, e.g. scrambled.
◆ Introduce finger foods and raw soft fruit, e.g. banana, melon, cheese fingers, soft cooked carrot, and fingers of toast, chapatti or pitta bread.
◆ Encourage food with a stronger flavour. In fact, many family foods are suitable if blended to a texture containing some soft lumps. Mild spices can be added to soft cooked lentils or dahl.

Process

◆ Offer solids three times daily.
◆ Decrease volume of milk to provide 55% of energy intake; increase solids to provide 45% of energy intake.
◆ Decrease milk feeds to three to four times daily.
◆ Encourage drinks from a feeder beaker.
◆ Infants must never be left unsupervised with finger foods.

Stage 3: 10 to 12 months

At this stage foods should be minced or chopped.

Suitable food

◆ Meat can be minced or finely chopped.
◆ Cooked vegetables need only be chopped and some sautéed vegetables can be included at each meal so the infant is encouraged to self-feed.
◆ Introduce pasta dishes with small shaped pasta.
◆ By the age of 1 year, the infant should be eating similar foods to the rest of the family.

Table 3.9 Example of a weaning plan (0–6 months)

Age	Solids/drinks to introduce	6.00 am	10.00 am	2.00 pm	6.00 pm	10.00 pm
4 months	1–2 teaspoons of puréed baby food	✔	✔ ●	✔	✔	✔
4½ months	3–4 teaspoons of puréed baby food	✔	✔ ●	✔	✔ ●	✔
5 months	6 teaspoons of puréed baby food	✔	✔ ●	✔ ●	✔ ●	✔
		8.00 am	12.00 pm	5.00 pm	9.00 pm	
5½ months	3–4 tablespoons of puréed baby foods	✔ ●	✔ ●	✔ ●	✔	
6 months	5–6 tablespoons of mashed baby food	✔ ●	✔ ●	✔ ●	✔	

✔ = infant feeds (breast or formula)
● = solids

Process

- Offer three main meals.
- Milk should supply 40 to 45% of energy intake.

Choice of weaning foods

Home-made weaning foods

Approximately 40% of infants are given home-made weaning foods at the age of 4 to 5 months (Foster et al 1997). There are several advantages to using home-made foods, and they should be encouraged because:

- they accustom the infant to the taste of adult-based food
- they are cheap to prepare – wastage is low if a batch of bulk meals is prepared at one time and frozen in ice cube trays or other suitable containers
- meat-based halal weaning dishes can be prepared for Muslim infants
- they are easy to prepare and require little specialist equipment.

Drawbacks of home-made weaning foods include:

- preparation time
- nutritional quality – home-made solids have been shown to be low in energy, iron and zinc (Stordy et al 1995).

Commercial weaning foods

Most mothers use dried weaning food or jars or tins of weaning food at some stage during the weaning process because they are so convenient. Manufacturers have to conform to strict regulations governing their safety, composition and added vitamins and minerals. They are not allowed to contain artificial colourings, flavourings or preservatives. Such foods are, however, relatively expensive, wastage is high, and the range of vegetarian meals is limited. However, the first commercial halal baby meals have recently been produced.

Box 3.5 lists some of the equipment which is useful for the preparation of home-made baby food. Some of this equipment is shown in Figure 3.2.

Box 3.5 Useful equipment for preparation of home-made baby food

- Metal sieve.
- Mouli: this hand-turned food mill with variable cutting discs purées the food, separating it from the seeds and skin which can be difficult for the baby to digest. It is best used for fruit, vegetables, fish and the softer textured meats such as chicken.
- Baby mouli (a smaller version of the mouli): useful for puréeing small amounts of fresh food.
- Blender or food processor: this is useful for puréeing larger quantities. However, foods for young babies will often need to be sieved afterwards to remove any seeds and skin.
- Hand blender: useful for puréeing small quantities of food. Foods will still need to be sieved afterwards to remove any seeds and skin.
- Ice cube trays: pour prepared, puréed food into plastic, pop-out ice cube trays. Freeze immediately. Pop out the frozen cubes and transfer them to plastic freezer bags. Label and date. The food cubes can be stored for up to 2 months.

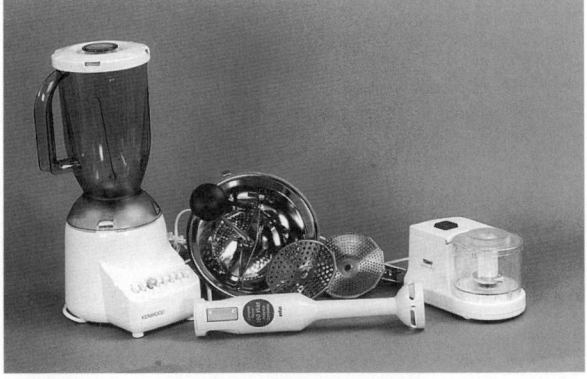

Figure 3.2 Weaning equipment

Weaning the vegetarian infant

Table 3.10 lists some of the problems which can be associated with a lacto-vegetarian weaning diet and identifies some of the solutions to these problems. Table 3.11 lists some of the problems associated with vegan diets.

BABY DRINKS

KEY POINTS

◆ Infants are now more likely to be given water than baby juice or other drinks as an additional drink to milk (Foster et al 1997).
◆ Sugar levels in baby juices and herbal infant drinks vary from 3 g/100 ml to 10 g/100 ml.
◆ Baby drink composition (i.e. juices and herbal drinks) is controlled by EU regulations for weaning foods.

Baby juices and herbal drinks are unnecessary. This is because breast or infant formula should provide the majority of fluid given, and if an infant is thirsty or needs extra fluid, water only should be offered. If baby drinks are given, they should be:

– given sparingly
– well diluted
– given from a feeder beaker
– given at mealtimes only.

It is important to note that the infant should not be allowed to fall asleep or be left alone with a bottle or feeding reservoir in the mouth.

◆ Natural fruit juices should only be offered very diluted and at mealtimes. Their natural acidity can contribute to dental caries.
◆ Adult squashes and aerated drinks are unsuitable for infancy. Colas and several other drinks contain stimulants such as caffeine. Soft drinks contain additives and artificial

Table 3.10 Problems associated with a lacto-vegetarian weaning diet

Problems	Solutions
Low energy density	Add extra cereal, breast or formula milk, margarine or oil to weaning foods
Risk of iron deficiency	Use iron-enriched cereals, pulses and bread
	Use iron-enriched commercial baby foods
	Continue with infant formula or follow-on formula from 6 months
	Do not give breast-feeds with solids
	Give a source of vitamin C (e.g. fruit or fruit juice) with meals to facilitate iron absorption
Risk of vitamin D deficiency	Give vitamin D supplements (from Mother & Children's vitamin drops)
	Continue use of infant formula milk or follow-on formula

Table 3.11 Problems associated with a vegan weaning diet

Problems	Solutions
Low energy density	Add extra cereal, breast or fortified soya milk, soya margarine or vegetable oil to weaning foods
Risk of iron deficiency	Encourage iron-enriched cereals, pulses and bread
	Use iron-enriched commercial vegan baby foods
	Do not give breast-feeds with solids
	Encourage vegan infant soya formula e.g. Farleys Soya
Risk of calcium deficiency	Give frequent breast-feeds or at least 500 ml infant soya-based formula
	Encourage soya yoghurt and other soya desserts, tofu and bread
Risk of zinc deficiency	Encourage use of infant soya milk
	Encourage legumes, bread, fortified cereals, tofu, nut butters, and chopped meat substitute products: e.g. vegeburgers
Risk of vitamin B_{12} deficiency	Vitamin supplementation with B_{12}
Risk of vitamin D deficiency	Vitamin supplements – e.g. Mother & Children's vitamin drops
	Encourage use of infant soya formula

sweeteners such as aspartame, which should not be given to infants.
◆ Tea should not be given. It contains tannin and may inhibit iron absorption.
◆ Natural mineral water should not be given to infants. This is covered by less comprehensive regulations than tap water. It may contain higher concentrations of solutes such as nitrates, sodium, fluoride and sulphate.

VITAMIN SUPPLEMENTS

KEY FACTS

◆ At 9 months of age, only 17% of infants are being given vitamin supplements (Foster et al 1997).
◆ At least twice as many Asian mothers as white mothers give their infants vitamin supplements (Avery & Thomas 1997).
◆ Infants and children under 5 years, whose families are on Income Support or Job Seekers Allowance, are entitled to free Mother & Children's vitamin drops.
◆ Mother & Children's vitamin drops contain vitamins A, D and C.

Recommendations for vitamin supplementation in infancy

The Department of Health COMA report on 'Weaning and the weaning diet' makes the following recommendations.
For breastfed infants:

◆ Breastfed infants under 6 months do not need vitamin supplementation provided the mother had an adequate vitamin status during pregnancy.

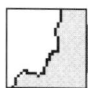

Box 3.6 Children's vitamin drops

Recommended dose: 5 drops per day. This contains:

Vitamin A – 200 µg
Vitamin D – 7 µg
Vitamin C – 20 mg

◆ From 6 months, they should be given A, D and C vitamin drops.

For formula-fed infants:

◆ Infants on formula milks do not need vitamin supplements if intake of formula or follow-on milk is more than 500 ml per day. If they are taking less than this, they should be given vitamins A, D and C.

The prevention of food allergy in infancy in high-risk infants

There are few proven guidelines for preventing food allergy, but for infants who have a strong family history of allergy, the following may be advisable:

◆ Breastfeeding should be encouraged for at least 6 months.
◆ A milk, egg and nut free exclusion diet for a mother during lactation may be helpful – but supporting evidence is inconclusive.
◆ Weaning should be discouraged before 4 months of age.
◆ Avoid 'allergenic' weaning foods before 6 months: i.e. cow's milk, wheat and eggs.
◆ Avoid peanuts until 3 years of age (Department of Health 1998).
◆ A dietitian should supervise any diet used in infancy or lactation.

NUTRITIONAL REQUIREMENTS OF PRETERM INFANTS

Table 3.12 summarizes the nutritional requirements of preterm infants weighing less than 2500 g.

KEY FACTS

◆ Preterm infants have a high nutritional requirement because of their rapid growth.
◆ Preterm infants born at 28 weeks' gestation double their birth weight in 6 weeks and treble it in 12 weeks, whereas term babies double their weight in 4.5 months and treble it in a year.

Table 3.12 Nutritional requirements of preterm infants weighing less than 2500 g. (From Lawson 1994 with permission.)

Nutrient		Requirements per kg of body-weight per day
Fluid	ml	150–200
Energy	kcal	130
	kJ	543
Protein		3.0–4.0
Calcium	mmol	2.0–6.25
Iron	μmol	35–45

Energy

Requirements for energy are very variable and depend on the individual infant, postnatal age, degree of prematurity, diet, activity and amount of handling.

Energy requirements are increased by:

◆ prematurity – preterm infants have a higher surface area to body weight ratio, so have an increased requirement.
◆ intrauterine growth retardation.
◆ metabolic state – e.g. stress, poor temperature control.

Protein

Requirements are high but intakes over 6.0 g/kg/day have caused long-term neurological impairment (Lawson 1994). The amino acids – cysteine, glycine and taurine – are considered essential.

Fat

◆ Fat digestion is impaired.
◆ Evidence suggests preterm infants require a dietary source of long-chain polyunsaturated fatty acids: i.e. docosahexaenoic acid and arachidonic acid.

Carbohydrate

◆ Levels of lactase are lower than in a term infant.
◆ Minimum needs are 12 to 14 g/kg/day of carbohydrate to prevent hypoglycaemia.

Vitamins and minerals

◆ Exact requirements for many micronutrients are unknown.
◆ Sodium requirements are high in infants of less than 34 weeks' gestation, due to increased sodium losses and an increased growth velocity.
◆ Preterm infants have low stores of iron, copper, zinc, magnesium and phosphorus.
◆ Infants fed on expressed breast milk need extra vitamin A supplements in order to meet requirements.

MILKS SUITABLE FOR PRETERM INFANTS

Breast milk

Preterm breast milk is slightly more concentrated nutritionally during the first 2 weeks of lactation than mature human milk. It contains more of the following:

◆ protein
◆ sodium
◆ calcium
◆ iron
◆ zinc.

The energy content is not increased.

Although infants fed preterm breast milk have been shown to have a higher intelligence quotient at the age of 7 years (Lucas et al 1992b), they still have a reduced growth velocity when compared to infants fed a more energy-dense formula.

Increasing the nutritional density of breast milk

To improve the energy and nutritional profile of breast milk it may be supplemented with:

◆ hydrolyzed protein infant formula
◆ commercially produced breast milk enhancers
◆ low birth-weight formula.

Preterm infant formulae

A number of preterm infant formulae are available. They have a higher nutrient density than

Table 3.13 Guidelines for the composition of preterm formula. (From ESPGAN 1987 with permission.)

		per 100 kcal	per 100 ml assuming 80 kcal/100 ml
Energy	kcal		80
	kJ		336
Protein	g	2.25–3.1	1.8–2.5
Fat	g	3.6–7.0	2.9–5.6
Carbohydrate	g	7.0–14.0	5.6–11.2
Calcium	mmol	1.75–3.5	1.4–2.8
Sodium	mmol	1.0–2.3	0.6–1.5
Iron	μmol	27	21
Vitamin C	mg	7.0	5.6

standard milks and contain all necessary vitamins, minerals and trace elements. They all contain long chain polyunsaturated fatty acids.

FEEDING THE PRETERM INFANT AT HOME

Usually, a preterm infant formula or supplemented breast-feed is stopped when an infant reaches 2.0 kg, and the infant is then given unsupplemented breast milk or normal infant formula. However, there are infant formulae available – Nutriprem 2 (Cow & Gate) and Premcare (Farleys) – whose composition falls between standard infant formulae and preterm formulae. There is some evidence that preterm infants grow better on these formulae than on standard formulae, although preterm infants have been shown to drink large volumes of normal formula post-hospital discharge (Lucas et al 1992a). The preterm infant formula powders are neither prescribable nor available on milk tokens, but this position may change. At present, they must be purchased from retail chemists and are 20% more expensive than standard infant formula.

Weaning the preterm infant

There are few firm guidelines when solids should be introduced. The Department of Health recommends that solids should only be introduced when:

◆ infant weighs 5 kg
◆ infant has lost extrusion reflex
◆ infant is able to eat from a spoon.

Parents are often keen to introduce solids at an early stage because many preterm infants consume large volumes of feed.

HEALTH CARE SUPPORT ON INFANT FEEDING

There is much need for standardized, accurate and practical information about infant feeding. Most parents want to discuss appropriate nutrition but frequently receive conflicting advice. The following should be implemented in all local health care areas to try and improve quality of information.

◆ Local infant feeding policy. This should be developed by a multidisciplinary team involving key members of the primary health care team and the hospital team, and should be produced in partnership with parents and local voluntary organisations.
◆ Development of undergraduate and postgraduate programmes on infant feeding for all health professionals involved in childcare. Ideally, these should be compulsory for all paediatric workers and updated at least biannually. This includes health visitors, doctors, paediatric nurses, midwives, link workers, ward assistants, primary care assistants and nursery workers.
◆ Local health care trusts should provide breastfeeding training to all paediatric health care workers.
◆ There should be good continuity of care by health professionals for individual mothers so conflicting advice is minimized.
◆ The personal child health record should be maximized to communicate information and advice given on infant feeding.

SUMMARY

◆ Infants are vulnerable to poor nutrition owing to low nutritional stores, rapid growth and development and immature body systems.

- The majority of infants in the UK are still given infant formula milk at some stage.
- If a modified infant formula is used, bottle-feeding is a safe and nutritionally satisfactory alternative to breastfeeding.
- Only about one quarter of first-time mothers have been shown how to make up a bottle of formula at antenatal classes.
- Unmodified cow's milk is not recommended as the main drink before 1 year of age.
- Early weaning before 4 months is associated with increased risk of food intolerance, persistent cough, obesity and poor neuromuscular coordination.
- Vegan weaning diets could result in low calorie intake, as well as iron, zinc, calcium, vitamin D and B_{12} deficiency.
- All formula-fed infants should be given clinic vitamin drops when the formula milk decreases below 500 ml daily. Breastfed infants should be given vitamin drops from 6 months but earlier if the mother is not eating a good mixed diet.

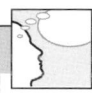

Questions

Answers are given in Appendix 2.

1. Plan a suitable feeding plan for a 4-week-old baby girl on formula feeds. She weighs 4 kg.

2. What factors are important for successful breastfeeding?

3. Describe the weaning pattern of a 6-month-old baby girl weighing 7.5 kg.

FURTHER READING

Barker M 1996 Nutrition and dietetics for health care. Churchill Livingstone, New York

British Paediatric Association Nutrition Standing Committee 1988 Vegetarian weaning. Archives of Disease in Childhood 63:1286–1292

Forsyth S J, Ogston S A, Clark A, Florey C du V, Howie P W 1993 Relation between early introduction of solid food to infants and their weight and illnesses during the first two years of life. British Medical Journal 306:1572–1576

Thomas B 1996 Nutrition in primary care. Blackwell Science, Oxford

Tyson T E, Lasky M, Miz C E 1983 Growth, metabolic response and development in very low birthweight infants fed banked human milk or enriched formula. Journal of Pediatrics 103:95–104

REFERENCES

Avery A, Thomas M 1997 Infant feeding in Asian families 1995. HMSO, London

Brown G A, Berger H M, Brueton M J, Scott P H, Wharton B A 1989 Nonlipid formula components and fat absorption in the low birth-weight newborns. American Journal of Clinical Nutrition 49:55–61

Department of Health 1991 Dietary reference values for food energy and nutrients. (Report on Health and Social Subjects No. 41.) HMSO, London

Department of Health 1994 Weaning and the weaning diet. (Report on Health and Social Subjects No. 45.) HMSO, London

Department of Health 1998 Peanut allergy. Committee on toxicity of chemicals in food, consumer products and the environment. HMSO, London

European Society of Paediatric Gastroenterology and Nutrition 1987 Nutrition and feeding of preterm infants. Acta Pediatrica Scandinavica, Suppl. 536

Foster K, Cheesbrough S, Lader D 1997 Infant feeding. HMSO, London

Lawson D 1994 Principles of paediatric dietetics. In: Shaw V, Lawson D (eds) Clinical paediatric dietetics. Blackwell Scientific, London, pp 3–12

Lucas A, King F, Bishop N B 1992a Post-discharge formula consumption in infants born preterm. Archives of Disease in Childhood 67:691–692

Lucas A, Bishop N J, King F J, Cole T J 1992b Randomised trial of nutrition for preterm infants after discharge. Archives of Disease in Childhood 67:324–327

Moya F R 1993 In: Suskind R M, Lewinter-Suskind L (eds) Textbook of pediatric nutrition. Raven Press, New York

Stordy B J, Redfern A, Morgan J B 1995 Healthy eating for infants – mothers' actions. Acta Paediatrica 84:733–741

Taitz L, Scholey E 1989 Are babies more satisfied by casein based formulas? Archives of Disease in Childhood 64:619–621

Wardley B L, Puntis J W L, Taitz L S 1997 Handbook of child nutrition. Oxford University Press, Oxford

Wells J 1998 Infant and follow-on formulas: the next decade. In: Wharton B (ed.) Nutrition in infancy – policy, practice and problems in Britain. BNF Nutrition Bulletin 23, Suppl. 1:23–34

Wharton B 1997 Nutrition in infancy. British Nutrition Foundation Briefing Paper. British Nutrition Foundation, London

World Health Organization 1981 International code of marketing breast-milk substitutes. World Health Organization, Geneva

World Health Organization 1995 Energy and protein requirements. Report of a Joint FAO/WHO/UNU Meeting. WHO Technical Report Series No. 724. World Health Organization, Geneva

4

The pre-school child

Anita MacDonald

INTRODUCTION

In this age group, food and mealtimes:

- help establish good eating habits
- enhance communication skills and language
- set dietary patterns for later life
- provide a useful medium for learning and play.

Factors in this age group, which can impede good nutrition, include:

- faddiness
- toddlers too busy to eat
- continuous snacking or poor mealtime routine
- laziness in chewing
- small appetites
- erratic food intake
- preference for drinks rather than food.

Pre-school children have high nutrient requirements relative to their size, as they are still undergoing quite rapid growth and development and are usually physically active. They should be offered small meals at regular times as well as small, suitable, snacks in between meals.

NUTRITIONAL REQUIREMENTS

Energy

Young children require energy for basic metabolic functions, for keeping warm, for activity and for growth. Table 4.1 shows the energy requirements of pre-school children (Department of Health 1991).

| Age (years) | Daily energy requirements (kcal) | |
	Boys	Girls
1 to 3	1230	1165
4	1715	1545

Protein

The UK reference nutrient intake (RNI) for protein for children aged 1 to 3 years is 14.5 g per day, and for children aged 4 to 6 years it is 19.7 g per day. This can easily be achieved by drinking 300 ml of cow's milk and eating two portions of higher protein foods such as meat, yoghurt, eggs or fish.

Fat

- ◆ The Committee on Medical Aspects of Food Policy report on nutritional aspects of cardiovascular disease recommends that the population aged 5 years and older should consume no more than 35% of calories from fat (Department of Health 1994). This does not apply to children before the age of 2 years.
- ◆ Between the ages of 2 and 5 years a flexible approach is recommended to the timing and extent of reduction in fat intake from 50% to 35% of energy. Appetite and growth will determine this.

Carbohydrate

- ◆ It is recommended for the population as a whole that 50% of energy should be supplied by carbohydrate. 39% should come from intrinsic and milk sugars and starch (e.g. in fruit, vegetables and milk) and no more than 11% should come from non-milk extrinsic sugars (e.g. in table sugar and honey).
- ◆ Such a high carbohydrate intake from starch and intrinsic sugars is inappropriate for children under 2 years of age. Although starch is well tolerated and efficiently absorbed, this type of carbohydrate intake is bulky and may inappropriately lead to a low energy intake.
- ◆ From the age of 2 years, there should be a gradual increase in energy derived from starchy foods with an equivalent decrease in energy from fats.

Fibre

- ◆ There are no UK recommendations for the amount of fibre appropriate for small children. In the United States recommendations are that children over 2 years of age should consume a minimum amount of dietary fibre equivalent to age (in grams) plus 5 g per day. For example, a 3-year-old child should consume 8 g per day and a 4-year-old should consume 9 g per day (Williams et al 1995, Wardley et al 1997).
- ◆ It should be noted that a diet too high in fibre and phytate may compromise energy intake or bio-availability of micronutrients, particularly in children under 2 years.

Calcium

- ◆ The calcium reference nutrient intakes for children aged 1 to 4 years are less than in the first year of life.
- ◆ Between 1 and 10 years, average daily calcium retention needed for skeletal growth has been estimated to rise from 70 to 150 mg per day. Only approximately 35% of dietary calcium is absorbed. (Table 4.2 shows the calcium requirements of pre-school children.)

Iron

Table 4.3 shows the iron requirements of pre-school children.

Age (years)	Calcium requirements mg/day
1 to 3	350
4	450

Table 4.3 Iron requirements of pre-school children. (DoH 1991. Crown copyright material is reproduced with the permission of the Controller of Her Majesty's Stationery Office.)

Age (years)	Iron dietary reference values mg/day
1 to 3	6.9 mg
4	6.1 mg

◆ Young children have relatively high iron requirements for tissue growth and to build up iron stores.
◆ Iron deficiency anaemia is particularly common in young children.
◆ Particular attention is needed to ensure pre-school children consume haem iron sources in appropriate quantity.
◆ Iron absorption from a diverse diet containing meat is assumed to be 15%, but is lower when little or no meat is consumed.

Vitamin C

Table 4.4 shows the vitamin C requirements of pre-school children.

◆ This is an important nutrient in young children. It is an antioxidant, aids wound healing, and assists in the absorption of non-haem iron.
◆ Dietary reference values for children have been scaled down proportionately from those of adults.
◆ Between 1 and 5 years, it is recommended vitamin C should be given in the form of Mother & Children's vitamin drops to all children, unless adequate vitamin status can be assured from a diverse diet.

Table 4.4 Vitamin C requirements of pre-school children. (DoH 1991. Crown copyright material is reproduced with the permission of the Controller of Her Majesty's Stationery Office.)

Age (years)	Vitamin C dietary reference values mg/day
1 to 3	30 mg
4	30 mg

Vitamin D

Table 4.5 shows the vitamin D requirements of pre-school children.

◆ Vitamin D has an important role in maintaining bone mineralization by enhancing calcium and phosphorus absorption and depositing calcium in bones and teeth.
◆ Children between 1 and 3 years are particularly vulnerable to vitamin D depletion because of the rate at which calcium is being laid down in bone.
◆ There are few dietary sources of vitamin D and the chief source is derived from the action of UV radiation on 7-dehydrocholesterol in the skin.
◆ There is limited availability of UV radiation for many children.
◆ After 3 years, children (apart from Asian and Afro-Caribbean children) usually have a satisfactory vitamin D status and have no vitamin D requirement.
◆ However, it is recommended for all children between 1 and 5 years that vitamin D should be given in the form of Mother & Children's vitamin drops.

WHAT DO PRE-SCHOOL CHILDREN ACTUALLY EAT?

In the past 10 years there have been a small number of studies, which have investigated the food and nutritional intake of young children in detail. In 1995, a DOH/MAFF comprehensive survey of the diet and nutritional status of children between the ages of $1\frac{1}{2}$ and $4\frac{1}{2}$

Table 4.5 Vitamin D requirements of pre-school children

Age (years)	Vitamin D dietary reference values μg/day
1 to 3	7
4	0*

*except Asian and Afro-Caribbean children

years was published. It found that children are taller and heavier, but not fatter than in 1967/8. However, energy intakes are lower, indicating that children are now more sedentary and that energy needs for keeping warm are less because most homes are better heated. This survey indicated a number of dietary quality issues, particularly with respect to sugar, fat, fibre and micronutrient intake (Gregory et al 1995).

Sugar

Sugar intake was high. In children aged $2\frac{1}{2}$ to $3\frac{1}{2}$ years, it provided 19.3% of the total energy intake. In this national study and in a smaller study of 153 pre-school children in Edinburgh (Payne & Belton 1992), chief sugar sources were beverages, mainly soft drinks.

Fat

In the DOH/MAFF national study, about 36% of total energy was from fat sources, with saturated fatty acids providing just less than half of this. The main source of fat was milk and milk products, with fried potatoes and savoury snacks also contributing significant amounts.

Fibre

The average daily intake was only 6.1 g daily from the national survey. Cereals and smaller amounts of fruits and vegetables mainly provided this. The most frequently consumed fruit and vegetables were potato crisps, peas, baked beans, carrots, bananas, apples and pears. The survey indicated that children with a higher average intake of fibre had more frequent bowel movements.

Micronutrients

Vitamin A

50% of $1\frac{1}{2}$ to $4\frac{1}{2}$-year-old children have intakes below the RNI, with a further 8% below the LRNI.

Vitamin C

38% of $1\frac{1}{2}$ to $4\frac{1}{2}$-year-old children have intakes below the RNI. Lower intakes were more likely to be reported in children of lower socioeconomic status and children living in Scotland.

Iron

84% of $1\frac{1}{2}$ to $4\frac{1}{2}$-year-old children have been shown to have iron intakes below the RNI. The same study demonstrated that 1 in 12 children overall, and 1 in 8 of those aged $1\frac{1}{2}$ to $2\frac{1}{2}$ years had low haemoglobin levels.

Calcium

The majority of children aged from 1 to 5 have adequate calcium intakes.

Zinc

Over 70% of $1\frac{1}{2}$ to $4\frac{1}{2}$-year-old children have been shown to have zinc intakes below the RNI. A large proportion of children had very low intakes: 14% of under-4s and 37% of 4 to 6-year-olds.

WHAT IS THE IDEAL TODDLER DIET?

Pre-school children need to be offered a variety of foods from all food groups (MAFF 1997). However, the diet of toddlers is notoriously monotonous and based on a limited range of foods. Parents are frequently unwilling to experiment with new foods which may be rejected and thrown away. In addition, because of their innate preference for sweet foods, consistent exposure to sweet foods may lead to rejection of other tastes. Parents need to encourage tastes of all foods, as this will increase the likelihood that a child will eventually eat them. It is also important to continue to offer different textures and colours to help maintain a child's interest in food and mealtime.

Milk and dairy foods

Toddlers should have two to three servings per day of these. Suitable foods include full fat milk, cheese, yoghurt and fromage frais.

◆ A minimum of 300 ml daily of cow's milk should be encouraged, but no more than 600 to 700 ml daily. Full fat cow's milk should be given until a child is at least 2 years old, but semi-skimmed milk can be introduced from this age providing a good variety of foods are being eaten.
◆ On average, milk and milk products provide about two thirds of the calcium and a third of the protein intake.

Meat, fish, eggs and pulses

Toddlers should have two servings of these daily. Suitable foods include beef, lamb, pork, fish, eggs, baked beans, lentils and dahl.

◆ Meat and meat products provide about one quarter of all protein intake.
◆ Encourage lean meats and use little or no fat when cooking meats.
◆ Red meat is a good source of haem-iron.

Bread, other cereals and potatoes

Toddlers should have four servings daily. Suitable foods include bread, potatoes, pasta, rice and breakfast cereals.

◆ Encourage at least one serving at each mealtime.
◆ Wholewheat bread and wholewheat cereals can be given and are helpful in preventing constipation in young children.
◆ Limit high-fat foods such as crisps, savoury snacks and pastry.

Fruit and vegetables

Toddlers should have four or more servings daily. Suitable fruits include pears, bananas, apple slices, orange segments, kiwi fruit, strawberries, raspberries, melon and raisins. Suitable vegetables include cooked carrot, peas, broccoli, cauliflower florets, cucumber slices and green or red pepper slices. It is better to grate or partially cook vegetables for younger children. Fruit and vegetables that are too hard and do not dissolve can cause choking and should not be given to children under 3 years of age.

◆ Vegetables like spring greens and cabbage are good sources of iron, but are often disliked by young children.
◆ Add vegetables to soups and casseroles.
◆ Try and make vegetables fun: use vegetables such as carrot slices and peppers to make faces on pizzas; refer to broccoli as 'little trees'.

Fatty and sugary foods

◆ Foods which are high in sugar provide calories but few other nutrients. This is particularly true for drinks such as squashes, fizzy drinks, sweets and sugar added to drinks and cereals.

Box 4.1 Guidelines on eating and mealtimes in toddlers

◆ Give meals at regular times so a good routine is established. Children should not be too tired to eat.
◆ Although families increasingly do not sit together as a family unit, encourage at least one carer to eat with the child.
◆ Mealtimes should be a happy time and family arguments should be minimized when eating.
◆ The child should be sitting comfortably at a table at a suitable height. Utensils should be appropriate to the child's age.
◆ Allow plenty of time for the meal, but ensure it is not prolonged beyond 30 minutes.
◆ Offer small portions.
◆ Do not use sweets as bribes or treats.
◆ Encourage self-feeding as much as possible. Too much assisted feeding may result in food refusal or a lazy eater.
◆ Accept mess as a normal part of the feeding process. Allowing children to play with food helps ensure mealtime is fun.

Table 4.6 Useful ways of incorporating foods into a toddler's diet

Cheese	Macaroni cheese, cauliflower cheese, cheese spread on toast fingers, pizza slices, cheese cubes.
Yoghurt/fromage frais	As a dessert, mixed with puréed fruit, to top fruit, fruit salad.
Milk	Milk puddings, custard, white sauces, cereal.
Potatoes	Yams and sweet potato are palatable alternatives to potato.
Bread	Offer small sandwiches or toast fingers as snacks between meals. Try fruit bread, crumpets, teacakes, fruit buns, bagels, pitta bread and breadsticks.
Vegetables	Disguise in stews, add to mashed potato, use to top pizza or add to pasta dishes. Offer brightly coloured vegetables such as carrots or sweetcorn or give raw celery or carrot sticks or cucumber pieces.
Biscuits	Offer plain biscuits (e.g. rich tea, oatcakes, cream crackers) or plain popcorn between meals.

◆ Sweet intake should be limited and kept to after mealtimes if possible.
◆ Fizzy drinks, squashes and fruit juices should be given with meals only and not given at bedtime. Water or milk are suitable alternatives.
◆ Limit the intake of fatty foods such as chips, cream, chocolate and ice cream.

Box 4.1 gives some guidelines on eating and mealtimes in toddlers, and Table 4.6 suggests ways of incorporating food into a toddler's diet.

EFFECT OF DIET ON LATER LIFE

The effect of childhood diet on long-term health is a topic that has caused much debate. The full relationship between childhood nutrition and adult disease is not established and there is concern that over-zealous application of adult healthy eating recommendations in early childhood may affect growth and nutritional status.

In 1992, the government produced a White Paper 'The Health of the Nation' in an attempt to reduce mortality from conditions such as coronary heart disease (Department of Health 1992). It identified nutrition as playing a key role in health promotion and helping reduce serum cholesterol levels, obesity and hypertension. This has helped to fuel the arguments over the importance of healthy eating in pre-school children. At the very least, it is accepted that dietary patterns common in childhood, such as regular consumption of high-fat and sugar-containing foods, and low fruit and vegetable intake, are associated with a poor diet later in life.

Fat

It has been observed that the arterial lesions of atherosclerosis have their origins in childhood. Lesions have been seen in the aorta and coronary arteries of children, and blood lipid profiles indicative of a greater than average risk of heart disease have been identified at an early age. There is evidence that semi-skimmed milk has been given to 2-year-old children in Sweden and Canada without harmful effects, and that dietary modifications of fat and fibre have not had a detrimental effect on the growth of pre-school children (Payne & Bolton 1992). However, there is still widespread concern that the over-restriction of fat may reduce energy intake at a time when children are particularly vulnerable nutritionally.

Sugar

There is much support for reducing sugar consumption in pre-school children to reduce the risk of dental caries and obesity. There is also agreement that foods and drinks containing artificial sweeteners should be minimized in pre-school children. Their use helps reinforce the liking for sweet foods.

Other carbohydrates

Foods containing fibre-rich carbohydrates such as bread, breakfast cereals, vegetables and fruit are important in the diet. However, too many fibre-containing foods are bulky and may inhibit the appetite for other foods or cause diarrhoea or abdominal discomfort. Some cereals contain phytate and this may inhibit iron absorption.

Salt

Moderation in salt intake is advisable for the pre-school child. There is a small but significant relationship between sodium intake and blood pressure in infancy. As it is highly unlikely that healthy pre-school children will become sodium depleted in a normal diet, it is sensible to limit salty snacks such as crisps and avoid adding salt to the food at the table.

FOOD REFUSAL AND FEEDING PROBLEMS

Food refusal and feeding problems are remarkably common in pre-school children. The incidence of feeding problems has been estimated to vary from 16% to 75% (Eppright et al 1969, Minde & Minde 1986). This is a time of growing individuality for any child, when the child's personality and temperament is demonstrated. Most cases of food refusal and feeding problems are minor and have no effect on growth and weight gain of the child, but occasionally the problems can be very severe.

Reasons for common feeding problems

Excessive intake of drinks, particularly squash and milk. This reduces the appetite for solid foods (Houlihane & Rolls 1995).

Prolonged use of semi-solid foods in the second year of life. Children may not be faddy, but refuse to eat food with more texture or lumps. Poor chewing skills are common in children not offered 'lumpier' foods from 6 to 7 months. Parents are left with the dilemma of offering suitable food textures with probable food refusal, or staying with a familiar food but inappropriate consistency to ensure their children at least eat something.

Failure to increase variety of foods offered. Some young children are highly selective in what they will eat. They may only eat a small range of foods – but the variety of these may change from month to month. It is tempting and quicker for parents to only offer the foods which they know will be eaten.

Poor routine. Giving snacks close to mealtimes or not spreading meals at regular time intervals throughout the day may suppress appetite.

Limited food appeal. Small children may be overwhelmed by a large plate of food. Small portions of colourful, attractively presented food are more tempting.

Parental anxiety. Parents are often very anxious about what their children eat. They often have an unrealistic expectation of what should be eaten. They become upset when the child refuses to eat the expected amount and this may be reflected in parental behaviour at mealtimes, with undue pressure, bribery and even force being used.

Adverse food reaction or emotional upset. A toddler may have vomited or choked with a food. Any remembered negative experience with food might result in food refusal. Transient food refusal may occur after the birth of a sibling or other event in an attempt to redirect attention to themselves (Harris & Booth 1992).

Manipulative behaviour. Some children are more easily distracted, non-compliant and generally difficult to control at mealtimes. Generally, parents do not have the appropriate child management skills to persuade their child to sit down quietly. This problem does not usually exist on its own, but is associated with other types of feeding difficulty (Harris & Booth 1992).

Assessment of food refusal and feeding problems

Regular weight and height (or length) checks should be made. Prolonged food refusal, even due to non-organic causes, can result in impaired growth. If growth is poor, referral should be made to a paediatrician.

An important part of any assessment will involved the taking of a detailed history. This should include:

- a food diary describing all food and drink consumed, with details of meal patterns, location of eating, time and duration of meals, and supervision received
- onset and duration of feeding problems and potential 'trigger' events
- parents' response to food refusal
- type of feeding utensils used.

Management of food refusal and feeding problems

The parents require support, education and direction on how best to encourage their children to eat and enjoy food (Thompson 1998). Providing growth is satisfactory and there is no physiological cause for the loss of appetite, parents need reassurance that their child is unlikely to come to any harm. It is important that nutritional requirements of toddlers and normal behaviour patterns of young children are explained. Although most food refusal is transient, parents should understand that patience, consistency (both by the main carer and

Box 4.2 Simple strategies for management of food refusal

- Offer small well-spaced meals and snacks.
- To start with, give foods known to be well accepted.
- Set a time limit for mealtimes, e.g. 30 minutes.
- Give lots of praise, even if the smallest quantity of food is eaten.
- Take away uneaten food without comment at the end of the meal.
- Do not discuss eating and food with others in front of the child.
- Do not coax, force or use bribery to persuade a child to eat.
- Keep calm.

other carers), encouragement and happy mealtimes are key factors. Eating with the child, inviting a friend for tea, and changing the venue to a picnic can all help. Useful strategies for encouraging children to eat are given in Box 4.2.

FAILURE TO THRIVE IN PRE-SCHOOL CHILDREN

Failure to thrive (FTT) is a common problem in primary care and paediatrics in young children. Skuse (1985) suggests that up to 5% of children suffer from FTT and 3% of children were found to have FTT in a large study in Newcastle upon Tyne (Wright et al 1998). The vast majority of these children will have non-organic FTT (94%), although for some children there is overlap between lack of feeding and physiological causes. There is evidence that 33% of children with FTT remain undiagnosed. This is due to lack of consensus over definitions, failure to plot growth on centile charts, inaccurate plotting of measurements and even subjective interpretation according to social class (Batchelor & Kerslake 1990).

Causes of FTT in pre-school children

Failure to thrive usually results from a range of dietary, organic and social factors leading to undernutrition. The main cause is lack of food intake and reasons include:

- food refusal
- poor routine
- lack of food due to ignorance, poverty or neglect
- poor appetite
- parental misconceptions and health beliefs
- inappropriate dietary restriction, e.g. factitious food allergy
- squash drinking syndrome
- chronic illness causing anorexia
- inability to feed due to mechanical feeding problems
- vomiting
- infections
- dental caries.

Problems observed in children with FTT

Long-term effects associated with FTT include stunting, developmental delay, poor weight gain and even heart disease in later adulthood. In a group of young children with FTT from the north of England, Rayner & Rudolf (1996) reported 55% had developmental delay, and other problems included eating difficulties, poor growth, low energy intakes, iron deficiency and behavioural and sleeping difficulties. The majority of the children were from families living in poverty with many from divorced, separated or single-parent families.

Assessment of FTT in pre-school children

Failure to thrive must be recognized and accurately defined for rational decisions to be made about management. Evaluation is divided into assessment of past and present dietary intake, clinical history, social and family history, past history, and anthropometric and laboratory assessments. The feeding history must include information about feeding routine, parental understanding of feeding, food restrictions and even maternal attitude to food and nutrition. Ideally mealtimes should be observed by video, preferably more than once. This is time-consuming but is useful for identifying feeding and behaviours that need to change.

Dietary management of FTT in pre-school children

The type of dietary management will vary according to the reason for FTT in the young child. However, for the majority of children it will involve behavioural management strategies, basic nutrition education, advice about feeding on a budget, encouraging regular meals and snacks, and increasing the nutrient and energy density of meals and snacks. It may be necessary to recommend additional vitamin and mineral supplements.

The role of health visitors in FTT in pre-school children

Although there have been few successful trials of intervention, studies have suggested that home-based nurtured support may improve growth and outcome. In a randomized, controlled trial, home visiting by health visitors led to a successful outcome in 75% of the children with FTT (Wright et al 1998).

The health visitor is, undoubtedly, a key worker in the management of FTT in the community. Roles include:

◆ screening children
◆ giving advice on diet, feeding and parenting
◆ providing parental support and reassurance
◆ monitoring growth.

Table 4.7 Useful sources of nutrients for pre-school children on a vegetarian diet

Nutrient	Sources
Protein	Soya protein, pulses, baked beans, grains, seeds, soya cheese, ground nuts
Calcium	Fortified soya milk, fortified soya desserts and soya yoghurts, tofu, seeds, green leafy vegetables, nuts, bread, dried fruit
Iron	Fortified breakfast cereals, bread, pulses, green vegetables, dried fruit, nuts, plain chocolate, raisins, curry powder
Zinc	Tofu, fortified cereals, ground nuts, beans and lentils, wholemeal bread, plain popcorn, sesame seeds and tahini
Vitamin B_{12}	Fortified soya milk, some margarines, textured vegetable protein products
Vitamin D	Fortified margarine, fortified soya milk, fortified breakfast cereals, sunshine
Vitamin A	Yellow or orange vegetables (e.g. carrots), sweet potato, yellow or orange fruit (e.g. mangoes and apricots), fortified margarine, red peppers

VEGETARIAN DIETS IN PRE-SCHOOL CHILDREN

A well-constructed vegetarian diet is theoretically suitable for young children, and normal growth and development have been demonstrated. The average growth of Caucasian vegetarian children parallels that of Caucasian omnivores and, although lower rates of early growth are seen in vegan children, catch-up growth occurs by 10 years of age (Sanders & Manning 1992). However, vegetarian diets vary considerably in the extent to which they exclude animal products. The more restrictive the diet, the greater the risk of nutrient deficiencies. Faddy children, already on a limited diet, are particularly vulnerable. Table 4.7 shows some useful sources of nutrients for vegetarians.

The following are particular issues:

◆ A vegetarian diet is generally higher in fibre. This is bulky and very filling and may decrease energy intake. This may lead to failure to thrive and to toddler diarrhoea, and may reduce the availability of some nutrients.

◆ Vegetable and pulse proteins have a lower concentration and range of essential amino acids than protein from animal sources, and careful planning of menus with pulse and cereal combinations is therefore necessary to ensure the correct balance of amino acids.

◆ Iron deficiency is a potential problem, particularly as iron sources from plant foods have a low bioavailability. Foods which are rich in vitamin C should be taken at the same time as iron plant sources to maximize iron utilization.

◆ Calcium intake may be low if cow's milk and milk products are avoided. Vegan children should be encouraged to drink at least 300 to 400 ml daily of fortified soya milk. Calcium intake should be regularly assessed, and if necessary a calcium supplement may be necessary to ensure calcium requirements are met.

◆ Vitamin B_{12} is low in vegan diets. Yeast extracts such as Marmite are high in vitamin B_{12} but do not have the biological activity of the vitamin so it is usually necessary to give an extra supplement.

◆ Vitamin D deficiency and rickets have been described commonly in young Asian and Rastafarian children. They not only have little exposure to sunlight, but a low vitamin D intake if they are on a vegetarian diet. All young children are recommended to take the Mother & Children's vitamin drops to ensure they receive adequate vitamin D.

◆ Other potential deficiencies include zinc, riboflavin and essential fatty acids, normally derived from fish and egg sources. Vegetable oils such as walnut oil with a good linoleic:α-

Table 4.8 Common diets used by ethnic minority groups

Group	Dietary customs and problems
Asian	
Sikh	Common nutritional problems: iron deficiency anaemia, rickets and failure to thrive. No beef. Often no pork. Some are vegetarian, but some eat chicken or lamb.
Hindu	No beef. Mainly vegetarian or vegan.
Muslim	No pork. Halal meat only. No fish without scales. Usually eat chicken or lamb.
Rastafarian	Usually exclude all meat, fish and preserved foods. Some are strict vegans while others will drink milk. Common nutritional problems: iron deficiency anaemia, rickets and megaloblastic anaemia.
Vietnamese	No forbidden foods, but unfamiliar foods such as lamb, ox liver, tinned or cooked fruit and some root vegetables are avoided. Little fresh milk, butter, margarine or cheese are used due to lack of availability in Vietnam and high incidence of lactose intolerance. Common nutritional problems: risk of calcium deficiency and rickets, if little milk and milk products are eaten.

linolenic acid ratio should be encouraged on a vegan diet.

◆ The growth and nutrient intake of all young children on a vegan diet should be regularly assessed. If there is any concern about nutrient intake, children should be referred to a paediatric dietitian for appropriate advice.

Cult diets used in pre-school children

Other extreme vegetarian diets such as Zen macrobiotic and fruitarian diets have reportedly been used in young children. They are particularly restrictive and nutritional adequacy is virtually impossible, placing the health and growth of young children at risk.

Zen macrobiotic diets

The Zen macrobiotic principle originates from Japan. There are 10 levels of dietary elimination. Animal products, fruit and vegetables are gradually removed from the diet until the final stage when only brown rice is eaten. Fluids may also be severely restricted. This diet is thought to maintain spiritual, mental and physical well-being. Not surprisingly, many nutritional problems have been reported including poor growth, muscle wasting, and deficiencies of iron, calcium, vitamin B_{12}, vitamin D and thiamin.

Fruitarian diets

These diets are based on fruit, uncooked fermented cereals and seeds. Nutritional problems identified include severe protein energy malnutrition, anaemia and a wide range vitamin and mineral deficiencies.

CONSTIPATION

Constipation is common in pre-school children, especially when toilet training is in progress. It is the painful passage of hard, infrequent stools (Booth 1997). It covers a wide spectrum of problems from the mildly affected to severe problems of encopresis. The causes of constipation include:

◆ fear of the toilet or potty
◆ distress or pain associated to the appropriate signals
◆ faddy eaters who eat little fibre and drink large volumes of milk (a poor appetite has been described in as many as 47% of children referred for constipation, Clayden 1992)
◆ a naturally sluggish bowel.

Management of constipation

Management of constipation depends on its severity. Important principles of treatment include:

◆ evacuation of the bowel at regular intervals following meals
◆ use of laxatives such as Lactulose.

Such laxatives should not be seen as a long-term solution, but as a stepping stone to the establishment of a normal bowel habit. Overuse will exacerbate the problem of a sluggish bowel by creating dependency on their use.

It is particularly important to increase dietary fibre:

◆ encourage a high fibre breakfast cereal, e.g. Weetabix, Shredded Wheat
◆ replace white bread with wholemeal or granary bread, but encourage the rest of the family to do the same (high fibre white bread is an acceptable alternative)
◆ offer wholemeal pasta and brown rice
◆ give high fibre snacks e.g. cereal bars, digestive biscuits, wholemeal scones, fruit cake and raisins
◆ encourage plenty of unpeeled fresh fruit and dried fruits such as prunes
◆ encourage jacket potatoes, baked beans and other pulse vegetables
◆ increase fluid intake (other than milk)
◆ use behaviour modification techniques and star charts.

DENTAL CARIES

Dental decay is common in young children. In 1995, an Office of Population Censuses and Surveys national survey indicated that 17%

of $1\frac{1}{2}$ to $4\frac{1}{2}$-year-olds had some dental decay. The proportion increased with age, was more common in children living in the north of England and Scotland, among children living in lone-parent families, and in households where the head was unemployed or in receipt of Family Credit (Hinds & Gregory 1995).

Children's teeth are particularly vulnerable to dental caries, when tooth enamel is relatively soft and easily damaged. Dental caries result from the action of bacteria on fermentable carbohydrate, from sugars and starches in foods resulting in the production of acid. The latter attacks tooth enamel, making it more porous and susceptible to further attack and tooth decay. Dental caries may also occur as a result of chemical action from acid present in some drinks such as fruit juice and coke.

Prevention of dental caries

The following steps will help to prevent dental caries:

◆ Reduce cariogenic plaque bacteria – this is achieved by brushing the teeth twice daily, including last thing at night. Parents should do this initially to ensure thorough cleaning.

◆ Reduce the frequency of consumption of foods which contain sugar, particularly those of a sticky or chewable nature. Sticky chewable foods will remain in the mouth longer and may leave small residues between the teeth where bacterial production can continue. Children from manual backgrounds have been found to be more frequent consumers of sugar confectionery than those from non-manual backgrounds.

◆ Reduce the total amount of sugars. If children are having sugary foods, these should be given with meals rather than between meals.

◆ Limit the consumption of acidic drinks. Diet cola, which is highly acidic, may be just as damaging to teeth as ordinary cola, despite the absence of sugar. Fruit juice and fruit-flavoured drinks are also highly acidic, especially citrus varieties.

◆ Discourage the use of baby bottles in children over 1 year, particularly to give a drink in bed late at night. Thirty one per cent of $1\frac{1}{2}$ to $2\frac{1}{2}$-year-old children are still given a bottle at night (Hind & Gregory 1995). When milk or a sucrose-containing drink is given, fluid collects around the upper anterior and posterior teeth, which become extensively damaged. Because of reduced salivation and swallowing during sleep, clearance and neutralization of acids is reduced.

◆ Encourage the use of fluoride toothpaste. Only a tiny smear is necessary – the size of a small pea.

◆ Fluoride supplements can be given if the local water supply does not have added fluoride.

◆ Children should visit the dentist regularly by 3 years of age. Dental check-ups and treatments are free up to the age of 18, or up to 19 years if they are in full-time education.

◆ Use sugar-free medicines where possible.

OBESITY

There is little information on the prevalence of obesity in pre-school years. In general, there are no agreed criteria to assess relative fatness in children, but a weight of more than two centiles higher than height constitutes obesity (Shaw & Lawson 1994). Obesity is more frequently associated with overweight parents, poor diet, low level of physical activity and low income.

Restrictive low-calorie diets are not suitable for young children because they may compromise nutritional quality and growth. Instead the diet should maintain a stable weight but still promote normal linear growth.

General dietary advice

◆ Limit chips and fried foods – give potatoes, rice, pasta or bread instead at mealtimes.
◆ Give 300 to 600 ml of semi-skimmed milk instead of whole milk. Low fat yoghurts and low fat cheese can be given as an alternative if milk is disliked.
◆ Limit crisps, sweets and high sugar foods.
◆ Limit sugar-containing drinks.
◆ Replace sugar-containing snacks with fruit, dried fruit, cereal and skimmed milk, crackers

and savoury spread or small sandwiches. Try and limit snacks to one daily.

◆ Give vegetables at every meal. Vary the choice and give them raw or cooked.
◆ Do not demand that food is finished, and do not give snacks in replacement of meals.
◆ It is supportive to the child if the whole family follows this dietary advice.

Other advice

Physical activity should be increased among the less active families. Children should be encouraged to walk rather than ride in pushchairs.

NUTRITION IN PRE-SCHOOL CHILDREN IN CHILDCARE

An increasing number of children under the age of 5 years spend some time being cared for away from the family home. It is estimated that 12% are cared for by childminders, 6% attend registered private nurseries, and less than 1% attend local authority day nurseries. In addition, many other children are cared for by nannies (Department of Health 1998).

Day care providers, therefore supply an increasing proportion of the total food eaten by children in their care. A new report by the Caroline Walker Trust (1998), sets out practical nutritional guidelines for the food offered during childcare. Based on current dietary recommendations, the guidelines are intended for use by all those involved in the care of children under 5. The recommendations are set as percentages of the total daily intake of nutrients that an average child requires. The recommendations consider the needs of the following groups of children (Table 4.9):

◆ children in childcare for a full day (8 hours or more)
◆ children in half-day care which includes lunch
◆ children in half-day care which includes tea.

The authors recommend that these guidelines become standards for childcare and that government departments include reference to these guidelines in legislation on childcare.

Learning through food

Childcare provides the opportunity for children to learn about food, food sources, nutrition, seasons and other people's way of life. Learning how to choose and enjoy many different nutritious foods in early childhood can provide the foundation for a lifetime of wise food choices. Box 4.3 shows some ideas for food-related activities.

Table 4.9 Nutritional guidelines for children in childcare. (Caroline Walker Trust 1998.)

	Nutritional guidelines for food prepared for children in:		
Nutrient	**Full-day care (8 hrs or more)**	**Half-day care including lunch and a snack**	**Half-day care including tea and a snack**
Energy	70% of the EAR	40% of the EAR	30% of the EAR
Protein	Not less than 70% of RNI	Not less than 40% of RNI	Not less than 30% of RNI
Fat	About 35% of food energy	About 35% of food energy	About 35% of food energy
Carbohydrate	About 50% of food energy	About 50% of food energy	Not less than 30% of RNI
Thiamin	Not less than 70% of RNI	Not less than 40% of RNI	Not less than 30% of RNI
Riboflavin	Not less than 70% of RNI	Not less than 40% of RNI	Not less than 30% of RNI
Niacin	Not less than 70% of RNI	Not less than 40% of RNI	Not less than 30% of RNI
Vitamin C	Not less than 70% of RNI	Not less than 40% of RNI	Not less than 30% of RNI
Vitamin A	Not less than 70% of RNI	Not less than 40% of RNI	Not less than 30% of RNI
Iron	Not less than 80% of RNI	Not less than 45% of RNI	Not less than 35% of RNI
Calcium	Not less than 70% of RNI	Not less than 40% of RNI	Not less than 30% of RNI

Box 4.3 Ideas for food-related activities

◆ Cutting out food pictures from magazines for collages or mobiles.

◆ Making pictures with food, e.g. dried pasta, pulses or seeds.

◆ Food prints: halved small potatoes, carrots and parsnips.

◆ Papier-mâché fruit and vegetables.

◆ Growing vegetables.

◆ Food tasting.

◆ Having a pretend cafe or shop.

◆ Pretend cooking with playdough.

◆ Food related songs.

SUMMARY

◆ In pre-school children, food and mealtimes help establish good eating habits, set dietary patterns for later life, and enhance communication skills and language.

◆ Energy and nutrient requirements are high in relationship to the body size of pre-school children.

◆ There should be no restriction of fat intake before 2 years. Between 2 and 5 years, fat intake should gradually decrease from 50% to 35% of energy. There are no recommendations for fibre intake.

◆ Iron deficiency anaemia is very common in young children.

◆ Sugar intakes are high in pre-school children. Vitamin C, vitamin A, iron and zinc intakes are commonly low.

◆ Food refusal and feeding problems are common in pre-school children.

◆ Up to 5% of young children suffer from failure to thrive and the majority of this is inorganic.

◆ Vegan pre-school children are at risk from poor growth, iron deficiency, and vitamins B_{12} and D deficiency.

◆ Constipation, dental caries and obesity are all common problems for the pre-school child.

◆ An increasing number of young children are given food by day food providers and nutritional guidelines are now issued for pre-school childcare.

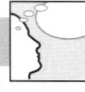

Question

Answer is given in Appendix 2.

The following is a healthy, but low calorie diet for a 2-year-old girl. Adapt this meal plan to make it more suitable.

Breakfast	Energy kcals/day
1 Weetabix	70
100 ml skimmed milk	35
100 ml natural orange juice	36
Mid-morning	
Sugar-free squash	–
Apple	47
Midday meal	
2 slices wholemeal bread	129
15 g very low fat margarine	41
Tuna	57
Tomato/cucumber	15
Low fat/low sugar yoghurt	50
Sugar-free squash	–
Mid-afternoon	
Sugar-free squash	–
Evening meal	
60 g jacket potato	46
30 g chicken	44
Carrots	12
Gravy	62
1 banana	64
150 ml skimmed milk	53
Total	**761**

FURTHER READING

Harriet A 1999 Feeding your baby and toddler. Dorling Kindersley, London

Tedstone A, Aviles M, Shetty P, Daniels L 1998 Effectiveness of interventions to promote healthy eating in pre-school children aged 1 to 5 years: a review. Health promotion effectiveness reviews. Health Education Authority, London, pp 1–65

REFERENCES

Batchelor J, Kerslake A 1990 Failure to find failure to thrive. Whiting and Bush, London

Booth I W 1997 Gastroenterology. In: Lissauer T, Clayden G (eds) Illustrated textbook of paediatrics. Mosby, London

Caroline Walker Trust 1998 Eating well for under-5s in child care. Caroline Walker Trust, St Austell, www.cwt.org.uk

Clayden G S 1992 Management of chronic constipation. Archives of Disease in Childhood 67:340–344

Department of Health 1991 Dietary reference values for food energy and nutrients for the United Kingdom. Report on Health and Social Subjects No. 41. HMSO, London

Department of Health 1992 The Health of the Nation – a strategy for health in England. HMSO, London

Department of Health 1994 Nutritional aspects of cardiovascular disease. Report on Health and Social Subjects No. 46. HMSO, London

Department of Health 1998 Children's day care facilities at 31 March 1997 (A/F 97/6). HMSO, London

Eppright E S, Fox H M, Fryer B S, Lamkin G H, Vivian V M 1969 Eating behaviour of pre-school children. Journal of Nutrition Education 1:16–19

Gregory J R, Collins D L, Davies P S W, Hughes J M, Clarke P C 1995 National Diet and Nutrition Survey: Children aged $1\frac{1}{2}$ to $4\frac{1}{2}$ years. Volume 1: Report of the Diet and Nutrition Survey. Office of Population Censuses and Survey. HMSO, London

Harris G, Booth I W 1992 The nature and management of eating problems in pre-school children. Monographs in Clinical Pediatrics 5:61–84

Hinds K, Gregory J 1995 National Diet and Nutrition Survey: Children aged $1\frac{1}{2}$ to $4\frac{1}{2}$ years. Volume 2: Report of the Dental Survey. HMSO, London

Houlihane J O B, Rolls C J 1995 Morbidity from excessive intake of high energy fluids: the 'squash drinking syndrome'. Archives of Disease in Childhood 72:141–143

Ministry of Agriculture, Food and Farming 1997 Healthy diets for young children: a guide for health professionals. Ministry of Agriculture, Food and Farming / Department of Health / Health Education Authority, London

Minde K, Minde R 1986 Infant psychiatry: an introductory text. Sage, London

Payne J A, Belton N R 1992 Nutrient intake and growth in pre-school children. 1. Comparison of energy intake and sources of energy with growth. Journal of Human Nutrition and Dietetics 5:299–304

Rayner P, Rudolf M 1996 What do we know about children who fail to thrive? Child Care Health Development 22:241–250

Sanders T, Manning J 1992 The growth and development of vegan children. Journal of Human Nutrition and Dietetics 5:11–12

Shaw V, Lawson M 1994 Clinical paediatric dietetics. Blackwell Science, Oxford

Skuse D H 1985 Non-organic failure to thrive: a reappraisal. Archives of Disease in Childhood 60:173–178

Thompson J M 1998 Nutritional requirements of infants and young children: practical guidelines. Blackwell Science, Oxford

Wardley B L, Puntis J W L, Taitz L S 1997 Handbook of child nutrition. Oxford University Press, Oxford

Williams C L, Bollella M, Wynder E L 1995 A new recommendation for dietary fiber in childhood. Pediatrics 96:985–988

Wright C M, Callum J, Jarvis S 1998 Effect of community based management in failure to thrive: randomised controlled trial. British Medical Journal 317:571–574

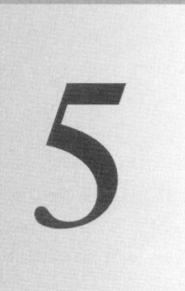

5

Feeding school-age children and adolescents

Carolyn Patchell

INTRODUCTION

The health of school-age children and adolescents is generally good, and dietary deficiency states are rarely seen. Children from poor social circumstances are more likely to have inadequate intakes and exhibit impaired growth, but even in these groups it is rare. Children have relatively high requirements for nutrients in relation to size, and adolescents have higher requirements for protein, vitamins and minerals per unit of energy consumed. For this reason, a high quality diet is needed to achieve adequate intakes of all nutrients. Dietary excesses of fat and energy are commonly seen, resulting in obesity. Nutrition education is essential to enable children to make informed choices about food and understand the relationship between diet and health.

Adolescence is a time of dramatic change. The uniform growth of childhood is taken over by a rapid growth spurt. It is also a time of hormonal, psychosocial and developmental change and as a result is a nutritionally vulnerable period of life. There is a greater demand for nutrients, due to the dramatic increase in physical growth and development, and there is a change of lifestyle and food choices which will affect intakes.

Adolescents have a great need to exert independence and make their own choices. There is a need to conform with their peer group regarding food choices. Incidence of smoking is high during teenage years and this affects nutrient intake. The nature of adolescence also means that advice given by parents and health professionals is likely to be ignored and tolerance is needed to guide teenagers towards a more sensible lifestyle.

THE NUTRITIONAL REQUIREMENTS OF SCHOOL-AGE CHILDREN

Nutrient intakes are high in young children in relation to their size. Many children have small appetites, and selective food refusal and food fads are frequently seen. For this reason, a high-quality diet is required in order to achieve adequate intakes of nutrients, particularly calcium and iron.

Dietary recommendations for school children are based on the Department of Health dietary reference values (DRVs) (1991). These give guidelines for population intakes and should not be considered as recommendations for individuals. Girls and boys have different requirements. Tables 5.1 and 5.2 summarize DRVs for boys and girls aged 4 to 18 years.

Reference values for starch, sugar and fats are given as a percentage of total energy intake. No figures are given for young children for non-starch polysaccharide (NSP) or fibre, but it is considered that children need a proportionately lower amount than adults (adult requirements are 12 to 24 g/day). There are no values for vitamin D because most people obtain the majority of vitamin D from sunlight. The DRVs need to be translated into advice on what to eat. These are given in the government's eight guidelines for a healthy diet (Department of Health 1990):

◆ Enjoy your food.
◆ Eat a variety of different foods.

Table 5.1 Dietary reference values for boys aged 4 to 18 years. (DoH 1991. Crown copyright material is reproduced with the permission of the Controller of Her Majesty's Stationery Office.)

Age (years)		4–6	7–10	11–14	15–18
Energy	(kcal)	1715	1970	2200	2755
	(MJ)	7.16	8.24	9.27	11.51
Fat	% food energy	35	35	35	35
Saturated fat	% food energy	11	11	11	11
Starch	% food energy	39	39	39	39
Non-milk intrinsic sugar	% food energy	11	11	11	11
Fibre (non-starch polysaccaride)	g			18	18
Protein	g	19.7	28.3	42.1	55.2
Minerals					
Iron	mg	6.1	8.7	11.3	11.3
Calcium	mg	450	550	1000	1000
Zinc	mg	6.5	7	9	9.5
Magnesium	mg	120	200	280	300
Phosphorus	mg	350	450	775	775
Sodium	mg	700	1200	1600	1600
Vitamins					
Vitamin A	μg	500	500	600	700
Vitamin B_1	mg	0.7	0.7	0.9	1.1
Vitamin B_2	mg	0.8	1.0	1.2	1.3
Nicotinic acid	mg	11	12	15	18
Vitamin B_6 (pyridoxine)	mg	0.9	1.0	1.2	1.5
Vitamin B_{12}	μg	0.8	1.0	1.2	1.5
Folate	μg	100	150	200	200
Vitamin C	mg	30	30	35	40

Table 5.2 Dietary reference values for girls aged 4 to 18 years. (DoH 1991. Crown copyright material is reproduced with the permission of the Controller of Her Majesty's Stationery Office.)

Age (years)		4–6	7–10	11–14	15–18
Energy	kcal	1545	1940	1845	2110
	MJ	6.46	7.28	7.92	8.83
Fat	% food energy	35	35	35	35
Saturated fat	% food energy	11	11	11	11
Starch	% food energy	39	39	39	39
(Non-milk intrinsic sugar)	% food energy	11	11	11	11
Fibre (non-starch polysaccaride)	g			18	18
Protein	g	19.7	28.3	41.2	45
Minerals					
Iron	mg	6.1	8.7	14.8	14.8
Calcium	mg	450	550	800	800
Zinc	mg	6.5	7	9	7
Magnesium	mg	120	200	280	300
Phosphorous	mg	350	450	625	625
Sodium	mg	700	1200	1600	1600
Vitamins					
Vitamin A	µg	500	500	600	600
Vitamin B$_1$	mg	0.7	0.7	0.7	0.8
Vitamin B$_2$	mg	0.8	1.0	1.1	1.1
Nicotinic acid	mg	11	12	12	14
Vitamin B$_6$ (pyridoxine)	mg	0.9	1.0	1.0	1.2
Vitamin B$_{12}$	µg	0.8	1.0	1.2	1.5
Folate	µg	100	150	200	200
Vitamin C	mg	30	30	35	40

◆ Eat the right amount to be a healthy weight.
◆ Eat plenty of foods rich in starch and fibre.
◆ Don't eat too much fat.
◆ Don't eat sugary foods too often.
◆ Look after the vitamins and minerals in your food.

WHAT SCHOOL-AGE CHILDREN EAT

A number of surveys have investigated the diet and health of young people. The 'Diets of British School Children' report gives the most comprehensive picture (Department of Health 1989). Some of the surveys give limited information on nutrient intakes, some are very small scale, and comparisons between the surveys may not be possible. Table 5.3 lists some recent UK surveys from which nutrient data have been derived.

Table 5.3 Dietary surveys of school children in the UK. (After Nelson 1993, reproduced with permission.)

Author	Year	Age of children	Number of children
Hackett et al	1979–81	11–14	405
Bull	1982	15–25	913
Department of Health	1989	10–11, 14–15	3296
Crawley	1986–87	16–17	4746
Nelson	1988	7–10, 11–12	227
McNeill et al	1988	12	61
Adamson et al	1990	11–12	379

There have been major changes in food consumption in the UK over recent years relating to economic changes, changes in lifestyle and the changing expectations of young people. One of the purposes of the 'Diets of British School Children' survey was to look at the effect on children's diets of the change in the 1980 Education Act, which removed the control of nutritional standards for school meals. The survey looked at 3296 children aged 10 to 11 years and 14 to 15 years. The results are summarized in Box 5.1.

Subsequent surveys, including those listed, confirm a trend away from family mealtimes and towards 'grazing' and eating out. Younger children have less opportunity to purchase food and so their consumption more closely follows family dietary patterns. Surveys using 24-hour recall and food frequency questionnaires confirm that the eating patterns of five- to seven-year-olds follow adult patterns. Children in manual socioeconomic groups eat less fruit and vegetables and more chips, and families in lower income groups eat more potatoes, bread, meat and sugar.

Nutrient intakes of school children based on data collected for the 'Diets of British school children' report are summarized in Box 5.2.

Food choices

The principles of a healthy diet apply to school age children; however, many factors affect children's choice of food and so their nutrient intake. The availability of appropriate foods at home, in schools and in fast food restaurants is essential to achieve adequate nutrient intakes and achieve a healthy diet in relation to energy and saturated fat intakes. The provision of good quality school meals is important, but it must be remembered that the majority of a child's meals are the

Box 5.1 Conclusions of the 'Diets of British school children' survey (DoH 1989)

◆ Children eat many foods which are high in sugar and fat, and eat less fruit and vegetables than is desirable.

◆ Bread, chips, milk, biscuits, meat products, cake and puddings were major contributors to energy intake.

◆ Almost all children ate chips, crisps, cake and biscuits.

◆ Children from manual socioeconomic groups were more likely to eat chips and less likely to drink milk.

◆ Children receiving free school meals had poorer diets. School meals were an important source of vitamin C.

◆ Boys ate more chips, milk, breakfast cereal and baked beans.

◆ Girls ate more fruit and drank more fruit juice.

◆ Older children drank more tea and coffee.

◆ Older girls drank less milk and ate less breakfast cereal.

◆ Yoghurt, fizzy drinks and sweets were popular with younger children.

Box 5.2 Summary of the nutrient intake of school children (DoH 1989)

◆ Children consumed 90% of the recommended energy, although they were of a normal nutritional status, reflecting a relative inactivity.

◆ The main sources of energy were bread, chips, milk, biscuits, meat products, cake and pastry.

◆ About 75% of children ate more fat than recommended.

◆ Intakes of protein, thiamin, nicotinic acid and vitamin C were above the recommended amounts for 10 to 11 and 14 to 15 year-olds.

◆ Average consumption of retinol, vitamin B_6, folate, magnesium and zinc were low.

◆ Intakes of riboflavin were lower than recommended in older girls.

◆ About 60% of older girls consumed less than the requirement for calcium.

◆ Average intakes of iron were below recommended intakes for girls.

responsibility of the parent, and so nutrition and health education to parents for their children is required. The biggest determinant of a child's food choice is the availability of appropriate food in the home, and so parents must be educated themselves regarding appropriate food choices both for themselves and for their family.

Social pressures, advertising and personal preference also play a role. Many advertising strategies are used to encourage children to eat particular foods; these strategies include the use of music, singing, jingles, promotions for toys and endorsements by celebrities or fictional characters. Parents must resist the pressure of advertising and not buy foods they do not wish their children to consume. Once again, education of parents is vital to enable them to select appropriate foods on their child's behalf.

Attitudes to food and eating are formed early in life but may be modified. Factors which influence eating habits can be classified as socioeconomic and personal. Socioeconomic influences include:

- economic status
- education of parent
- family structure
- ethnic origin
- social attitudes
- media influence.

Personal influences include:

- personal preferences
- personal relationships
- media.

Young children's attitudes to food are heavily influenced by what they eat at home. As children grow older, peer pressure affects their attitudes to food.

SCHOOL MEALS

In 1980 statutory obligations of local education authorities to provide meals of a set quality and price were removed. Prior to this it was expected that a school meal would provide 33% of a child's requirements for some nutrients. The requirement is now that a school provides a meal for children in receipt of free school meals and provides a place for children to eat a packed lunch brought to school. If meals are provided, local authorities are now able to charge whatever they wish. The hours of catering staff working in school canteens have been reduced to save money, resulting in more convenience foods being used. Fast foods are increasingly used to tempt children to eat and so guarantee a good income to the school.

The regulations regarding the provision of school meals have also changed in recent years. Free school meals are currently only provided for children of parents in receipt of family income support or supplementary benefit. Some families have been offered cash alternatives to a free school meal, and this may not always be spent on food for the child. The changes in the regulations regarding school meals have meant that there is no obligation on education authorities to provide a nutritionally adequate meal. Foods offered are frequently those which are seen as being popular with children, and these foods may be high in fat and sugar; children previously in receipt of free meals may no longer get them; and children may spend their dinner money on other items and miss their midday meal completely. The school meal may for some children be their first meal of the day, as breakfast is often missed. It is therefore essential that this meal is nutritionally adequate. The onus must, however, also be on parents to ensure an adequate intake outside school as less than 25% of a child's food intake will occur in school.

There are several types of meal service available in school. Prices vary and are set by the local education authority. At primary schools the service is generally of a cafeteria style in which there may be choice from one or two items or no choice at all, some guidance may be offered regarding appropriate choices, and prices are generally fixed. At middle school again there may be guidance, but individual items are generally priced. A wider range of foods will normally be available. A cash cafeteria system is also generally operated in secondary schools, where there may be no guidance regarding choice. A wide variety of foods will be offered and there is no limit on spending by the children.

Guidance on meal choices is therefore only usually offered at primary schools. A range of systems are used, including a 'traffic light' system in which foods which are high in fibre are colour-coded green, foods which are high in fat, sugar and salt are coded red, and other foods are coded amber. Children are encouraged to select fewer foods from the red group and choose amber or green foods in preference.

Menus may be coded according to food groups, and children are encouraged to choose three or more different colours to achieve a balance of food groups, or a unit choice system may be used in which foods are allocated a unit number depending on the nutritional value of that food. The least desirable foods are given the highest unit value, and a meal must be of 5 units maximum. Children are encouraged to choose foods of a lower unit value because they can eat more of them. However children may prefer to have a smaller amount of the least nutritionally suitable foods.

There remain many problems with the school meal service which must still be addressed. Some schools offer little guidance on food choice, and school meal supervisors may themselves not be adequately informed to offer advice regarding nutrition. There may be little time available for children to eat – this is a particular problem for younger children, who may be slow eaters – and there may be little choice for those children who are given their meal last. Many schools do not have adequate facilities for the provision of meals for Asian children and children from other ethnic backgrounds. It is, however, essential that parents are informed about the food choices available at school and are given guidance on the foods to include at home. Many parents rely on the school meal to provide the main meal of the day. However, this meal is frequently not nutritionally adequate.

In 1998, Gardner-Merchant published a school meals survey looking at the attitudes towards school meals and eating habits of children aged 8 to 16 years (Gardner-Merchant 1998). It revealed the following points:

◆ 18% of 15 to 16-year-old girls and 12% of 15 to 16-year-old boys do not have breakfast.
◆ Children spend an average of £1.00 on snacks such as sweets, canned drinks and crisps on the way to and from school.

◆ This grazing behaviour continues at home, particularly in the first hour after getting home.
◆ Consumption of yoghurt and fruit has increased.
◆ 74% of children have a cooked meal in the evening.
◆ Chips are eaten less frequently, with an average of 2.48 times per week compared to 2.9 times per week in 1996.
◆ Chips are most popular in 11 to 12-year-old boys.
◆ Meat consumption has increased.
◆ School meals are eaten an average of 2.54 times per week.
◆ Average expenditure is £1.28 per meal at school.
◆ The most popular school meal is pizza and chips with cake for dessert.
◆ Packed lunch favourite foods are crisps (57%), meat or cheese rolls (37%) and apples (34%).
◆ 14% of children believe their diet is 'very healthy'.
◆ The reasons for not having school meals are:
  – taste of the food
  – choice of food
  – smell of the food
  – temperature of the food.

The lifting of the statutory obligation of education authorities to provide meals of a set quality in 1980 has had major implications on the nutritional intakes of children in the UK. The government proposes to reintroduce national nutritional standards for school meals by May 2002. This proposal forms part of the government's health strategy to improve the health of the population as a whole, and to reduce inequalities by particularly targeting those in lower socioeconomic groups.

'Ingredients for Success' (Department for Education and Employment 1998), a consultation paper on nutritional standards for school lunches, highlights the following concerns regarding the nutrition of school children in the UK:

◆ Children are getting taller.
◆ Children are getting heavier.
◆ Children are getting fatter.

◆ Children consume too much sugar and fat.
◆ Children's diets have insufficient vitamins and minerals.

The government aims to set standards for all school lunches, including cooked and sandwich meals. For pupils in primary school the preferred option is to apply food-based standards specifying that each meal should contain a portion of specific size of vegetables, meat or fish, carbohydrate and dairy product.

In secondary schools all pupils should be offered:

◆ a carbohydrate which is not chips or fried potato
◆ at least one vegetable or salad
◆ fruit or fruit juice
◆ a protein item
◆ reduced-fat dairy products.

Schools will have a duty to provide free lunches to some pupils and paid lunches for those not eligible for free meals. The government hopes to improve the overall nutritional intake of children in the UK by example in school.

NUTRITION EDUCATION FOR SCHOOL-AGE CHILDREN

The National Curriculum has 10 foundation subjects, three of which – English, mathematics and science – are core subjects. A child's years at school are divided into four key stages, and children are expected to attain a certain level at each stage. Table 5.4 shows suggested attainments for nutrition by primary school pupils.

Nutrition was traditionally taught in home economics, but this is not a foundation topic. It can, however, be incorporated into science, which is a core subject, and also into technology, which is another foundation subject. Health education has been identified as an essential part of the curriculum, and it is recommended but not mandatory that this is covered. Food and nutrition can be incorporated into this. A food and nutrition policy for the entire school is recommended so that knowledge acquired in the classroom is supported by the food choices in the snack shop

Table 5.4 Suggested attainment targets for food and nutrition for pupils aged 5 to 11 years. (From National Curriculum Council 1990, with permission of the Qualifications and Curriculum Authority.)

Key stage	Attainment targets
Key stage 1 (5–7 years)	Know that there is a wide variety of food to choose from and that choice is based on need and culture. Know that food is needed for health, and that some foods are better than others.
Key stage 2 (7–11 years)	Know that a diet is a combination of foods with differing nutrient content. Know that different nutrients have different effects on the body, and the amounts in the diet and their balance can influence health. Know how to handle food safely.

and at school meals. Health education, however, is not statutory and many schools may opt to omit it in preference for other topics.

The aims of nutrition education will be to allow children to understand the relationship between diet and health, to recognize the nutritional content of different foods, to understand factors affecting children's food choice, and to teach children food hygiene and food preparation. It is possible to link nutrition into science and technology foundation subjects so that all pupils will have access to some basic nutrition education to help them to make informed choices about food.

NUTRITIONAL PROBLEMS AMONG SCHOOL-AGE CHILDREN

Obesity

Obesity for children is identified by plotting weight and height on percentile charts. Obesity is usually related to a sedentary lifestyle and low energy expenditure rather than excessively high energy intakes. There is a hereditary tendency to obesity due both to genetic factors and family lifestyle. Food for many children is a source of comfort; it may be used as a bribe or reward and sweets and chocolates are often given to gain favour and confidence. Children who are overweight are less likely to participate in games and sports, either in school or at home, due to lack of confidence and embarrassment regarding their physical appearance. Obesity contributes to the development of a poor body image and low self-esteem. Children who are obese in primary school are more likely to be obese in later life; this in turn has a negative effect on physical and mental health. Treatment of obesity is only successful if both the child and the family are motivated. The aim should be to maintain body weight rather than lose weight so that the child will grow into his or her weight. The emphasis should be on family eating habits and lifestyle, and parents should be encouraged to make changes for the whole family. Box 5.3 shows some dietary recommendations for overweight children.

Iron deficiency anaemia

Iron deficiency anaemia is a particular problem in children from low-income families and children who are excessively fussy regarding food. Iron-rich foods, such as red meat, may not be popular with many children. Iron may be encouraged in alternative forms, such as iron-enriched breakfast cereals, or from red meat in more popular forms such as beefburgers, sausages, pâté or meatballs. An adequate vitamin C intake should be encouraged in the form of fresh fruit and vegetables. If these are not popular, fresh fruit juice or squashes with a high vitamin C content may be used.

Dental caries

Dental caries result from demineralization of enamel by acids produced from dietary sugars. A cavity will appear as mineral disappears from the surface of the tooth. Bacterial growth in the cavity can speed the loss of enamel and dentine, and may result in the loss of the tooth.

Dental caries require the presence of appropriate bacteria in the mouth plus a sugar substrate (sucrose or glucose). Cariogenic conditions are produced by an acid pH in the mouth, and acid foods such as citrus fruit, fruit juice and fizzy drinks enhance conditions. Dental caries can be reduced by good oral hygiene, reduction in sucrose and glucose consumption, particularly between meals, and avoidance of sticky or slowly sucked sugary food. Fluoridation of drinking water in some areas has reduced dental caries. Fluoride supplements can be given to children in areas with water of a low fluoride content. This will help to reduce the incidence of caries.

Poor eating habits and undernutrition

Undernutrition is identified by poor growth rates as shown by plotting weight and height on the percentile chart. Children require a wide range of foods in order to achieve a good quality diet. This may be difficult as many children are limited in their food preferences, may be reluctant to try new foods, and go through periods of food fads and food refusal when dietary intakes may be far from ideal. Children tend to adopt the food habits and preferences of the family. It is important that the whole family has a varied and balanced diet and that there is a healthy attitude to food. Children with limited food intakes or fussy, faddy eaters can be encouraged to eat through various methods. Food should be presented in an attractive manner and the whole family should be encouraged to eat

Box 5.3 Dietary recommendations for the mealtimes of overweight children

- A low-sugar, low-fat, high-fibre diet.
- Increased fruit and vegetable consumption.
- Fried foods, crisps and sweets are allowed in moderation.
- An increase in exercise is encouraged.
- Packed lunches may be preferable to a school meal.

Table 5.5 Requirements of major nutrients in adolescence. (DoH 1991. Crown copyright material is reproduced with the permission of the Controller of Her Majesty's Stationery Office.)

| | Male | | Female | |
	11–14 yrs	15–18 yrs	11–14 yrs	15–18 yrs
EAR Energy kcal/day	2200	2755	1845	2110
RNI Protein g/d	42.1	55.2	41.2	45.4
RNI Calcium mg/d	1000	1000	800	800
RNI Iron mg/d	11.3	11.3	14.8	14.8

together to make mealtimes a pleasant occasion. New foods should be served without comment, and if they are rejected they should be given without comment again a few weeks later. This should be repeated, and eventually the child will develop a liking or tolerance for that food. If a meal or food is rejected, it should be removed without comment and no alternative should be offered until the next meal time. Bribes, force-feeding, punishment and coaxing to eat rarely work and are more likely to exacerbate the problem. Children will often eat better if they eat out with friends and they may be more willing to try new foods in this environment than with the family at home.

THE NUTRITIONAL REQUIREMENTS OF ADOLESCENTS

The nutrient requirements of adolescents are relatively high, with particularly high requirements for protein, vitamins and minerals per unit of energy. Boys show a greater adolescent growth spurt and so have a higher nutritional need. Many boys become thin during this time prior to muscular development in their late teens. Table 5.5 details requirements for major nutrients.

Requirements correlate poorly with chronological age and are more closely linked to biological age as indicated by bone age or sexual maturity ratings. However, recommendations are given for chronological age due to the difficulty in determining biological age. Particular attention must, however, be paid to early or late maturers whose nutritional requirements may differ dramatically from those stated for their chronological age.

Energy

Adolescents have high energy requirements, particularly boys aged 15 to 18 years when energy expenditure has been shown to be high. Many adolescent boys may consume in excess of estimated average requirements at levels of 3000 to 4000 kcal per day. This is often achieved by substantial meals plus frequent snacking between meals. The high energy requirements of adolescents, particularly boys, mean that compliance with a low-fat, high-fibre diet may make achieving required energy intakes impossible as the diet becomes bulky.

Protein

Protein requirements again correlate more closely with biological age than chronological age. Intake of protein for the majority of adolescents is in excess of requirements. Extreme calorie restriction, for example as seen in some teenage girls, may mean that protein is diverted as an energy source, and this may in the long term result in a reduction in growth rate and lean body mass.

Iron

Iron requirements increase dramatically in both boys and girls. In boys the increase is due to the expanding blood volumes and increase in haemoglobin level which accompanies sexual maturation. The requirement for boys decreases after the growth spurt and sexual maturation. In girls the requirement reaches the highest level during the peak growth spurt, but remains high to compensate for the losses during menstruation. Iron deficiency anaemia is common in girls due to a dislike or avoidance of iron-rich foods (particularly red meat), and is extremely likely in girls who become pregnant. Anaemia may limit growth and impair the immune response.

Calcium

The accelerated muscle, skeletal and hormonal development means that calcium needs are highest during puberty and adolescence. During the peak of the growth spurt, deposition of calcium may be twice the daily deposition at other stages of adolescence.

Calcium requirements are easily met if milk and dairy products are taken in the diet on a daily basis. They are extremely difficult to achieve if there is an avoidance of milk and milk products due to dislike or avoidance for other reasons. Calcium absorption is more efficient during adolescence and this may partly compensate for poor intakes. Teenage boys are more likely than girls to have adequate calcium intakes, due to the inclusion of milk and dairy produce in their diets.

Other nutrients

The need for vitamins is increased. Due to the increased energy needs, requirements for thiamin, riboflavin and nicotinic acid are high. There is an increased need for folic acid and vitamin B_{12} due to greater tissue synthesis, and requirements for vitamin D are high due to rapid skeletal growth.

NUTRIENT INTAKES AMONG ADOLESCENTS

There have been four major dietary surveys in the UK to include adolescents (Bull 1988, Department of Health 1989, Barker et al 1988, Lee &

Box 5.4 Summary of the findings of the 'Diets of British school children' survey for adolescents

- ◆ A low energy and nutrient intake has been shown in girls who claim to be dieting or who see themselves as overweight.

- ◆ Overall, 35% of girls consider themselves to be overweight, 5% claimed to be dieting and 15% claimed to be careful about what they eat.

- ◆ In these groups, iron, thiamin and riboflavin intakes were low.

- ◆ The study identified iron, riboflavin and calcium intakes to be low in girls, with the poorest intake seen in girls who do not have a school meal, but preferred instead to eat out of school at cafes, takeaway or fast food outlets.

- ◆ Scottish teenagers were shown to have lower intakes of vitamins C and A than English teenagers.

Cunningham 1990). These provide information on nutrient intakes, foods consumed and eating habits.

The most comprehensive survey is the 'Diets of British school children' survey. Its findings with regard to adolescents are summarized in Box 5.4.

Eating habits

Adolescents are maturing physically and psychosocially. The strive for independence and acceptance, the need to show their own identity, and concern regarding their physical appearance affect eating habits and food choices. Meals may be skipped, there is an increase in snacking and eating away from home, and an increased interest in vegetarianism and dietary fads.

There is a common belief that teenagers consume a large proportion of junk foods. However, the Department of Health report shows that a wide variety of foods are eaten. Children tend to eat three meals a day, with 30% of energy coming from lunch, 30% from an evening meal and the remainder from snacks and breakfast.

Missed meals

If meals are missed, it tends to be breakfast or lunch. Lunch may be missed due to social activities during the lunchtime period at school. Breakfast is the most commonly missed meal, particularly in teenage girls. Missing meals is not of concern if adequate food is available, as most children eat sufficient for their needs. However, skipping breakfast may make it more difficult to concentrate on school work during the morning.

Snacking

People aged from 16 to 25 are more likely to have a diet based on chips, nuts, sweets, soft drinks, meat or savoury pies. Snacks eaten by teenagers may provide substantial amounts of nutrients other than energy, including iron, calcium, thiamin, vitamin C and riboflavin.

The incidence of snacking is thought to be an average of 6.8 occasions per day for 11 to 12-year-olds.

Snack foods preferred by 14 to 16-year-old Scottish girls are summarized in Table 5.6 (Cresswell et al 1983).

NUTRITION EDUCATION FOR ADOLESCENTS

There is a direct link between diet in adolescence and long-term health. Other lifestyle factors such as alcohol, drug abuse, exercise and smoking are also linked. Adolescents, however, do not take a long-term view, and any discussion regarding their future health will have little impact. Instead, nutrition education must motivate the teenager by relating lifestyle or dietary changes to immediate benefits.

Nutrition education can be included within the National Curriculum key stages 3 and 4. Attainment targets are shown in Table 5.7.

The study of food and nutrition is currently a component of the key stage 3 science programme of study.

Technology in the National Curriculum includes some aspects of food and diet; the emphasis is on design and production, looking at aspects of food preparation, food safety, food preservation and the nutritional value of foods.

Many important aspects of health education go beyond the curriculum, such as the facilities in the school and the messages conveyed by the school environment. Hidden messages are conveyed by the nature of school meal provision, attitudes to snacks, and the foods available in vending machines. It is therefore important that the school policy on health education extends to these areas.

In secondary schools subjects are taught by specialist teachers, meaning that there may be fragmentation in teaching about food and nutrition. With care and planning, however, all aspects of food and nutrition can be covered. A well-formulated policy of health education can also promote nutrition and education as part of the more general social and personal development programmes.

Table 5.6 Adolescents' preferred snacks. (From Cresswell et al 1983, with permission.)

Snack	% reporting
Crisps/savoury snack	56
Soft drinks	50
Chocolate	39
Sweets	31
Chewing gum	15
Ice cream	7
Cakes	6
Biscuits	2
Fruit	<1

NUTRITIONAL PROBLEMS AMONG ADOLESCENTS

Vegetarianism

Adolescents may adopt a vegetarian or vegan diet for a variety of reasons including their reaction to animal slaughter, for health benefits and as a way of expressing individuality. Vegetarian and vegan diets can be a healthy way of eating, but teenagers may try to follow diets without guidance and may fail to replace animal products with suitable vegetable alternatives. Poor intakes of energy, iron, vitamin B_{12} and protein may result unless advice is sought.

Table 5.7 Suggested attainment targets for food and nutrition for pupils aged 11 to 16 years. (From National Curriculum Council 1990, with permission of the Qualifications and Curriculum Authority.)

Key stage	Attainment targets
Key stage 3 (11–14 years)	Know that individual health requires a varied diet. Understand malnutrition and relationship of diet to health and fitness, and understand food microbiology, food production and processing.
Key stage 4 (14–16 years)	To be able to analyse and evaluate diet and recognize adjustments which take account of the availability of food and social, cultural and financial influences. Know that various types of diet promote growth for different groups. Understand consumer aspects of food hygiene and food legislation including labelling. Understand the relationships between food, body image and self-esteem. Have information to be able to distinguish between fact and propaganda in dietary issues.

Teenage pregnancy

Pregnancy makes considerable nutritional demands, particularly for iron, calcium, zinc, folate and vitamin D. These demands are additional to the already high demands in the teenage girl. Other considerations include the following:

◆ Poor nutrient intake during pregnancy is associated with increased morbidity and mortality in the baby.
◆ Pregnant teenagers may have considerable social and financial difficulties.
◆ Knowledge about food preparation and food hygiene may be poor, and education should focus on practical aspects of food choice and preparation.
◆ Some girls may be unaware that they are pregnant or may try to disguise the pregnancy, and the need for a good diet during pregnancy may then go unrecognized, affecting the health of both the baby and the mother.

Sports and athletic training

Teenagers who adopt sports and athletic training schedules may adopt inappropriate dietary habits. In particular:

◆ high doses of vitamin and minerals may be taken
◆ high-protein dietary supplements may be used

◆ mealtimes may be limited by training schedules, and snacks may replace meals in the interests of speed.

A high-protein diet is not necessary, and vitamin and mineral intakes can be achieved without the use of expensive supplements. Adequate fluid intake and a relatively high carbohydrate intake should be encouraged, particularly before and during exercise. A range of complete liquid diets are promoted for athletes. These are unnecessary and expensive, and their use should be discouraged.

Slimming diets

About 5% of 14 to 15-year-old girls who took part in the Department of Health survey were dieting to lose weight (Department of Health 1989). The regime may be extremely restrictive and consist of two or three foods only. It will also clearly be nutritionally inadequate with nutritional consequences if followed for long periods. Slimming drinks may be used. These are expensive and do not sustain weight loss in the long term as they do not encourage a change in eating habits and lifestyle.

It is important to set targets for the teenager wishing to lose weight, and to advise not only on diet but also to encourage an increase in activity. Advice must be individually adapted and practical to fit in with the teenager's lifestyle.

SUMMARY

◆ The composition of diet in childhood is important in the short term to sustain growth and health, and in the long term to reduce the risk of chronic disease in adult life.

◆ The dietary guidelines set out in 'The Health of the Nation' should be implemented in school age years.

◆ Children's ideas about health and diet are influenced by parents, peers and the media, and schools have an important role to play in promoting health and good dietary habits.

 FURTHER READING

Health Education Authority 1995 Diet and health in school age children. Nutrition Briefing Paper. Health Education Authority, London

School Meals Campaign 1996 Healthy school food: a guide for school governors and school boards. School Meals Campaign, London

Winick M 1982 Adolescent nutrition. John Wiley, Chichester

REFERENCES

Adamson A, Rugg-Gunn A, Butler M R, Appleton D, Hackett A F 1992 Nutritional intake, height and weight of 11 to 12-year-old Northumbrian children in 1990 compared to 1980. British Journal of Nutrition 68(3): 543–563

Barker M E, McClean S, McKenna D G, Reid N G, Strain J J, Thompson K A, Williamson A P, Wright M E 1988 Diet, lifestyle and health in Northern Ireland. Centre for Applied Health Studies, University of Coleraine

Bull N L 1988 Dietary habits of 15 to 25-year-olds. Human Nutrition: Applied Nutrition 39A (Suppl. 1):1–68

Crawley H F 1993 The energy nutrient and food intakes of teenagers aged 16 to 17 years in Britain. British Journal of Nutrition 70:15–26

Cresswell J, Busby A, Young H, Inglis V 1983 Dietary portions of third year secondary school girls in Glasgow. Human Nutrition: Applied Nutrition 37A:301–306

Department for Education and Employment 1998 Ingredients for success: a consultation paper on nutritional standards for school lunches. DfEE, London

Department of Health 1989 Diets of British school children. Sub Committee of Nutritional Surveillance Committee on the Medical Aspects of Food Policy Report on Health and Social Subjects 36. HMSO, London

Department of Health 1990 Health Education Authority / Ministry of Agriculture Fisheries and Food. Eight guidelines for a healthy diet. Food Sense, London

Department of Health 1991 Dietary reference values for food energy and nutrients in the UK. HMSO, London

Gardner-Merchant 1998 'What are today's children eating?' The Gardner-Merchant School Meals Survey 1998. Gardner-Merchant, Kenley

Hackett A F, Rugg-Gunn A J, Appleton D R, Eastoe J E, Jenkins G N 1984 A 2-year longitudinal nutritional survey of 405 Northumberland children initially aged 11.5 years. British Journal of Nutrition 51(1):67–75

Lee P, Cunningham K 1990 Irish National Nutritional Survey. Irish Nutrition and Dietetic Institute, Dublin

McNeill G, Davidson L, Morrison D C, Crombie I M, Keighran J, Todman J 1991 Nutrient intake in school children: practical considerations. Proceedings of the Nutrition Society 50:37–43

National Curriculum Council 1990 Curriculum guidance 5: health education. National Curriculum Council, York

Nelson M 1993 Children's diets – problems and solutions. Paper presented at National Dairy Council Conference

Nelson M 1993 Nutritional content of children's diets and the health implications. National Forum for Coronary Heart Disease Prevention, London

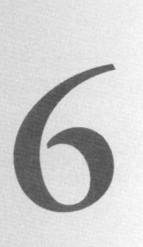

6

Vitamins and minerals in paediatrics

Anita MacDonald

INTRODUCTION

A vitamin is characterized as follows:

- an essential organic chemical compound
- present in plant and animal tissue in small quantities
- required only in tiny amounts
- it must be supplied in the diet or synthesized from essential dietary precursors
- a substance with specific biochemical functions in the human body.

Most vitamins have complex chemical structures and they do not belong to one chemical family. Disorders of vitamins include deficiency, toxicity and biochemical dependency states.

A mineral is characterized as follows:

- an inorganic chemical compound
- about 15 of them are known to be essential and they must be derived from food
- calcium, phosphorus, magnesium, sodium, chloride, potassium, iron and zinc are the eight major elements and are needed in the greatest quantities
- others, which are required in much smaller quantities (usually less than 1 mg daily) are known as trace elements.

A trace element is considered essential if a dietary deficiency of that element consistently results in physiological and structural abnormalities which are preventable and reversible by administration of the element. There are 13 trace elements, seven of which (copper, manganese, cobalt, chromium, selenium, molybdenum and iodine) are considered to be essential. Fluoride is considered to be semi-essential and although iron may be classified as a major element, requirements are small.

VITAMIN AND MINERAL REQUIREMENTS

Vitamin and mineral requirements are reviewed and defined in 'Dietary reference values for food energy and nutrients for the United Kingdom' (Department of Health 1991). In these recommendations, the reference nutrient intake (RNI) is the amount which meets the requirements of 97.5% of the population in health. An RNI is set for most vitamins and minerals. Unfortunately, there are inherent difficulties in the interpretation of these requirements. These include:

1. For children, reference values or requirements are frequently calculated from values for infants and adults. This is because few studies have examined the vitamin and trace mineral requirements for this age group. This applies to many of the vitamins and most trace elements.

2. For some vitamins and trace elements, due to insufficient data, no dietary reference values (DRV) are set. Instead, safe intakes are identified which define a level or range of intake at which there is no risk of deficiency, and below a level where there is a risk of undesirable effects. This applies to the following nutrients: pantothenic acid, biotin, vitamin E, vitamin K, manganese, molybdenum, chromium and fluoride.

3. An RNI applies to the requirements of vitamins and minerals for groups of healthy people, and is not necessarily appropriate for sick children or patients on synthetic diets. Gastrointestinal losses such as vomiting, diarrhoea and fistula losses, haemodialysis and skin losses, especially from exudate following severe burn injury, are likely to increase vitamin and trace mineral requirements. Anorexia, associated with a disease state, may lead to a prolonged inadequate vitamin and trace element intake and, therefore, a depleted micronutrient patient status, which is likely to increase requirements.

4. Standard RNIs assume a normal intake of other nutrients and this may not be the case for children on synthetic diets or enteral nutrition, in whom intake of some trace minerals or vitamins may be disproportionate. This is important because an imbalance of trace elements, in particular, may precipitate deficiencies of other trace elements due to minerals of similar physiochemical properties antagonizing one another, e.g. high doses of copper may affect zinc absorption and may induce zinc deficiency.

Bioavailability of vitamins and minerals

The bioavailability of many vitamins and trace minerals is low and often poorly predictable. Factors which influence bioavailability include the nature of the diet and nutrient itself, intestinal factors which influence luminal and mucosal digestion and absorption, and systemic factors which control intestinal absorption and systemic distribution of a nutrient (Department of Health 1991, Aggett 1994) (Box 6.1).

Box 6.1 Examples of factors influencing absorption and utilization of nutrients

Diet

Chemical form of nutrient: e.g. haem iron vs inorganic iron; carotene vs retinol.

Enhancers of absorption: e.g. ascorbic acid, lactic acid, fructose, amino acids.

Inhibitors of absorption: e.g. phosphate, oxalates, avidin, bran, tannins, competing metals.

Systemic factors

Anabolic demands: growth in infancy and childhood; pregnancy and lactation; post-catabolic states.

Genetic influences: inborn errors of metabolism.

Nutritional status of other nutrients.

Intestinal factors which affect luminal and mucosal digestion and absorption

Changes in mucosal structure and function.

Bacterial fermentation.

Efficiency of dietary hydrolysis.

Assessment of vitamin and mineral adequacy

The diagnosis of deficiency is difficult. No single test reliably indicates whether an individual child is at risk of deficiency. All data need to be interpreted in the context of the homeostatic mechanisms for the vitamins and minerals, an appreciation of the clinical state of the child and how this would alter the metabolism of the vitamin and mineral (Aggett 1994).

Biochemical markers

Maintenance of enzyme activity. Many micronutrients are required for enzyme activity, either as coenzymes or as part of metalloenzymes, and hence measurement of enzyme activity may be useful: e.g. tests of selenium status by red cell glutathione peroxidase activity, or intracellular vitamin B_6 by transaminase activation. Such tests only have limited application, as specific examples do not exist for most micronutrients (Shenkin 1994).

Maintenance of plasma concentration. The most widely used test of micronutrient adequacy is the plasma concentration, mainly because the sample is readily available. However, the relationship of plasma concentration to intracellular concentration is poor for most micronutrients, this being especially the case during illness, as values may be depressed (e.g. iron and zinc), or may even be increased by infections and stress (e.g. copper). Thus, measurement of plasma concentration is of only limited value in assessing the intracellular content and function of a micronutrient.

VITAMIN A

Functions

Vitamin A has the following functions:

◆ Its main function is in the control of cell differentiation and turnover. It is therefore essential for growth.

◆ It is essential for the normal function of the retina and development of epithelial surface in the retina.

◆ β-carotene, the precursor of vitamin A, is an antioxidant in its own right. It is the single most effective, naturally occurring quencher of singlet oxygen and can prevent oxidative damage to cells. Carotenes can react with radicals to form relatively stable unreactive radicals and this reduces radical damage to tissues, which can have a variety of serious effects, including damage to DNA, which may result in the development of cancer (Barker & Lees 1996).

Table 6.1 shows requirements for vitamin A up to the age of 18.

Risk of deficiency

The risk of vitamin A deficiency in infants and young children is small. However, almost 10% of normal children aged between $1\frac{1}{2}$ and $4\frac{1}{2}$ years have dietary intakes below the lower reference nutrient intake (Gregory et al 1995).

Risk areas include:

◆ children who are faddy eaters
◆ infants and children with fat malabsorption: e.g. cystic fibrosis and severe cholestatic liver disease
◆ very low fat diets: e.g. very long chain fatty acid defects, lymphangiectasia and adrenoleukodystrophy.

Table 6.1 Vitamin A requirements (DoH 1991)

Age	Reference Nutrient Intake (µg/day)
0–12 months	350
1–6 years	400
7–10 years	500
11–14 years	600
Male	
15–18 years	700
Female	
15–18 years	600

It has long been recommended that all children under 5 years take supplements of vitamins A, D and C. The only exceptions are:

◆ breastfed babies less than 6 months of age, providing the mother was in good vitamin status during pregnancy
◆ bottle-fed infants who are consuming 500 ml daily of infant formula.

Children with cystic fibrosis, cholestatic liver disease or on very low fat diets require vitamin A supplementation.

Worldwide, vitamin A deficiency is a major problem in children, and the most important preventable cause of blindness. It is widespread in south-east Asia, the Middle East and Africa. In the UK, vitamin A deficiency is rarely seen, but has been reported in a number of children with cystic fibrosis.

Symptoms of deficiency

Impaired vision

There is a loss of sensitivity to green light; this is followed by impairment of the ability to adapt to dim light, followed by night blindness. More prolonged or severe deficiency leads to xerophthalmia, which causes blindness.

Reduced resistance to infection

Vitamin A deficient humans are more susceptible to infection, and epidemiological studies indicate that low vitamin A status is frequently associated with increased disease incidence and mortality rates. Vitamin A deficiency affects immunity in several ways, but retinoids in particular act on the differentiation of immune cells, increasing mitogenesis of lymphocytes and phagocytosis of monocytes and macrophages.

Rough, scaly skin

In the skin, vitamin A deficiency results in keratinization, which blocks the sebaceous gland with plugs, producing a condition known as follicular keratosis.

In general, vitamin A deficiency can cause loss of appetite, retarded growth, drying and keratinization of membranes and even death. Table 6.2 shows some important dietary sources of vitamin A.

Risk of toxicity

Children are more sensitive than adults to a high vitamin A intake. Excessively high intakes lead to accumulation in the liver. Intakes should not exceed the following:

Infants – 900 μg daily
1 to 3 years – 1800 μg daily
4 to 6 years – 3000 μg daily
6 to 12 years – 4500 μg daily
Adolescents – 6000 μg daily.

Symptoms of toxicity include liver and bone damage, hair loss, vomiting and headaches. β-carotene is not toxic, but high intakes lead to a yellow appearance. An excess intake of food rich in carotenoids can result in a distinct orange yellow colour of the skin, called hypercarotenaemia. This is a benign condition, but the persistence of this change in colour is dependent upon continued intake of carotenoids. It is more common in young children.

Table 6.2 Dietary sources of vitamin A (Holland et al 1991)

Vitamin A is obtained from two sources: it is found in retinol, and it can be synthesized from carotenoids.

Retinol sources	Retinol (μg) per 100g
Liver – lamb	19895
Full cream milk	52
Cheese	325
Butter	815
Cod liver oil	18000

Carotenoids	Retinol equivalent (μg) per 100g
Carrots	1353
Tomatoes	107
Red peppers	640
Mangoes	300
Sweet potato (orange)	655

VITAMIN D

There are two main forms of vitamin D:

◆ Cholecalciferol (vitamin D_3) occurs naturally and is formed by the action of sunlight on 7-dehydrocholesterol, which occurs naturally in the skin of humans and other animals.
◆ Ergocalciferol (vitamin D_2) is a synthetic source of vitamin D. This is made by exposing the compound ergosterol, found in funghi and yeasts, to ultraviolet light. This form of vitamin is prepared commercially and is used in vitamin supplements and for the fortification of foods such as margarine.

Vitamin D has an important metabolic role in the control of calcium homeostasis. Its role includes:

◆ enhancing the absorption of calcium and phosphorus
◆ deposition of calcium in bones and teeth.

Table 6.3 shows requirements for vitamin D up to the age of 18.

Risk of deficiency

Children under 3 years are particularly vulnerable to poor vitamin D status because of demands resulting from the high rate at which calcium is being laid down in the bone. The risk of deficiency is particularly high in Asian children and some childhood disease states. Mean dietary intake in pre-school children has been shown to be less than 2 µg daily (Gregory et al 1995). Vitamin D is present in few foods, and sunlight is the main source.

Table 6.3 Vitamin D requirements (DoH 1991)

Age	Reference Nutrient Intake (µg/day)
0–6 months	8.5 µg
7–12 months	7 µg
1–3 years	7 µg
4–18 years	0 *

* Certain at-risk individuals or groups may require dietary vitamin D.

Risk areas include:

◆ children with increased skin pigmentation: e.g. Asian, African and Afro-Caribbean
◆ children wearing concealing clothing
◆ children living a predominantly indoor life: e.g. for religious and cultural reasons
◆ children living in northern latitudes with cloudy skies and not taking vitamin D supplements
◆ poor maternal diet, without vitamin D supplementation, leading to reduced maternal–fetal transfer of vitamin D during pregnancy
◆ prolonged breastfeeding into late infancy without vitamin D supplementation
◆ children on vegan diets with little exposure to sun, or with dark skin pigmentation
◆ children with fat malabsorption such as liver disease or cystic fibrosis
◆ children with chronic renal disease
◆ children on very low-fat diets, or on synthetic diets without vitamin supplementation.

Symptoms of deficiency

Prolonged deficiency of vitamin D in children results in rickets. The main symptoms include skeletal deformity, delayed dentition, bone pain, muscle weakness, hypocalcaemia, misery and failure to thrive or short stature. Biochemical features of the disease include increased serum alkaline phosphatase, low serum concentrations of 25-hydroxycholecalciferol and secondary hyperparathyroidism leading to hypophosphataemia. Although frank rickets is now uncommon, new cases are still being reported (Mughal et al 1999). However, low serum 25-hydroxycholecalciferol concentrations have been noted in 20% of Bangladeshi, 34% of Pakistani and 25% of Indian 2-year-old children living in England. All these children were apparently healthy and none had been clinically diagnosed as having rickets (Lawson & Thomas 1999). The clinical significance of this is unknown (Wharton 1999). Table 6.4 shows some dietary sources of vitamin D.

Table 6.4 Dietary sources of vitamin D (Holland et al 1991)

Food	Quantity per 100 g (µg)
Margarine	7.94
Low fat margarine	8.0
Herring	22.5
Kipper	25.0
Sardines	7.5
Pacific salmon	12.5
Eggs	1.75
Cod liver oil	210

All infants and children at high risk of vitamin D deficiency should be encouraged to take supplements throughout the first five years (Department of Health 1994). This should include children who are poor eaters, children on vegan diets, as well as diets that exclude food items for the management of allergy or other disorders.

Risk of toxicity

Infants are particularly vulnerable to vitamin D toxicity, with intakes as low as 50 µg per day causing hypercalcaemia. During the 1950s, rickets was more or less totally eradicated, but over-enrichment of fortified infant foods and vitamin D supplements led to an epidemic of infant hypercalcaemia (Wharton & Darke 1982). The consequences of vitamin D toxicity include an increase in plasma calcium concentration, tetany, electrocardiogram changes, convulsions and occasionally death.

VITAMIN C

Functions

Vitamin C has several important functions:

◆ It is important in the synthesis of collagen proteins. It is important for wound healing. The requirements for vitamin C increase after trauma or surgery when the rate of collagen synthesis increases.

◆ It has important roles in several hydroxylases involved in the metabolism of neurotransmitters, steroids, drugs and lipids. It acts as a co-factor in the synthesis of carnitine, which is required for the transport of fatty acids into the mitochondria for oxidation to provide energy for the cell.

◆ It increases the bioavailability of iron in foods. The effect is associated with increased enteric absorption. With non-haem iron, it reduces the ferric to the ferrous form, improving its absorption. With haem iron, it is thought to involve enhanced incorporation of iron into the intracellular form, ferritin.

◆ It has been found to affect immune function in several different ways, including stimulating the production of interferons (the proteins that protect cells against viral attack).

◆ It acts as an antioxidant.

Table 6.5 shows requirements for vitamin C up to the age of 18.

Risk of deficiency

The risk of deficiency is high in some groups of children, although dietary intake is generally good. However, a survey of pre-school children indicated that the mean vitamin C intake was 52 mg/day (Gregory et al 1995). Only 1% of children had vitamin C intakes below the lower reference nutrient intakes. Even so, the majority of children did not eat fruit and vegetables (excluding potatoes and snacks) during the survey. The chief sources of vitamin C were soft drinks and fruit juice. Daly et al (1998) found that in a group of children, predominantly from low income single-parent families, the purchase

Table 6.5 Vitamin C requirements (DoH 1991)

Age	Reference Nutrient Intake (mg/day)
0–12 months	25
1–3 years	30
4–6 years	30
7–10 years	30
11–14 years	35
15–18 years	40

of fresh fruit was rare due to high wastage and transport difficulties. In addition, storage, preparation and prolonged cooking can result in much loss of ascorbic acid.

Risk areas include:

◆ faddy eaters
◆ children from low income families
◆ chronic illness
◆ cult diets
◆ low sucrose and fructose diets
◆ long term hospitalization with low fruit and vegetable intake
◆ teenage smokers (smokers have an increased turnover of vitamin C and requirements are estimated to be 80 mg/day).

Deficiency

Severe deficiency causes scurvy. This is probably the most well-known deficiency disease, but is now only occasionally seen in the UK. Symptoms include:

◆ failure of hair follicle eruption
◆ poor wound healing
◆ lowered resistance to infection
◆ bleeding gums, fragile capillary blood vessels
◆ damage to bone and connective tissue.

In infancy, scurvy is characterized by painful, swollen joints. The limbs are tender and the baby cries when being handled. Bone degeneration may give rise to deformities resembling those seen in rickets. Spontaneous haemorrhages can also occur (Barker & Lees 1996). Table 6.6 shows some dietary sources of vitamin C.

Risk of toxicity

The risk of vitamin C toxicity is low, as surplus vitamin C is excreted in the urine. However, continual megadoses of vitamin C (in excess of 1 g/day) can cause diarrhoea, increased production of oxalate and kidney stones. Sudden cessation of a high intake may cause scurvy due to an enhanced turnover of the vitamin.

Table 6.6 Dietary sources of vitamin C (Holland et al 1991)

Food	Content per 100 g (mg)
Oranges	54
Kiwi fruit	59
Mango	37
Boiled potatoes – old	11
Chips	9
Crisps	27
Green peppers	120
Natural orange juice	39
Ribena – undiluted	78

FOLIC ACID

'Folate' is the generic descriptor for folic acid and related compounds exhibiting qualitatively the biological activity of folic acid.

Functions

The primary biochemical function of folate coenzymes is in the transfer and utilization of one-carbon units in a variety of essential reactions involved in amino acid interconversions, biosynthesis of the nucleic acids, purines and pyrimidines and certain methylation reactions.

Folic acid is also involved in:

◆ maturation of red blood cells
◆ embryonic development of the nervous system.

Table 6.7 shows requirements for folic acid up the age of 18.

Risk of deficiency

The risk of deficiency in children is low. The average daily intake of folate from dietary sources

Table 6.7 Folic acid requirements (DoH 1991)

Age	Reference Nutrient Intake (µg/day)
0–12 months	50
1–3 years	70
4–6 years	100
7–10 years	150
11–18 years	200

for pre-school children was 132 µg and mean folate intake increased with age (Gregory et al 1995).

Risk areas include:

- poor diet – particularly in children from low income families
- secondary malabsorption: e.g. coeliac disease
- interference with folic acid metabolism: e.g. anticonvulsant therapy
- increased cell proliferation: e.g. lymphoproliferative disorders
- patients on haemodialysis
- teenage pregnancies
- inborn errors of folic acid metabolism.

Deficiency

Deficiency symptoms include:

- poor growth in children
- megaloblastic anaemia (immature red blood cells)
- diarrhoea
- smooth, atrophic tongue
- splenomegaly.

Table 6.8 shows some dietary sources of folic acid.

Table 6.8 Dietary sources of folic acid (Holland et al 1991)

Food	Amount (μg/100 g)
Broccoli	90
Spinach	150
Brussels sprouts	135
Oranges	31
Grapefruit	26
Bananas	14
Natural orange juice	20
Enriched breakfast cereals	250
Wholemeal bread	39
Yeast extract (e.g. Marmite)	1010
Baked beans	22
Peas	62
Peanuts	110
Almonds	48
Liver	320
Kidney	79
Beef	17

Risk of toxicity

The risk of toxicity in children is small. Toxicity symptoms may include:

- mood changes, although there is little evidence to support this
- reduction of zinc absorption.

Folate supplements given to patients with developing vitamin B_{12} deficiency may obscure a correct diagnosis and delay appropriate treatment. Relatively large doses of folic acid (over 1000 µg/day) may antagonize the beneficial effects of anticonvulsants.

VITAMIN B_{12}

The structure of vitamin B_{12} is complex. Compounds with vitamin B_{12} actively consist of a corrinoid ring surrounding an atom of cobalt. The synthesis of vitamin B_{12} is limited almost exclusively to bacteria so the vitamin is found only in foods that have been bacterially fermented and those derived from the tissue of animals that have obtained it from their intestinal microflora.

Functions

Its metabolic function is closely linked with that of folic acid:

- It is essential for the synthesis and methylation of DNA, metabolism of lipids and maintenance of tissue integrity.
- It is important in red blood cell formation.
- It also has an important role in the maintenance of myelin in the nervous system.

Table 6.9 shows requirements for vitamin B_{12} up to the age of 18.

Risk of deficiency

Dietary deficiency of vitamin B_{12} is rare. Potential risk areas include:

- Vegan diets.
- Very low natural protein diets: e.g. phenylketonuria.

Table 6.9 Vitamin B$_{12}$ requirements (DoH 1991)

Age	Reference Nutrient Intake (µg/day)
0–6 months	0.3
7–12 months	0.4
1–3 years	0.5
4–6 years	0.8
7–10 years	1.0
11–14 years	1.2
15–18 years	1.5

◆ Secondary to gastric, intestinal and ileal resection. Vitamin B$_{12}$ is normally absorbed in the terminal ileum, but first must bind to salivary haptocorrin and then the 'intrinsic factor', a protein co-factor which is secreted by the parietal cells of the stomach.
◆ Secondary to tapeworm infestation or bacterial overgrowth: these assimilate vitamin B$_{12}$ for their own use.

Deficiency symptoms

Deficiency results in pernicious anaemia which is characterized by large, immature red blood cells (megaloblastic anaemia). Glossites, stomatitis and diarrhoea may occur. Prolonged deficiency leads to irreversible neurological damage with degeneration of the spinal cord.

Dietary sources

Food sources of vitamin B$_{12}$ include almost all animal products, and certain algae (e.g. seaweed)

Table 6.10 Dietary sources of vitamin B$_{12}$ (Holland et al 1991)

Food	Amount (µg/100 g)
Milk	0.4
Cheese	1.1
Eggs	2.5
Beef	2.0
Liver	81.0
Cod	2.0
Fortified breakfast cereals	1.7
Marmite	0.5

and bacteria, which can synthesize it. It does not occur in plant foods unless added artificially. Table 6.10 shows some dietary sources of vitamin B$_{12}$.

Risk of toxicity

This is low. No toxic symptoms have been documented in humans.

IRON

Functions

Iron has several important functions:

◆ It is necessary for the structure of the haem part of haemoglobin which is central to oxygen transport.
◆ It is involved in the formation of myoglobin in muscle which provides a reservoir of oxygen for muscle metabolism.
◆ It is an integral part of haem protein cytochromes, which are involved in electron transfer.

Table 6.11 shows requirements for iron up to the age of 18.

Risk of deficiency

Iron deficiency is common, particularly in ethnic and socioeconomically deprived toddlers in the UK. In a national survey, 1 in 12 pre-school children have been found to have anaemia (i.e.

Table 6.11 Iron requirements (DoH 1991)

Age	Reference Nutrient Intake (mg/day)
0–3 months	1.7
4–6 months	4.3
7–12 months	7.8
1–3 years	6.9
4–6 years	6.1
7–10 years	8.7
Males	
11–18 years	11.3
Females	
11–18 years	14.8

haemoglobin concentration below 11.0 g/dl) (see Table 6.11); 84% of pre-school children have iron intakes below the RNI (Gregory et al 1995).

In adolescents, about 11% of white 11 to 14-year-old girls in London have been found to be anaemic, compared with 22% of Indian girls (Nelson et al 1994). A third of girls aged 10 to 11 years have been shown to have low iron intakes.

KEY POINTS

◆ Iron deficiency anaemia affects 1 in 8 toddlers in the UK.
◆ It is associated with poor weaning diets, low-iron toddler diets, and early introduction of pasteurized cow's milk before 1 year.
◆ Iron deficiency anaemia may cause delayed psychomotor development.
◆ The use of iron-fortified formula may be useful in preventing iron deficiency in children over 1 year.
◆ There is a need for appropriate and effective dietary education in nutritionally at-risk groups.

Causes of iron-deficiency anaemia

Prolonged breastfeeding

Although the level of iron in breast milk is low, it has a good bioavailability and about 50% of iron is absorbed from this source, so in the early stages of weaning it makes an important contribution to iron intake. However, after the age of 6 months, the amount of iron in breast milk is inadequate and alternative dietary iron sources are needed.

Early introduction of pasteurized cow's milk

Pasteurized cow's milk contains only 0.5 mg of iron per litre and this is poorly absorbed. Mothers have commonly given pasteurized cow's milk to infants after the first few months because it is easy to use. However, the ONS 1995 survey (Foster et al 1997) indicated that the situation had improved and that only 16% of infants were given cow's milk as the main drink at 8 to 9 months of age.

Inadequate iron intake during weaning

A MAFF survey (Mills & Tyler 1992) investigating the iron intake of 10- to 12-month-old infants, found both mean and median iron intakes below the Department of Health reference nutrient intake (RNI), with 21% having a daily intake below the lower reference nutrient intake (LRNI). Infants given family foods had lower iron intakes than infants eating commercial baby foods. This finding was confirmed by Daly et al (1996) who found in a group of deprived inner city 6- to 8-month-old infants, iron content was low and common foods given included mashed potato, tinned spaghetti and baked beans. These are cheap and convenient but low in dietary iron.

Inadequate iron intake in pre-school years

Many toddlers eat tiny food portions and are fussy, but no longer drink iron-fortified milks. Meat is a rich source of iron, but is often disliked by toddlers, and the proportion of mothers offering this to their children is gradually decreasing (Foster et al 1997), partly due to vegetarianism and concerns over BSE and Creutzfeldt–Jakob disease.

Inadequate iron intake during adolescence

In teenage girls, low haemoglobin levels have been associated with vegetarian diets (in white girls only), slimming diets, families who are manual workers, and early menarche (Nelson et al 1994).

Poor availability of dietary iron

Although the most readily absorbed iron source is haem, the majority of dietary iron is non-haem. Absorption can be impaired by high intakes of fibre, oxalates, phytates, phosphates and tannin in tea, which is commonly given to toddlers. Ascorbic acid increases the absorption of ferric to ferrous iron and so increases iron absorption. Ideally, foods rich in vitamin C should accompany non-haem sources, but fruit and vegetables are not popular with children and are expensive.

Increased losses of iron

There is some evidence that infants who are given pasteurized cow's milk from 6 months of age may suffer from significant blood loss (Ziegler et al 1990), although other workers (Fuchs et al 1993) have not confirmed this.

Table 6.12 shows some statistics on the prevalence of anaemia.

Effects of deficiency

Iron deficiency is defined as a diminished total body iron content. It may range in severity from reduced body stores with no effect on functional iron to severe anaemia with multiple deficiencies of tissue iron enzymes. Haemoglobin is probably the most widely used screening test for iron deficiency anaemia and the World Health Organization definition of anaemia is when haemoglobin is less than 110 g per litre.

Iron deficiency ultimately results in defective erythropoiesis, leading to normocytic anaemia (Figure 6.1). Infants and children are usually asymptomatic until the anaemia becomes marked, when pallor and tiredness are noted. However, many studies have now indicated that psychomotor development is adversely affected in children with iron deficiency and unfortunately

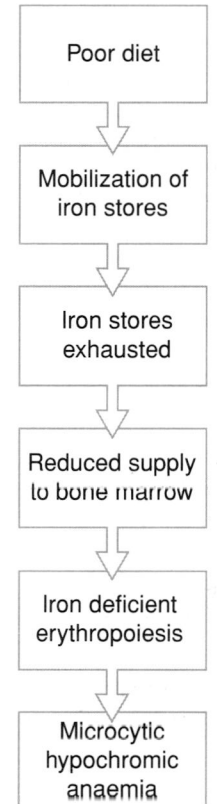

Figure 6.1 Iron deficiency anaemia

there is evidence to suggest that deficits may not be fully reversible in the long term (Williams et al 1999). Box 6.2 shows some of the symptoms of iron deficiency.

Table 6.12 Prevalence of anaemia (Aukett et al 1986, Ehrhardt 1986, DoH 1994, Gregory et al 1995, Daly et al 1996)

Year	Location	Age (months)	Sample group	% of sample with anaemia
1983/4	Bradford	6–48	European	12
			Asian	28
1984/5	Birmingham	21–23	European	18
			Asian	27
1998	Newcastle	9–15	Affluent	11
			Deprived	16
1992/3	United Kingdom	18–29	National	12
1997	Birmingham	18	European	19
			Asian	27
			Afro-Caribbean	29

Box 6.2 Symptoms of iron deficiency

◆ Poor appetite
◆ Fatigue/listlessness
◆ Decreased physical activity
◆ Decreased resistance to infection
◆ Pallor
◆ Irritability
◆ Reduced attention span
◆ Impaired psychomotor development

Sources of dietary iron

Dietary iron is present in two forms:

◆ haem iron, derived from animal muscle or blood tissue, which is readily absorbed
◆ non-haem iron, an inorganic form of iron, which is less easily absorbed.

Between 10 and 15% of dietary iron is absorbed to compensate for daily losses. Table 6.13 shows some dietary sources of iron.

Prevention of iron deficiency

Finding an acceptable method of preventing iron deficiency anaemia has been difficult. A number of methods have been explored. Some of these are described below.

Screening

Despite the high incidence of iron deficiency, screening is not common practice in the UK. Unanswered questions include the ideal age of screening, the most appropriate laboratory tests, whether to screen all children or just high-risk groups, and measurable benefits from identifying and treating iron deficiency anaemia (Department of Health 1994).

Health education

Innovative dietary education methods of promoting iron-rich foods are urgently needed. Although

Table 6.13 Dietary sources of iron (Holland et al 1991)

Food	Amount (mg /100 g)
Haem sources	
Beef	3.4
Mince	3.1
Pork	1.3
Liver	10.0
Non-haem sources	
White bread	1.5
Wholemeal bread	3.5
Fortified breakfast cereals	6.0
Biscuits	2.0
Baked beans	1.4
Egg	1.9
Spinach	1.6

health education has been shown to be successful in small, highly motivated general practices, large-scale dietary education by health visitors has failed. A health education programme encouraging the use of iron-rich food failed to show a decrease in anaemia (Childs et al 1997).

Iron supplementation

Although iron supplements are used to treat iron deficiency and are used prophylactically in pre-term infants, there are several concerns about routine iron supplementation. These include accidental poisoning, iron overdose and gastro-intestinal disturbance (Wharton 1997).

Iron fortification of feeds

In the UK, some infant cereals and other weaning foods are fortified with iron, but no accurate data exist on the effective absorption of iron from these foods. In addition, difficulties are found in fortifying these foods due to rancidity and discoloration (Wharton 1997).

Use of iron-fortified formula in children over 1 year

The use of iron-fortified formula is one strategy which has been shown to be successful in preventing iron deficiency anaemia in older infants and toddlers. In Birmingham in an 18-month prospective study in infants aged 6 months to 2 years, the use of follow-on formula when compared to pasteurized cow's milk resulted in higher dietary iron intakes, improved haemoglobin concentrations and a lower incidence of iron deficiency anaemia. At 18 months, one third of the cow's milk group were anaemic compared with 2 per cent of the follow-on formula group. The benefit of follow-on formula was still present 6 months after it was stopped (Daly et al 1996).

A follow-on formula, in particular, provides a concentrated source of nutrition. It contains more protein, iron and vitamin C than ordinary infant formula and is designed to compliment a weaning diet from the age of 6 months. There is a strong rationale in continuing iron-enriched milk until the age of 2 years. Children in the second year of life are particularly vulnerable to nutritional deficits. They are beginning to feed themselves, have learnt to say no, and food wastage is consequently high. Unfortunately, families receiving income support are unable to obtain free iron-fortified formula beyond the age of 1 year. However, it would now appear appropriate to extend the age limit of free fortified formula so it is available to all high-risk groups. A similar approach has proved effective in the USA (Yip 1989).

Risk of toxicity

Most cases of iron poisoning occur in children, with over-dosage from iron supplements. An acute toxic dose in infants is calculated to be 20 mg (0.4 mmol) per kg/day. A lethal dose in infants is calculated to be 200 to 300 mg (3.6 to 5.4 mmol) per kg/day.

The main problem associated with iron toxicity is haemochromatosis. This is usually genetic, but it can be acquired due to prolonged ingestion of medicinal iron.

ZINC

Functions

Zinc is a component of 70 mammalian enzymes active in many metabolic pathways. These include:

- DNA synthesis
- cell division
- carbohydrate, fat and protein synthesis
- immune function
- wound healing
- insulin production
- growth.

Table 6.14 shows requirements for zinc up to the age of 18.

Risk of deficiency

There is no overt evidence of zinc deficiency in the UK. However, the majority of pre-school children have been shown to have zinc intakes below the RNI levels.

The following children are at risk:

- children who dislike meat
- children from low income families
- children who are faddy eaters
- children on vegan diets
- older children eating a diet based on chips, crisps and fizzy drinks
- children on low protein diets.

There is also a risk of zinc deficiency secondary to malabsorption syndromes, and secondary to widespread burns.

Table 6.15 shows some dietary sources of zinc.

Table 6.14	Zinc requirements (DoH 1991)
Age	**Reference Nutrient Intake (mg/day)**
0–6 months	4
7–12 months	5
1–3 years	5
4–6 years	6.5
7–10 years	7.0
11–14 years	9
Males	
15–18 years	9.5
Females	
15–18 years	7.0

Table 6.15 Dietary sources of zinc (Holland et al 1991)

Food	Amount (mg/100 g)
Beef	5.0
Chicken	1.5
Milk	0.4
Cheese	2.3
Eggs	1.9
Baked beans	0.5
White bread	0.6
Wholemeal bread	1.8

Symptoms of deficiency

In infants, features of zinc deficiency include:

◆ anorexia
◆ failure to thrive
◆ weight loss
◆ tremor
◆ jitteriness
◆ dermatitis
◆ stomatitis
◆ glossitis
◆ nail dystrophy.

In older children, additional symptoms include:

◆ pica
◆ impaired taste and smell
◆ poor growth
◆ depression
◆ intention tremor
◆ photophobia
◆ night blindness
◆ delayed puberty
◆ hypogonadism.

Zinc toxicity

Zinc has low toxicity and does not accumulate in the body. Acute intoxication may occur as a result of ingesting relatively large quantities of zinc salts and symptoms include:

◆ nausea
◆ vomiting
◆ fever
◆ dizziness
◆ lethargy.

Habitual high intakes may suppress copper nutrition.

CALCIUM

Functions

Calcium's diverse functions include maintaining skeletal integrity, as well as regulating nerve excitability, muscle contraction and blood coagulation. During childhood and adolescence adequate dietary calcium builds the skeletal endowment and helps to prevent skeletal disorders. More than 99% of the total body calcium is in the skeleton, and bone mass continues to increase up to the third decade of life (Levenson & Bockman 1994). Between 40 and 50% of the skeletal mass is deposited during adolescence. Table 6.16 shows requirements for calcium up to the age of 18.

Risk of deficiency

There is a moderate risk of deficiency in children. Two per cent of children have been shown to have calcium intakes below the lower reference nutrient intake (Gregory et al 1995). Bone density has been related to calcium intake in adolescent females (Valimiki et al 1994) and about 1 in 4 teenage girls have low calcium intakes.

Risk areas include:

◆ vegan diets – without a calcium-fortified milk substitute
◆ milk-free diets

Table 6.16 Calcium requirements (DoH 1991)

Age	Reference Nutrient Intake (mg/day)
0–12 months	525
1–3 years	350
4–6 years	450
7–10 years	550
Male	
11–18 years	1000
Female	
11–18 years	1000

◆ dislike of milk and dairy products
◆ poor and faddy diets
◆ anorexia nervosa
◆ low protein diets
◆ adolescents.

Symptoms of deficiency

The symptoms of calcium deficiency include:

◆ Neonatal hypocalcaemia – jittery movements, convulsions, and occasionally apnoea (associated with failure of calcium control).
◆ Rickets – caused by low calcium intakes or impaired calcium absorption in infancy.
◆ Osteopenia, osteoporosis, decreased skeletal integrity, and increased risk of fracture in later life – due to failure to reach peak bone mass. Several epidemiological studies in diverse populations have shown an inverse relationship between dietary calcium intake and fracture incidence.

Some dietary sources of calcium are shown in Table 6.17.

Risk of toxicity

The risk of toxicity is low. Body calcium metabolism is under close homeostatic control so that excessive accumulation in blood or tissue from overconsumption is virtually unknown and is more likely to be due to failure to control mechanisms. However, symptoms include:

◆ Hypercalcaemia – general malaise, failure to thrive, polyuria, vomiting, constipation and abdominal pain. Hypercalcaemia may occur in infants who have been given an excess of vitamin D.
◆ Hypercalciuria – sometimes leading to formation of renal stones.

FLUORIDE

Fluoride forms calcium fluorapatite in tooth and bone but no essential function has been proven in humans.

It may have a role in bone and tooth mineralization, and it protects against dental caries. When drinking water contains 1 mg/litre (1 ppm), there is a 50% reduction in tooth decay in children.

Requirements of fluoride

There is no reference nutrient intake for fluoride. However, because of its role in the prevention of dental caries, continued fluoridation of water supplies to achieve levels of 1 ppm is recommended.

Risk of deficiency

Fluoride deficiency has not been demonstrated in humans. In adolescents, the fluoride intake from drinks has been shown to be 0.96 mg/day. The only potential risk areas for deficiency are patients on long-term enteral feeds, if no fluoride is added to the enteral feed and if deionized water is used during preparation.

Dietary sources

The main dietary sources are:

◆ drinking water with a high natural or added level of fluoride
◆ fish
◆ tea
◆ fluoride toothpaste
◆ fluoride supplements.

If a water supply is not fluoridated and a high intake of sugar is taken, fluoride drops should be given from 6 months of age.

Table 6.17 Dietary sources of calcium (Holland et al 1991)	
Food	**Amount (mg/100 g)**
Milk	115
Cheese	720
Yoghurt	150
Fromage frais	89
White bread	110
Wholemeal bread	54
Baked beans	53
Pilchards	300
Sardines	460

Toxicity

The risk of toxicity is high. The maximum recommended intake of fluoride for infants and young children is 0.05 mg/kg per day. In an area with a water supply containing 1 mg/litre, 10% of children have tooth-mottling indicative of mild fluorosis. Intakes of 0.1 mg/kg per day in children under 12 years cause more pronounced enamel changes. Fluoride concentrations of 10 ppm cause loss of appetite, sclerosis of the spine, pelvis and limbs. There may be ossification of the tendon insertion of muscles.

SELENIUM

Functions

Selenium-dependent enzymes (e.g. iodothyronine, deiodinase and glutathione peroxidases) protect the cell from peroxidative damage and therefore act as an antioxidant. Selenium is also involved in the metabolism of the long chain fatty acid, arachidonic acid.

Table 6.18 shows requirements for selenium up to the age of 18.

Risk of deficiency

The risk of deficiency is low. Selenium nutrition has not been extensively investigated in children.
Risk areas include:

◆ very low natural protein diets: e.g. in phenylketonuria and other amino acid disorders
◆ synthetic diets not supplemented with selenium
◆ total parenteral nutrition – devoid of selenium
◆ under-nutrition.

The risk of selenium deficiency depends on the relative activity of other potential antioxidants such as vitamins A, C and E.

Symptoms of deficiency

The main condition is called Keshan disease. This is a cardiomyopathy. It is common in children in

Table 6.18 Selenium requirements (DoH 1991)

Age	Reference Nutrient Intake (µg/day)
0–3 months	10
4–6 months	13
7–12 months	10
1–3 years	15
4–6 years	20
7–10 years	30
11–14 years	40
Males	
15–18 years	70
Females	
15–18 years	60

China with selenium intakes below 12 µg/day. Other symptoms include:

◆ skeletal myopathy
◆ macrocytosis
◆ lightening of hair pigmentation.

Table 6.19 shows some dietary sources of selenium.

Toxicity

The risk of toxicity is low, but the margin between selenium requirements and toxicity is narrower than for many trace elements. Disturbed selenium homeostasis occurs at intakes above 750 µg daily, and symptoms occur at intakes over 900 µg daily.

Toxicity symptoms include:

Table 6.19 Dietary sources of selenium (Holland et al 1991)

Food	Amount (µg/100 g)
Cod	28
Plaice	36
Tuna	90
Beef	3
White bread	28
Milk	1
Chips	2
Red kidney beans	16

- dry brittle hair
- dermatitis
- malodorous breath
- alopecia
- discoloured tooth enamel
- neurological abnormalities.

USE OF VITAMIN AND MINERAL SUPPLEMENTS

These may be necessary in three specific situations:

1. **Poor diet.** Children at risk of developing vitamin and trace mineral deficiencies are those with feeding problems, on a vegan or vegetarian diet that may be low in iron and zinc, and children on bizarre diets such as Zenmacrobiotic diets. Preferably their diets should be reviewed by a paediatric dietitian to assess the need for vitamin and trace element supplementation. Vitamin and mineral supplementation should be used in conjunction with dietary advice; they do not convert a poor diet into a good one. Children with poor appetites as a result of a disease state (e.g. malignancy or renal disease) may need supplementation.

2. **Therapeutic diets.** The need for a specific vitamin and trace element to be provided will depend on the severity of the diet. However, diets excluding two or more staple foods used in the treatment of food intolerance, very low protein diets in the treatment of inborn errors of protein metabolism, and children on limited diet therapy in renal failure may need comprehensive supplementation. Diets excluding or reducing specific items such as milk or fructose and sucrose may need supplementation with calcium or vitamin C respectively; low-fat diets need routine supplements of fat-soluble vitamins. A complete trace element and vitamin supplement is needed with modular feeds used in liver and gastro-intestinal disease.

3. **To replace increased losses.** This may be to compensate for losses of nutrients due to disease state (e.g. fat-soluble vitamins in cystic fibrosis and cholestatic liver disease), or general nutrient loss in short bowel syndrome. Haemodialysis may lead to folic acid deficiency and there may be losses of zinc, copper and selenium in the exudate of burns patients which may need replacing by possibly four to six times the standard daily dose.

Unproven use of vitamin supplements in paediatrics

Effect of vitamin supplementation on IQ

There was a claim a few years ago that vitamin and mineral supplementation in children improved non-verbal intelligence. Carefully controlled studies have failed to substantiate these findings and there is no evidence that giving extra vitamins and minerals improves IQ in school children. However, it is well established that anaemia can impair psychomotor development in the early years and other vitamins and minerals have important effects on cognitive function. Therefore, if there are groups of children eating a poor diet, and intake cannot be improved by normal food intake, a comprehensive vitamin and mineral supplement may be helpful.

Vitamins and mineral supplements available on the NHS

There are only a limited number of vitamin and mineral supplements that can be prescribed on the NHS. Some may only contain a narrow range of vitamins or trace minerals, for children, whereas other preparations in powder or liquid form have strong and unusual tastes and children find these unpalatable. A few preparations are available in capsule form, and children may find these large and difficult to swallow. Trace element powders are particularly unpalatable and bulky, and children have difficulty in taking the full quantity prescribed. In some cases, formulations have not been updated for many years and may not contain all the necessary nutrients in the recommended quantities. Generally, there is little published evidence concerning the efficacy of these common vitamin and trace mineral preparations. The range

Table 6.20 Useful vitamin and mineral supplements available on the NHS

Type	Contains	Dose	Comments
Abidec *Warner Lambert*	Vitamins A, D, C, B_1, B_2, B_6, nicotinamide	<1 year: 0.3 ml daily >1 year: 0.6 ml daily	Useful as a routine vitamin supplement when the food intake is poor. Useful in cystic fibrosis as a vitamin A and D source.
Dalivit *Eastern*	Vitamins A, D, C, B_1, B_2, B_6, nicotinamide	<1 year: 0.3 ml daily >1 year: 0.6 ml daily	Useful as a routine vitamin supplement when the food intake is poor. Useful in cystic fibrosis as a vitamin A and D source.
Ketovite tablets and liquid *Paines and Byrne*	Tablets: Vitamins B_1, B_2, B_6, nicotinamide, pantothenic acid, vitamin C, E, inositol, biotin, folic acid, vitamin K	3 tablets daily	When both tablets and liquid are taken together they provide a complete vitamin supplement. Useful for metabolic diets and modular feeds.
	Liquid: vitamins A, D, B_{12}, choline	5 ml liquid daily	
Mother & Children's vitamin drops *Houghs*	Vitamins A, D, C	5 drops daily	Recommended for all children aged 1 to 5 years
Multivitamin capsules	Vitamins A, D, C, B_1, B_2, nicotinamide	1 daily	A general vitamin supplement. Unsuitable for young children in case of choking.
Paediatric Seravit *SHS*	All vitamins and trace minerals. Does not contain sodium, potassium or chloride	0–6 months: 14 g daily 6–12 months: 17 g daily 1–7 years: 17–25 g daily 7–14 years: 25–35 g daily	A powder available in plain or pineapple flavours. Useful as a complete vitamin and trace mineral supplement for modular feeds and metabolic diets.
Forceval Junior capsules *Unigreg*	Contains all vitamins and trace minerals. Does not contain sodium, phosphorus, chloride or calcium	>5 years: 2 daily	Not recommended for children under 5 years. A useful supplement for children eating poorly or on restricted diets.

of vitamins and minerals contained in common paediatric supplements, the conditions they are suitable for, and information concerning practical usage is given in Table 6.20. Care must be taken to match the dose of any supplements to the actual needs of the patient. Avoid preparations that contain unrecognized nutrients, nutrients in minute amounts or high potency products, as this increases the risk of toxicity.

In practice, compliance with vitamin and mineral supplements is a particular problem and children with malabsorption and on restricted dietary regimens will need careful monitoring of vitamin and trace element status. Furthermore, clear explanation of the dosage, method of administration, availability and length of usage is important. Parents should be instructed to use recommended preparations only and not purchase other preparations from chemists or health food stores as these may be given in addition to prescribed preparations. A study in a GP practice has shown that parental knowledge of vitamin supplements is poor and professional follow-up is inadequate (Ko et al 1992).

Other dietary supplements

There are numerous other dietary supplements which are promoted vigorously and can be purchased over the counter. Parents may wish to use them for their children. The evidence for the need for such supplements is often scanty, conflicting, inconclusive and based on uncontrolled clinical trials (Mason 1995). They have rarely been studied in children, and their use in paediatrics should be discouraged. A summary of some of the dietary supplements is given in Table 6.21.

SUMMARY

With the exception of iron deficiency, primary vitamin and mineral deficiency in paediatrics is rare. However, many children, particularly if they are faddy eaters or are on restrictive diet therapy, are at risk of developing deficiencies, and appropriate vitamin and mineral supplementation is required if dietary intake is poor. More information is needed on specific vitamin and mineral requirements in children, as well as additional published studies to support the

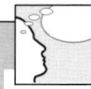

Questions

Answers are given in Appendix 2.

1. What advice would you give to a parent of a 14-month-old child on improving the iron intake?

2. What dietary advice would you give on improving the calcium intake of a 2-year-old child?

3. What dietary advice would you give on improving the vitamin C intake of a young child?

4. What advice would you give to parents of young children with well-pigmented skins to improve vitamin D intake?

Table 6.21 Unproven dietary supplements in paediatrics

Name	Description	Function	Dietary need
Bioflavonoids	Sometimes known as P substances. Do not belong to official group of vitamins.	A group of polyphenolic antioxidants.	No proof of a dietary need exists.
Coenzyme Q	A naturally occurring enzyme.	Involved in electron transport in the mitochondrial membrane.	Insufficient evidence to make recommendations for this as a dietary supplement.
Ginseng	Dried root of Panax ginseng. Ancient remedy for increasing stamina.	Has wide range of pharmaceutical effects but clinical significance in humans has not been fully investigated.	No proof of a dietary need exists.
Lacto bacillus	A genus of bacteria.	Has ability to ferment carbohydrate to produce lactic acid. Claimed to be useful for treatment of diarrhoea.	Random controlled trials failed to show protective effect against *E. coli* and diarrhoea.
Lecithin	An essential component of diet synthesized from choline.	Essential component of cell membranes.	No known dietary deficiency established. Supplements unnecessary.

efficacy of many of the existing vitamin and mineral preparations aimed at the paediatric population.

 FURTHER READING

Bender D A 1997 Introduction to nutrition and metabolism. Taylor and Francis, London

Bender D A, Bender A E 1997 Nutrition: a reference handbook. Oxford University Press, Oxford

Booth I W, Aukett M A 1997 Iron deficiency anaemia in infancy and early childhood. Archives of Disease in Childhood 76:549–554

Combs G F 1992 The vitamins: fundamental aspects in nutrition and health. Academic Press, San Diego

Department of Health 1998 Nutrition and bone health. Report on Health and Social Subjects. HMSO, London

Eastwood M 1997 Principles of human nutrition. Chapman and Hall, London

Landsdown R, Wharton B A 1995 Iron and mental and motor behaviour in children. In: Iron. Nutritional and physiological significance. Report of the British Nutrition Foundation Task Force. Chapman and Hall, London, pp 65–78

McLaren D S 1992 A colour atlas and text of diet related disorders. Wolfe Publishing, London

Thomas B (ed.) 1994 Manual of dietetic practice. Blackwell Science, Oxford

REFERENCES

Aggett P J 1994 Essential trace elements. In: Clayton B E, Round H M (eds) Clinical biochemistry and the sick child. Blackwell Science, Oxford

Aukett M A, Parks Y A, Scott P H, Wharton B A 1986 Treatment with iron increases weight gain and psychomotor development. Archives of Disease in Childhood 61:849–857

Barker H M, Lees R 1996 Nutrition and dietetics for health care. Churchill Livingstone, New York

Childs F, Aukett M A, Darbyshire P, Illett S, Livera L N 1997 Does nutritional education work in preventing iron deficiency in the inner city? Archives of Disease in Childhood 76:114–147

Daly A, MacDonald A, Auckett A, Williams J, Wolff A, Davidson J, Booth I W 1996 Prevention of anaemia in inner city toddlers by an iron supplemented cow's milk formula. Archives of Disease in Childhood 75:9–16

Daly A, MacDonald A, Booth I W 1998 Diet and disadvantage: observations on infant feeding from an inner city. Human Nutrition and Dietetics 11:381–389

Department of Health 1991 Dietary reference values for food energy and nutrients for the United Kingdom. Report on Health and Social Subjects No. 41. HMSO, London

Department of Health 1994 Weaning and the weaning diet. Report on Health and Social Subjects No. 45. HMSO, London

Ehrhardt P 1986 Iron deficiency in young Bradford children from different ethnic groups. British Medical Journal 292:90–93

Foster K, Cheesbrough S, Lader D 1997 Infant feeding 1995. HMSO, London

Fuchs G J, De Wier M, Hutchinson S, Sundeen M, Schwatz S, Suskind R 1993 Gastrointestinal blood loss in older infants impact on cow's milk versus formula. Journal of Pediatric Gastroenterology and Nutrition 16:4–9

Gregory J R, Collins D L, Davies P S W, Hughes J M, Clarke P C 1995 National diet and nutrition survey: children aged $1\frac{1}{2}$ to $4\frac{1}{2}$ years. Volume 1: Report of the Diet and Nutrition Survey. HMSO, London

Holland B, Welch A A, Unwin I D, Buss D H, Paul A A, Southate D A 1991 McCance and Widdowson's The composition of foods. The

Royal Society of Chemistry and Ministry of Agriculture, Fisheries and Food, London

Ko M L B, Ransell N, Wilson J A 1992 What do parents know about vitamins? Archives of Disease in Childhood 67:1080–1081

Lawson M, Thomas M 1999 Vitamin D concentrations in Asian children aged 2 years living in England: population survey. British Medical Journal 318:28

Levenson D I, Bockman R S 1994 A review of calcium preparations. Nutrition Reviews 52:221 232

Mason P 1995 Handbook of dietary supplements. Blackwell Science, Oxford

Mills A, Tyler H 1992 Food and nutrient intakes of British infants 6 to 12 months. HMSO, London

Mughal M Z, Salama H, Laing I, Mawer E B 1999 Florid rickets associated with prolonged vitamin D supplementation. British Medical Journal 318:39–40

Nelson M, Bakaliou F, Trivedi A 1994 Iron deficiency anaemia and physical performance in adolescent girls from different ethnic backgrounds. British Journal of Nutrition 72:427–433

Shenkin A 1994 Mineral and vitamin metabolism. In: Heatley R V, Green J H, Losowsky M S (eds) Consensus in clinical nutrition. Cambridge University Press, Cambridge

Valimiki MJ, Karkkainen M, Lamberg-Allardt C et al 1994 Exercise, smoking and calcium intake during adolescence and early adulthood as determinants of peak bone mass. British Medical Journal 309:230–235

Wharton B 1997 Nutrition in infancy. British Nutrition Foundation, London

Wharton B A (ed.) 1999 Low plasma vitamin D in Asian toddlers in Britian. British Medical Journal 318:2–3

Wharton B A, Darke S J 1982 Infantile hypercalcaemia. In: Jelliffe E F P, Jelliffe D B (eds) Adverse effects of foods. Plenum, New York

Williams J, Wolff A, Daly A, MacDonald A, Auckett A, Booth I W 1999 Iron supplemented formula milk related to reduction in psychomotor decline in infants from inner city areas: randomised study. British Medical Journal 318:693–698

Yip R 1989 The changing characteristics of childhood iron nutritional status in the United States. In: Filer L J Jr (ed.) Dietary iron: birth to two years. Raven Press, New York

Ziegler E E, Forman S H, Nelson S E et al 1990 Cow milk feeding in infancy: further observations on blood loss from gastrointestinal tract. Journal of Pediatrics 116:11–18

Section Two
Feeding sick children

Feeding problems in infants

John W L Puntis

KEY ISSUES

- Failure to thrive
- Posseting, vomiting and gastro-oesophageal reflux
- Colic and wind
- Constipation and acute diarrhoea
- Overfeeding
- Food allergy

INTRODUCTION

Failure to thrive, colic, vomiting and constipation are among the common feeding-related problems seen during infancy. Although the cause of much parental anxiety, serious underlying medical pathology accounts for only a small proportion of cases. In many situations thorough history taking and examination can be followed by simple advice and reassurance. Colic, innocent vomiting and food intolerance improve with time and providing support for the family may be the most important role of the health care professional. Sometimes, however, specific medical intervention is called for and may include dietary manipulation as well as the use of pharmacologic agents. Disturbance of the complex processes of parent–child interaction may produce symptoms or feeding difficulties in the child. Management of these situations often requires a multidisciplinary approach.

FAILURE TO THRIVE

KEY POINTS

- Defining 'failure to thrive' is difficult as it involves a discrepancy between predicted and actual growth rather than just being below the normal weight range.
- Failure to thrive is a common problem, resulting from a combination of dietary, organic and social factors which lead to undernutrition, the final common denominator.
- Only a small number of children will be found to have an underlying medical condition.

There is no universally accepted definition of 'failure to thrive' (FTT) and it is perhaps best regarded as a failure to gain weight appropriately. New growth charts available in the UK are based on growth surveys carried out between 1978 and 1990 and reflect current feeding practices. They differ from the older Tanner and Whitehouse charts, and nine centiles are now highlighted (0.4, 2, 9, 25, 50, 75, 91, 98 and 99.6). Clearly children who are above average weight may 'fail to thrive' yet remain within the normal reference range, making the old definition of FTT as 'less than the third centile' inadequate. A recent measure adopted in some community studies is a weight deviation downwards from the 'true centile' (defined as the maximum centile achieved between 4 and 8 weeks of age), crossing two or more of the nine centile lines and persisting for more than one month (Edwards et al 1990). A 'thrive index' which is a measure of the discrepancy between a child's predicted and actual growth can be derived (Wright et al 1994). If this approach is used, many more children are identified as showing FTT than when 'below the third centile' is taken as the definition.

However, by any definition FTT is a common problem both in primary care and hospital paediatrics and results from a combination of dietary, organic and social factors leading to undernutrition (Skuse 1985). Prospective studies indicate that only a small percentage of infants with FTT are found to have an underlying medical condition ('organic' rather than 'non-organic' FTT), and relatively few cases in the community are identified and referred for specialist assessment. The heterogeneity of children with FTT is evident from numerous studies, the aetiology including:

◆ neglect by parents or carers
◆ unintentional inadequate energy intake
◆ subtle oro-motor problems making food intake difficult, compromising energy intake
◆ children with difficult behaviour or food refusal
◆ disturbed parent–child interaction
◆ chronic illness or disability adversely affecting nutritional status – the minority.

It is possible that non-organic FTT represents one end of a continuum of problems with chronic food refusal at the other. If the interaction between child and parent is regarded as central to the difficulties, resolution clearly depends upon parental response. Children with chronic food refusal typically give strong, clear signals of dislike and refusal, whereas infants with FTT are not good at communicating their needs during mealtimes (Harris & Booth 1992). Ideally, management interventions should be community- rather than hospital-based. In a recent study from Newcastle upon Tyne, health visitor input, with limited specialist support, was shown to significantly improve growth compared with conventional management (Wright et al 1998).

POSSETING, VOMITING AND GASTRO-OESOPHAGEAL REFLUX

Posseting or 'innocent vomiting' is the repeated, effortless regurgitation of small quantities of milk soon after feeding. The child is otherwise well and thriving (like Shakespeare's infant, 'mewling and puking in the nurse's arms') and may be regarded as having what is 'physiological' gastro-oesophageal reflux (GOR) in this age group. Persistent posseting requiring changing of clothes and bedding is perceived by families as a major problem. In this case, treatment as for 'pathological' GOR may be warranted. Physiological GOR can almost always be expected to resolve itself over the first year of life, often improving with the introduction of solids. It results from an immaturity of the gastro-oesophageal sphincter mechanism, partly related to the short intra-abdominal segment of lower oesophagus in the small infant. Feeding technique should always be evaluated to make sure the baby is not being given too much milk, or swallowing a lot of air with feeds (Figure 7.1).

Vomiting

'Nervous vomiting' is a term which has been used to characterise vomiting which goes together with other behavioural symptoms of infant stress and impairment of maternal–infant interactions (Fleischer 1994). The mechanism involved may be trans-

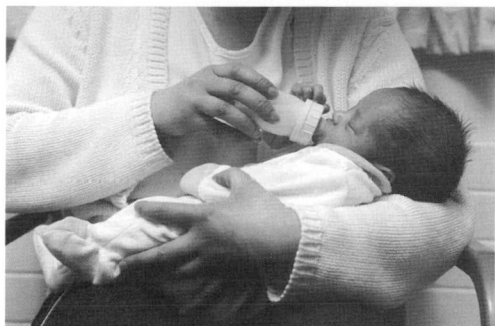

Figure 7.1 The correct position for bottle-feeding an infant. (Reproduced with permission of The General Infirmary at Leeds.)

mission of maternal anxiety to the infant provoking changes in gastrointestinal motility. Infant rumination syndrome is another functional vomiting disorder which occurs when the carer is emotionally distant, unable to sense the baby's needs and unresponsive to his or her signals (Fleischer 1994). The baby learns to bring up gastric content into the mouth for the purpose of self-stimulation and need-satisfaction that would normally be supplied by the carer. Rumination usually occurs after 3 months of age, does not cause distress to the infant, and does not happen during sleep or when the child is actively engaged with people or objects. The important point here is that recurrent vomiting may be a pointer to fundamental problems with parent–child interaction rather than underlying disease.

Persistent projectile vomiting developing around 2 weeks of age is suggestive of pyloric stenosis, particularly if associated with weight loss or cessation of weight gain. Urgent referral to a paediatric unit for further assessment is warranted. This often includes measurement of the electrolyte and acid-base status of the infant (looking for hypochloraemic alkalosis indicating considerable loss of stomach secretions), together with test feed, and ultrasound examination of the stomach and pylorus (Figure 7.2). Overfeeding and cow's milk protein intolerance are other causes of vomiting which form part of the differential diagnosis. Bile-stained vomiting indicates possible gastrointestinal obstruction and always requires an urgent surgical assessment. Persistent vomiting in an infant may be an indicator of serious disease, particularly if there is associated failure to thrive. Sometimes per-

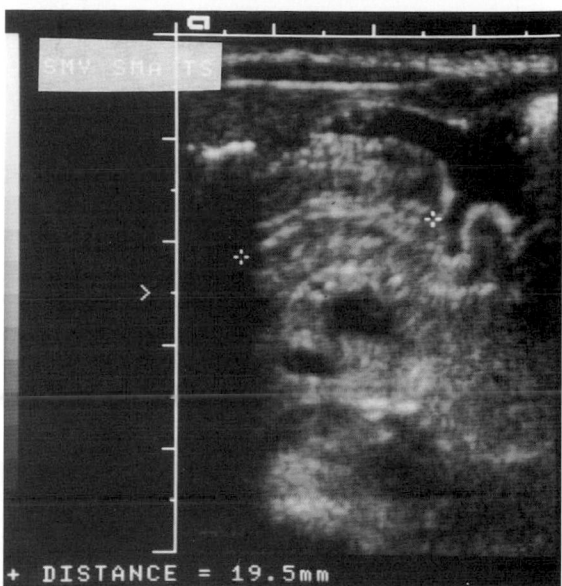

Figure 7.2 Ultrasound picture of pyloric tumour in baby with projectile vomiting. The white crosses mark each end of the pyloric canal, with the hypertrophic muscle on either side and the stomach lumen (black area) on the right. Reproduced with permission of The General Infirmary at Leeds.

sistent vomiting may be factitious and is a well-documented presentation of Munchausen's syndrome by proxy (Hyman 1995).

Gastro-oesophageal reflux (GOR)

Features indicating 'pathological' GOR and the need for further investigation and treatment include:

◆ inadequate weight gain (significant volumes of milk being regurgitated?)
◆ feed refusal or pain on feeding (heartburn, oesophagitis?)
◆ blood-streaked vomitus (oesophagitis?)
◆ recurrent cough, wheezing or choking (aspiration?)
◆ episodes of apnoea (vagal reflex triggered by acid reflux?).

Investigation and management of GOR

In pathological GOR the aim of medical management is to reverse or prevent the complications listed above. Investigation should include a barium

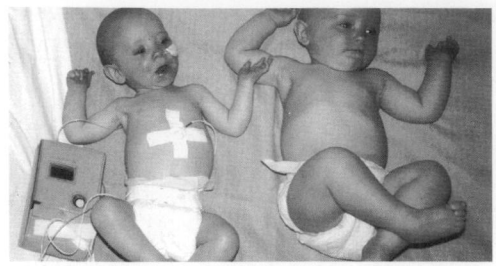

Figure 7.3 pH monitoring in one of twins with failure to thrive as a consequence of severe gastro-oesophageal reflux disease. (Reproduced with permission of The General Infirmary at Leeds.)

study to exclude an anatomical abnormality which might require surgical intervention such as hiatus hernia or malrotation of the small bowel. Twenty-four hour pH monitoring (Figure 7.3) is useful for confirming the diagnosis of GOR, giving an indication of severity and clarifying the relationship between reflux and symptoms such as apnoea. Upper gastrointestinal endoscopy is necessary to establish the presence and severity of oesophagitis.

Medical treatment for GOR consists of positioning in the young infant, thickening the feed (Table 7.1), and use of medications which promote stomach emptying (Drug and Therapeutics Bulletin 1997). The prokinetic agent cisapride is associated with important drug interactions and cardiac arrhythmias. Although it is now said to be contraindicated in the preterm infant for the first three months of life because of unpredictable

pharmacokinetics (Current Problems in Pharmacovigilance 1998), it may still be prescribed at the discretion of the doctor concerned. Although prone positioning used to be favoured for infants with GOR, this conflicts with the 'back to sleep' advice given to reduce the risk of cot death. The left lateral position appears to be a suitable alternative (Tobin et al 1997). When oesophagitis is present or suspected treatment with agents which suppress gastric acid secretion is also given.

Hopes that pH monitoring might prove sufficiently sensitive to reliably identify that group of children who would not respond to medical treatment and required anti-reflux surgery have proved largely unfounded. Should complications of GOR fail to respond to a trial of medical management there is a case for surgical intervention with a procedure designed to improve lower oesophageal sphincter competence. Surgery such as the Nissen fundoplication is complex and associated with its own morbidity and mortality (Oldham & Massey 1998). This means that every attempt should be made to manage the infant medically in the first instance including, if necessary, a trial of nasogastric or nasojejunal tube feeding, since with time and growth severe GOR may still resolve. After a trial of full medical management, the indications for surgery (Kiely 1990) are:

◆ failure to thrive
◆ recurrent aspiration pneumonia, severe asthma and chronic lung disease in the preterm infant
◆ episodic apnoea caused by acid reflux
◆ oesophageal stricture.

When surgical intervention is required, the Nissen fundoplication involves loosely wrapping the fundus of the stomach around the circumference of the intra-abdominal oesophagus in order to create an effective anti-reflux valve mechanism. This is usually performed as an open procedure, but is now also carried out laparoscopically by some surgeons.

Feeding problems relating to GOR

GOR in infants can cause heartburn and provoke excessive crying. Symptoms of oesophagitis

Table 7.1 Feed thickeners for use in gastro-oesophageal reflux

	Quantity required (per 100 ml feed)	Comments
Instant Carobel (Cow and Gate)	0.3–1.5 g	mainly non-digestible may cause bulky stool
Nestargel (Nestlé)	0.5–1 g	mainly non-digestible may cause bulky stool
Thixo-D (Sutherland)	1–3 g	4 kcal/g
Vitaquick (Vitaflo)	1–3 g	4 kcal/g
Thick and Easy (Fresenius)	1–3 g	4 kcal/g

In addition, there is a pre-thickened formula milk available, Enfamil AR (Mead Johnson).

include arching of the back and feed refusal, and may occur in the absence of vomiting (so-called 'occult' GOR). A hypothetical explanation for food refusal in some infants is that pain with swallowing (odynophagia) or heartburn as a consequence of peptic oesophagitis leads to the child associating feeding with painful consequences (Hyman 1994). A trial of feed thickening and treatment with drugs to suppress acid secretion and improve gastrointestinal motility may be worthwhile. However, an aversion to feeding can persist even when GOR has been effectively treated or resolved (Dellert et al 1993). It has also been suggested that GOR may lead to visceral hyperalgesia, a neuropathic condition in which prior experience changes sensory nerves so that previously innocuous stimuli (luminal distension and acid reflux) are perceived as painful (Hamilton & Zeltzer 1994). Occasionally, prolonged tube feeding is required. Some children who undergo a surgical anti-reflux procedure become feed refusers. This may occur because of dysphagia, gas-bloat syndrome (trapped wind in the stomach) or dumping syndrome complicating the surgery.

COLIC AND WIND

Colic

Infantile colic, or excessive crying in healthy, thriving infants, is a common problem during the first months of life. A baby with colic screams in pain and draws the knees up to the abdomen. This typically occurs from some time in the first 3 weeks of life until 3 to 4 months of age, often in the evening. The infant may not be able to settle after the afternoon or late evening feed or will suddenly wake from sleep soon after feeding. The cry may be high-pitched and the baby inconsolable, with repetitive bouts occurring over several hours until suddenly ceasing. Breastfed babies seem just as prone to colic as bottle-fed infants (Barr 1996).

The aetiology of infantile colic remains unknown, but the following explanations have been discussed in the literature:

◆ Cow's milk protein intolerance, lactose intolerance or excess gas produce painful gut contractions.
◆ Impaired parent–infant interaction results in behavioural disturbance manifesting itself as colic.
◆ Colic simply represents the extreme end of the normal spectrum of crying.
◆ Colic is a common presentation of aetiologically different entities that are difficult to distinguish clinically.

In addition, recent attention has been drawn to the fact that occult gastro-oesophageal reflux may present as colic and respond to medical therapy (Berkowitz et al 1997). Despite the fact that colic resolves spontaneously with most infants being symptom free by 4 to 5 months, many different treatments have been studied. These include use of soya milk or protein hydrolysate feeds, low lactose or fibre-enriched milk, herbal tea and drugs to reduce gut contractions (e.g. dicyclomine) or gas production (e.g. simethicone). Behavioural interventions have included attempts to modify parents' responsiveness. A systematic review of such interventions was carried out by Lucassen and colleagues (Lucassen et al 1998) who assessed 27 controlled clinical trials. Elimination of cow's milk protein was effective when a hypoallergenic hydrolyzed protein formula was used as the milk substitute, but not when soya milk was used. Dicyclomine was effective, but this treatment is undesirable because of serious side effects which include apnoea, syncope, seizures, hypotonia and coma. Advice to reduce stimulation of the child appeared to be beneficial whilst advice to increase carrying and holding seemed not to reduce crying. No benefit was shown for simethicone.

One of the key roles for health professionals when consulted about such symptoms is explanation and then parental reassurance that colic:

◆ is common during the first months of life, but its cause is unknown
◆ may be reduced in some infants by substituting a protein hydrolysate feed for cow's milk formula
◆ can improve if parents are taught to be more appropriately responsive to their infants and

give less overstimulation and more effective soothing

◆ should not be treated with dicyclomine because of the potentially serious side effects.

Wind

Babies normally swallow some air while feeding. When feeds are taken too slowly or too quickly for some reason, the amount of air swallowed may increase. It is possible that this might lead to gastric distension and discomfort in some infants, but 'wind' is a catch-all explanation for many symptoms including crying for a host of different reasons. Wind passed rectally will be regarded as excessive by some parents and yet will be accepted as normal by others. In the first few weeks of life, the breastfed baby may not be able to make a good lip seal around the areola and as a consequence swallows air during sucking. When the breast is distended, flow of milk is very rapid and causes the baby to gulp in both milk and air. For the first feed in the morning, it may be helpful for the mother to express some milk prior to putting the infant to the breast. Allowing the baby to suckle from one breast for too long so that there is no more milk left will also encourage air swallowing.

If a bottle-fed infant is thought to be swallowing excessive air, the teat should be checked to make sure the hole is neither too large nor too small. When the feed bottle is inverted, there should be a steady sequence of drips almost fast enough to make a continuous stream of milk. Once made up, the feed should not be shaken vigorously as this will trap air bubbles which the baby then swallows. During the feed the bottle should be tilted correctly and not held too horizontal or the baby will be able to ingest both air and milk through the teat. The teat should be removed from the infant's mouth periodically to stop it collapsing and encouraging the baby to gulp air. If it is difficult to remove the teat from the baby while feeding, a bottle with a collapsible disposable bag interior may be helpful. Babies who are fed in a near-horizontal position will tend to accumulate air in the stomach, whereas sitting them more upright encourages wind to pass through the gastro-oesophageal sphincter.

CONSTIPATION AND ACUTE DIARRHOEA

Constipation

Constipation accounts for around 2% of all new referrals of children under 5 years of age to the paediatric outpatient department. Onset in the newborn period should raise the possibility of a structural abnormality, but onset in infancy is not usually associated with a recognizable underlying cause. Poor fluid intake in the infant, or excessive milk intake in the toddler predispose. Medical management aims first to empty the rectum and then encourage regular passage of soft stools. Laxative treatment is safe and often required for at least a year if symptoms have been present for many months at the time of referral.

Anatomy and physiology

The internal anal sphincter smooth muscle activity is the most important factor for maintaining anal continence, together with the external anal sphincter and levator ani muscle. The internal sphincter is an extension of the rectum and is connected to it by the nervous pathways of the superficial Auerbach's plexus and the deeper lying Meissner's myenteric plexus. Whenever the rectum is distended enough with stool, it stimulates defecation by inhibiting the internal anal sphincter allowing the stool to enter the anal canal and be expelled. In constipation, the accumulation of hard bulky stools in the rectum causes rectal distension, and in long-standing constipation the rectum may be enormously enlarged (megarectum). In this situation rectal sensation is decreased and further retention of stools will occur. With severe stool retention, faecal incontinence or soiling may develop due to overflow of watery or loose faecal material around the hard, bulky stools in the rectum.

Management

Constipation (the difficult passage of hard stools) is a common complaint and one of the most frequent reasons for referral to a paediatric outpatient department. When the onset is in infancy a serious

Box 7.1   The management of constipation

If constipation is a problem in a young infant the following steps should be taken:

◆ Check that the overall fluid intake is adequate for the child's weight.
◆ Make sure the formula feed is not being over-concentrated.
◆ Offer drinks of boiled water or diluted fresh orange juice between feeds.
◆ Consider giving 2.5 ml of the non-absorbable sugar lactulose once or twice a day.

underlying pathology is unlikely to be found (Loening-Baucke 1993). In contrast, constipation in the newborn should raise the possibility of Hirschprung's disease (particularly if passage of meconium was delayed beyond the first 24 hours of life), or structural abnormality such as imperforate anus, anal stenosis or ectopic anus. Breastfed babies are rarely constipated, probably due to the more complete absorption of fats in breast milk leaving low levels of calcium soaps which otherwise act as stool hardeners. Typically, the breastfed infant passes a soft, watery stool after most feeds, while bottle fed infants may pass a firm stool only once a day.

The introduction of solids at 3 months may help constipation, starting with puréed fruits, vegetables and cereals. Wholegrain cereals can be introduced gradually from 6 months of age, and beans and pulses at a later stage. Pure bran is not recommended in infants and young children, and is not necessary if the fibre content of the diet is gradually increased using food naturally high in fibre. In fact, many infants seem to develop their constipation around the time of weaning (Gallagher et al 1998), and this may be associated with decreased fluid intake. Treatment with laxatives is often required in addition to dietary and behavioural interventions in order to re-establish a normal bowel habit (Clayden 1994). Blood in the stool is suggestive of an anal fissure. Severe constipation which is refractory to treatment or associated with failure to thrive requires further investigation for underlying conditions. Possible diagnoses include Hirschprung's disease, hypothy-

roidism and renal concentrating problems such as occur in hypercalcaemia or diabetes insipidus.

Acute diarrhoea

Acute diarrhoea is frequently due to a viral gastroenteritis and remains one of the most common reasons for admission to hospital of young children in the UK. In those who do not become dehydrated, normal food may be given in addition to fluids in the form of glucose and electrolyte solution. In the small percentage who present with clinical signs of dehydration, nutritional intake should be stopped only until rehydration has been achieved. The practice of 'starving the gut' and prolonged 'regrading' of feeds is unnecessary and potentially harmful in that it may further compromise nutritional status and delay recovery. Inappropriate use of anti-diarrhoeal drugs should be discouraged. Persistent diarrhoea may sometimes be caused by secondary lactose or cow's milk protein intolerance.

Diarrhoea in infants and young children is defined as the frequent passage of watery stools. Excessive loss of intestinal contents may have nutritional consequences through interruption of normal food intake, or as a result of maldigestion and malabsorption of nutrients. During short-lived episodes of acute onset diarrhoea the main risk to the child is dehydration and associated electrolyte disturbance. With more than a billion diarrhoeal episodes amongst children each year worldwide, diarrhoea is second only to malnutrition as a cause of infant death. In developed countries, particularly with improvements in infant feeding, it has become a much less severe condition than in the past, yet in the UK it still remains one of the most common reasons for admission to hospital for children under 5. Younger infants are at greatest risk of dehydration because:

◆ they have increased insensible fluid losses
◆ the large osmotic load from milk may promote osmotic diarrhoea
◆ the large protein load from milk results in a high renal solute load.

Breast milk provides protection against gastroenteritis not only because it is free of pathogens which cause diarrhoeal disease, but also because it contains anti-infective agents such as secretory IgA and lactoferrin. Bottle feeds and solid food can be contaminated with bacteria, particularly where there is a lack of refrigeration, poor hygiene and contaminated water supplies.

Causes of acute diarrhoea

Acute sickness and diarrhoea (gastroenteritis) is usually infectious in origin. The causative organisms are most commonly viral (e.g. rotavirus, adenovirus, Norwalk agent), but may be bacterial (e.g. salmonella, shigella, campylobacter, *E. coli*) or protozoal (e.g. *Giardia lamblia*). Around 50% of children admitted to hospital in the UK with gastroenteritis have no pathogen isolated from stools (Conway et al 1990). It should be remembered that in young children extra-intestinal sepsis, such as urinary tract infection, may be a cause of acute sickness and diarrhoea.

A number of different mechanisms contribute to infectious diarrhoea, including:

◆ disruption of normal cell transport processes in the gastrointestinal mucosa
◆ an osmotic load from non-absorbed solutes in the intestine
◆ deranged intestinal permeability
◆ disruption of normal bowel motility.

Nutritional effects

Acute diarrhoea in otherwise healthy infants generally does not affect nutrition, but in malnourished children it can lead to a further deterioration of nutritional status. Food intolerance may occur as a secondary complication of gastroenteritis and is an important cause of persistent diarrhoea. In countries where children may be chronically undernourished, malnutrition, compounded by specific deficiencies such as zinc, adversely affects immunity and predisposes to further infection, leading in time to impairment of pancreatic and gastric function. A cycle is thereby established where repeated infection predisposes to worsening malnutrition and further infection.

Management

Managing the child with acute diarrhoea involves prevention or treatment of dehydration with its associated electrolyte disturbance, together with maintenance or resumption of adequate nutritional intake. Risk factors for dehydration include failure to give glucose-electrolyte solution (GES) and discontinuation of breast milk during the illness. Dehydration as a consequence of diarrhoea is often categorized as mild, moderate or severe based on the percentage loss of body weight. Mild dehydration corresponds to a loss of less than 5%, moderate dehydration to a loss of 5 to 10%, and severe dehydration when more than 10% of body weight has been lost. However, accurate clinical assessment of dehydration is difficult and the severity tends to be overestimated (Mackenzie et al 1989); this results in unnecessary admission to hospital and use of intravenous rather than oral rehydration (Conway et al 1990). Box 7.2 shows some of the clinical features of dehydration.

If an accurate and recent pre-illness weight is available, comparison with current weight gives the best guide to the degree of fluid deficit. Loss of skin turgor, dry oral mucosa, sunken eyes or altered neurological state indicate dehydration requiring hospital admission. In general, only a very small proportion of children admitted to hospital in the UK with acute diarrhoea are in fact clinically dehydrated.

 Box 7.2 Clinical features of dehydration

◆ 2 to 3% – thirst, mild reduction in urine output.
◆ 5% – thirst, reduction in urine; slightly sunken eyes and fontanelle; alteration in skin turgor.
◆ 6 to 9% – sunken eyes with loss of eyeball tension; sunken fontanelle, loss of skin turgor; marked thirst and decrease in urine output; increasing apathy.
◆ 10%+ – all the above, plus poor perfusion, rapid heart rate, weak pulse, low blood pressure.

Box 7.3 Management of acute gastroenteritis in infants

If dehydration is absent:

- the aim is to prevent dehydration
- provide clear instructions to parents
- keep under careful observation during illness to check for signs of dehydration
- if there is vomiting, small volumes of fluid may need to be given (for example, using a teaspoon).

For breastfed infants:

- continue breast-feeds, stop solids
- offer GES after feeds (10 ml/kg for each diarrhoeal stool passed)
- if GES tolerated, reintroduce solids after 4 hours
- offer supplements of GES for duration of diarrhoeal episode.

For formula-fed infants:

- stop milk feeds, stop solids
- give maintenance fluids (per 24 hours: 100 ml/kg for the first 10 kg weight, 50 ml/kg for the next 10 kg, and 25 ml/kg thereafter)
- if GES tolerated, reintroduce normal full-strength formula
- if formula tolerated, reintroduce solids
- continue to offer GES supplements for the duration of the diarrhoeal episode.

If mild to moderate dehydration is evident:

- admit for oral rehydration using GES under supervision.

If there is evidence of shock, or uncontrolled vomiting:

- intravenous fluids are required
- admit to hospital for intravenous fluids
- recommence normal diet after 24 hours.

Management of acute gastroenteritis

An outline of management for acute gastroenteritis in infancy is given in Box 7.3. The majority of children without clinical dehydration can be managed safely at home, but there should be a lower threshold for admission of infants under 6 months. Glucose-electrolyte solution should be given and

Table 7.2 Some oral glucose and electrolyte preparations

Product (powder)	Glucose (mmol)	Na⁺ (mmol)	K⁺ (mmol)	Cl⁻ (mmol)	HCO3⁻ (mmol)	citrate (mmol)
Diocalm Junior	111	60	20	50	–	10
Dioralyte (effervescent tablets)	90 (90)	60 (60)	20 (25)	60 (45)	–	10 (20)
Electrolade	111	50	20	40	30	–
Gluco-lyte	200	34	20	37	18	–
Rapolyte	111	60	20	50	–	10
Rehydrat	91*	50	20	50	20	9

All concentrations are given for the product diluted to 1 litre according to the manufacturer's instructions. When preparing these products for infants all water should be freshly boiled and cooled.
* also contains 94 mmol sucrose and 1 to 2 mmol fructose

the desired fluid intake and feed schedule written down for parents. Small amounts of fluid given frequently are often tolerated even when vomiting (from gastric stasis) has been a prominent symptom. The various preparations available in the UK and which are suitable for home therapy are listed in Table 7.2. Solutions containing higher concentrations of sodium (e.g. World Health Organization solution – 90 mmol/L) are not widely used in Europe where viral gastroenteritis is most common and stool sodium losses are lower than they would be in countries where cholera is prevalent and WHO solution would be the first choice.

Indications for hospital admission include:

- clinical signs of dehydration
- vomiting of glucose-electrolyte solution, or inability to comply with oral rehydration advice for whatever reason
- persistence or recurrence of diarrhoea
- suspected surgical conditions (e.g. intussusception, appendicitis)
- poor social circumstances/lack of supervision
- short history of profuse diarrhoea
- pre-existing medical condition which may worsen with diarrhoea (e.g. diabetes, inborn error of metabolism, congenital adrenal hyperplasia).

Nutritional management of acute gastroenteritis

The practice of regrading feeds in children with gastroenteritis – a slow build-up in feed concentration over several days – is no longer regarded as appropriate (Murphy 1998). Normal formula feeds can be introduced following an initial four-hour period of rehydration. Breastfeeding should continue through rehydration and maintenance phases of treatment. If there is persistent diarrhoea after reintroduction of feeds, lactose intolerance should be looked for by testing the stool for lactose. This can be done simply by mixing 5 drops of stool fluid with 10 drops of water and adding one Clinitest (Ames) tablet. A colour-change in the specimen can be compared with a chart which indicates whether reducing sugars are present. The diagnosis of lactose intolerance is usually based on the finding of 1% or more of reducing substances. Lactose intolerance, if confirmed, should be managed by substituting a lactose-free formula feed.

Persistent diarrhoea without reducing substances may indicate secondary cow's milk protein intolerance. An extensively hydrolyzed protein feed should be given for a few weeks with cautious reintroduction of milk-based feed. Use of such formulas requires supervision by a paediatric dietitian and paediatrician.

OVERFEEDING

Overfeeding

Appetite and satiety mechanisms enable most babies to control the amount of energy ingested. Based on animal studies it used to be thought that overfeeding in infancy would predispose to later obesity by increasing the number of adipocytes. However, this is no longer considered to be the case (Rosenbaum & Leibel 1988) and overfeeding to the point of causing the infant to become obese is probably uncommon. Overfeeding is not, however, without its hazards and may cause vomiting. In addition, allowing the toddler continuous access to a bottle (or indeed to the breast at nighttime) can be a cause of severe dental decay (Figure

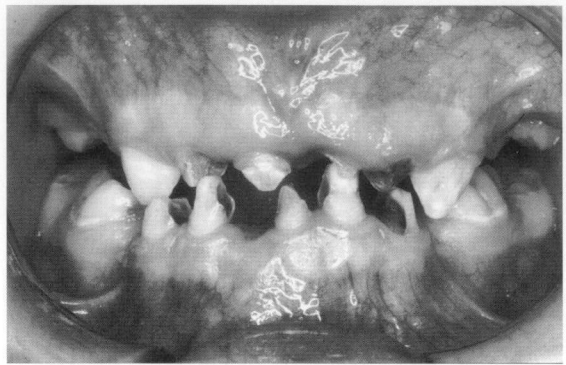

Figure 7.4 Severe breastfeeding caries. (Reproduced with permission of The General Infirmary at Leeds.)

7.4). Too much reliance on bottle feeding as the infant gets older will reduce his or her appetite for food, and a reduction of milk intake may be essential to encourage progress with eating.

FOOD ALLERGY

Adverse reactions to ingested foods cause a wide variety of symptoms and disease for which the general descriptive terms 'sensitivity' and 'intolerance' are useful. These terms can be applied to a reaction

 Box 7.4 Proposed definitions of food intolerance and food allergy (Ferguson 1992)

Food intolerance or sensitivity – a reproducible, unpleasant reaction, not psychologically based, to a specific food or ingredient.

Food allergy or food hypersensitivity – a form of food intolerance in which there are both reproducible food intolerance and evidence of an abnormal immunological reaction to food (mediated by antibody or T-lymphocytes, or both).

Psychologically based food reactions (food aversions) – this may be when the subject avoids food for psychological reasons, or when there is an unpleasant bodily reaction caused by emotions associated with the food (rather than by the food itself) and does not occur when the food is given in an unrecognizable form.

with an unknown mechanism as well as to a clearly defined metabolic, pharmacologic, or immunopathologic process. Box 7.4 shows a number of definitions which have been proposed (Ferguson 1992).

Mechanisms of food intolerance include enzyme deficiency (e.g. lactase deficiency), pharmacologic effects (e.g. those caused by caffeine), non-immunological histamine-releasing effects (e.g. those caused by certain shellfish) and direct irritation (e.g. by gastric acid in oesophagitis, or colonic flatus in carbohydrate intolerance).

Food intolerance

'Food intolerance' is the preferred term when referring to adverse reactions to food, as it does not imply any particular mechanism, whereas 'allergy' implies an underlying immunological mechanism, which may be food-specific antibodies, immune complexes or cell-mediated reactions. Food intolerance in general appears to be more common in infancy than in adult life and in atopic rather than non-atopic individuals. Cow's milk, eggs, nuts and fruit are the most frequently implicated foods. In a North American study 16% of children were said to have had reactions to fruit or fruit juice and 28% to other food by the age of 3 (Bock 1987). Peanut allergy is becoming increasingly common in young children and may relate to the trend towards earlier introduction of peanut protein in infancy. One problem with defining the frequency of food intolerance is that parents' reports often prove unreliable when compared with double-blind placebo-controlled food challenges. The latter are the gold standard for testing for food intolerance, but are difficult to perform and are not often employed in clinical practice.

Aetiology of food intolerance

The permeability of the gastrointestinal tract mucosa to food allergens is thought to be an important factor in the pathogenesis of antigenic food reactions. The integrity of the bowel mucosa is maintained in part by secretory IgA and the glycoprotein covering of enterocytes, as well as mucosal associated lymphoid tissues. Oral introduction of cow's milk proteins in early infancy elicits clear-cut antibody production to these antigens. The immune response is strongest when cow's milk antigens are introduced early during the neonatal period. The reactivity decreases with age suggesting the development of a systemic hyporesponsive state (tolerance) to ingested antigens. Allergen exposure and sensitization can occur during fetal development, although the mechanism is uncertain. It has recently been suggested that fetal swallowing of IgE in amniotic fluid is an important factor, amnion transmission of IgE having evolved as a mechanism for sensitizing and thereby protecting the fetus from parasites infecting the mother (Jones et al 1998).

A recent cohort study in Dundee suggested that exclusive breastfeeding for 15 weeks and no introduction of solids during this time significantly reduces the probability of respiratory illness at any time during childhood (Wilson et al 1998). Thus breastfeeding and late introduction of solids may have a beneficial effect on childhood health and subsequent adult disease. In babies in general, and those from allergic families in particular, in order to reduce the risk of food intolerance it may well be prudent to:

◆ exclusively breastfeed for the first 4 to 6 months of life
◆ avoid early introduction of foods which have a high potential for sensitisation (e.g. egg, nuts)
◆ consider excluding these foods (and milk) from the diet of the atopic mother during lactation (Chandra et al 1989).

Although it is commonly stated that early exposure to cow's milk antigens (for example, by a single bottle-feed in the neonatal period) increases the risk of atopic disease, this viewpoint has been challenged (David 1998). A large randomized controlled trial in which 1533 breastfed neonates were randomized to receive either cow's milk protein or a placebo mixture of maltodextrin, glucose and mineral solution emulsified with vegetable fats was recently reported (de Jong et al 1998). Atopic disease in the first year was found in 10% of those who received the cow's milk and 9.3% of those who received the placebo. In the second year the figures were 9.6% and 10.2% respectively.

Acute reactions to food

Acute IgE mediated type I reactions to food do occur during infancy and are most likely to be due to cow's milk or egg protein sensitivity. Swelling, redness, or even blistering of the lips or skin around the mouth occur on contact, followed by vomiting and diarrhoea. Anaphylaxis is at the extreme end of the spectrum of reactions, with bronchospasm and circulatory collapse. Such reactions in infancy are relatively rare. Emergency treatment with adrenaline is required, and the precipitating food needs to be excluded from the diet.

Cow's milk protein intolerance

Reactions to foods are often delayed hours or even days after ingestion, and a number of different immunological mechanisms (e.g. cell-mediated or immune complex formation) are implicated. One example is cow's milk protein intolerance (CMPI), which affects around 2.5% of formula-fed infants (Høst 1995). CMPI is the clinical syndrome or syndromes resulting from sensitization of an individual child to one or more proteins in cow's milk. This may be a primary problem in which there appears to be no predisposing factors, or secondary to acute infective gastroenteritis. Primary CMPI is possibly due to a disturbance in the local immune response for antigen control, particularly antigen exclusion. The secondary syndrome can result when gastrointestinal damage following infection makes the mucosa abnormally permeable to antigen entry. An immunodeficiency state, such as transient IgA deficiency, may be an important predisposing factor for both syndromes.

In most children gastrointestinal symptoms (vomiting, diarrhoea, colic, failure to thrive, constipation) develop within the first 6 months of life. There may be a family history of atopy, except in cases secondary to gastroenteritis. Symptoms can come on acutely, mimicking acute infectious gastroenteritis, or may develop insidiously. In the breastfed infant, the disease may present following introduction of infant formula, and very occasionally an anaphylactic reaction is observed. Cow's milk proteins can be detected in breast milk in many mothers, which probably explains why

around 0.5% of exclusively breastfed infants develop CMPI. Other presentations of CMPI include:

◆ respiratory (wheeze, rhinitis, asthma)
◆ dermatological (atopic dermatitis, urticaria, laryngeal oedema)
◆ behavioural (irritability, crying, milk refusal).

Of those infants with predominantly gastroenterological symptoms, some present only with colic or constipation whilst others are well except for blood in the stools. The latter have an underlying colitis, and histological examination of colonic mucosa characteristically shows infiltration by eosinophils (Odze et al 1995). Gastro-oesophageal reflux secondary to CMPI may be relatively common; 24-hour pH studies showing a 'phasic' slow fall in pH after a feed are regarded by some authors as characteristic of CMPI (Cavataio et al 1996).

The diagnosis of CMPI is based largely on clinical history, and the following criteria are widely used:

◆ definite disappearance of symptoms after each of two dietary eliminations of cow's milk and cow's milk products from the diet
◆ recurrence of identical symptoms after one challenge
◆ exclusion of lactose intolerance and coincidental infection.

Box 7.5 Major foods to be excluded on a cow's milk protein free diet

Cow's milk – all types including skimmed, low fat, whole, dried, condensed, evaporated and buttermilk

Butter, ghee, most margarines, and low fat spreads (check label)

Yoghurt, fromage frais, cream, ice cream, frozen yoghurt

Cheese, cottage cheese, cream cheese, curds

Chocolate and some other sweets may contain milk solids

Many manufactured products have milk added, avoid these ingredients listed on food labels:
non-fat milk solids, whey, casein, sodium caseinate, lactoglobulin, lactalbumin

In children with chronic diarrhoea and CMPI, jejunal biopsy may show patchy abnormality with partial atrophy of the villi. The removal of cow's milk protein from the diet will lead to marked clinical improvement, usually within days and certainly within a fortnight. Box 7.5 shows foods which are excluded on a diet which is free of cow's milk protein.

Peanut allergy

Peanut allergy has received much recent attention, and the occasional death due to accidental ingestion is often widely reported. There is limited evidence that infants may be sensitized to peanut protein in the womb or during breastfeeding. It has been suggested that if a parent or sibling is atopic (has asthma, eczema, hayfever or other allergies) it may be a sensible precaution for the mother to avoid peanut products during pregnancy and while breastfeeding. There is no reason for pregnant or nursing mothers without a personal or family history of atopy or allergy to do this. In atopic or allergic children, peanuts or food containing peanut products are probably best not introduced into the diet until after 3 years of age. Whole peanuts should not be given to children under 5 years of age because of the risk of choking. Peanut oil, which is a highly refined product, does not produce reactions in susceptible individuals. Products containing refined peanut oil, but not raw pressed oils, can be considered safe.

Use of special milk substitutes

Swapping from one milk to another because of 'feeding problems', although a common practice, is unlikely to be of any benefit except in specific circumstances: for example, lactose intolerance following gastroenteritis requires a lactose-free formula such as Wysoy (Table 7.3). Routine use of a lactose-free feed in all infants following gastroenteritis is not necessary (Brown et al 1994). Although soya milks are often prescribed for suspected CMPI, there is a high chance (between 30–50%) of a child with genuine CMPI also being intolerant of soya protein (Jakobsson & Lindeberg 1979). When cow milk protein intolerance is suspected therefore, a

Table 7.3 Infant formulae suitable for use in lactose intolerance (soya milks) and CMPI (hydrolyzed formulae)

Soya formulae	Hydrolyzed protein formulae
Infasoy (Cow and Gate Nutricia)	Pepti Junior (Cow and Gate Nutricia)
Isomil (Abbot Laboratories)	Alfare (Nestlé)
Farleys Soya (Farley Health Products)	
Prosobee (Mead Johnson Nutritionals)	Nutramigen (Mead Johnson Nutritionals)
Wysoy (SMA Nutrition)	Pregestimil (Mead Johnson Nutritionals)

trial of protein hydrolysate feed should be given (Table 7.3). However, this will not resolve symptoms in all infants and an amino acid based feed may then be necessary (Vanderhoof et al 1997).

SUMMARY

◆ Children who are 'failing to thrive' are failing to reach their true growth potential although many will still fall within the normal distribution for weight and height for age. They are a heterogeneous group and few have an underlying medical condition.

◆ Regurgitation of stomach contents is normal in young infants; persistent vomiting and poor feeding may indicate disordered child–parent interaction and occasionally more serious underlying disease.

◆ Pathological gastro-oesophageal reflux may cause failure to thrive, feed refusal, recurrent respiratory symptoms and apnoea; medical treatment is usually effective, with surgery being reserved for a small minority of children when major complications persist despite medical therapy.

◆ Colic or excessive crying is poorly understood and occurs mainly in the first three or four months of life; a key role for health professionals is parental reassurance following thorough assessment and explanation.

◆ Constipation is common among toddlers, is usually idiopathic and has a good prognosis; treatment is aimed at emptying the large bowel and then maintaining regular passage of soft stools, often requiring prolonged treatment with laxatives.

◆ Acute gastroenteritis is one of the most frequent causes of hospital admission in young children, although the vast majority of cases will be looked after at home. Treatment is aimed at preventing dehydration and electrolyte disturbance by giving additional fluids or glucose and electrolyte solution; prolonged withholding of milk or food ('gut rest') should no longer be practised.

◆ Adverse reactions to ingested foods cause a widespread variety of symptoms, particularly in early life; exclusive breastfeeding for the first 4 to 6 months of life appears to protect against the development of atopic disease.

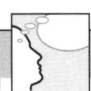

Questions

Answers are given in Appendix 2.

1. An atopic pregnant mother requests dietary guidance regarding how to minimize the risk of eczema and asthma in her baby. What advice would you give?

2. Following an apnoea at home requiring resuscitation, a 2-month-old infant is found to have severe gastro-oesophageal reflux. The parents wish to be reassured that the baby will not have a further life-threatening episode. What treatment options would you put to this family and how would you manage their anxiety?

3. A 6-month-old child admitted because of persistent vomiting is failing to thrive. After 3 weeks as an inpatient all investigations have been normal. The mother has experienced a cot death previously and spends all her time in the cubicle with the vomiting baby, giving feeds as well as filling in the nursing observation charts. How would you investigate the possibility of factitious vomiting?

4. A 2-year-old child is referred to the outpatient clinic with a 3-month history of straining and screaming when passing stool despite laxative prescriptions from the GP. Clinical examination including growth assessment is entirely normal. What are the possible reasons for treatment failure?

CASE STUDIES

1. An 11-month-old infant was referred to clinic with poor weight gain, vomiting and poor feeding. He had been born at 28 weeks' gestation but had few problems until he went home at around 3 months of age. He then developed both vomiting and colic which prompted a change to a protein hydrolysate milk in case his symptoms represented cow's milk protein intolerance. This made no difference to his symptoms, and treatment for gastro-oesophageal reflux was started with a feed thickener (Thixo-D) and Cisapride. He remained very miserable and Ranitidine was added to his treatment in case he had an underlying oesophagitis. Barium studies confirmed free gastro-oesophageal reflux but 24-hour pH monitoring showed that this was not severe. His weight fell to 1.5 kg below the third centile, vomiting continued and he became increasingly reluctant to take milk or solids. Nasogastric tube feeding was instituted and anti-reflux treatment continued in the hope that gastro-oesophageal reflux would resolve with time and growth of the infant. Although his weight improved and vomiting slowly decreased, he remained a difficult feeder causing much anxiety to his parents. Nasogastric feeding was stopped and the parents were encouraged to slowly introduce small amounts of different types of food, to let the child spoon or finger-feed himself, and to give family food and snacks in between meals. Over the next 4 months weight gain continued to improve and vomiting resolved such that all medical treatments were withdrawn without recurrence of symptoms. This child's feeding problems appeared to be secondary to gastro-oesophageal reflux which, even when

resolved, left him with an aversion to eating. A gradual behavioural approach to his eating difficulties successfully resolved the problem although a period of tube feeding was required to sustain growth.

2. A 2-year-old child was referred to clinic by her GP because of constipation. According to her parents she opened her bowels just once a week, passing a large, hard stool after much straining and crying. Sometimes fresh blood was seen on the surface of the stool. She had passed meconium in the first 24 hours of life and there were no problems with her bowels over the first 4 months when she was exclusively breastfed. Stools had changed from loose to hard around the time of weaning, from which time stool frequency slowly decreased. She ate a normal diet with adequate amounts of fibre, but still drank four bottles of whole cow's milk each day. There was no family history of constipation, although both parents came from atopic backgrounds. Clinical examination of the child showed her to be thriving; a posterior anal fissure was noted and hard stool was palpable per rectum. She was treated with lactulose 10 ml twice daily and senokot 5 ml each night. Cow's milk protein intolerance was considered a possible cause for her constipation in view of the atopic family background, but her symptoms responded to laxative treatment. Her high milk intake was thought to be a contributory factor to constipation and a reduction in intake was advised. Over the next year her symptoms waxed and waned in severity but tended to improve overall such that after 12 months of laxative treatment the dose was slowly reduced until discontinued altogether. This case of idiopathic constipation in a young child illustrates the fact that problems often begin around the time of weaning, and hospital referral may be very delayed. In such a young child, however, the overall prognosis is excellent although treatment is commonly needed for at least a year. Her normal growth, negative clinical findings and rapid response to treatment precluded the need for investigations but regular outpatient follow-up was arranged in order to emphasize the need for compliance with medication and to support and encourage her parents.

FURTHER READING

Cooper P J, Stein A 1992 Feeding problems and eating disorders in children and adolescents. Harwood Academic, Reading

Although encompassing the entire paediatric age range, the first three chapters of this book examine the nature and consequences of feeding problems in infants, the management of infant feeding problems, and the nature and management of eating problems in pre-school children. Useful features include a check list of possible problem behaviours to help pinpoint areas that require modification, and a questionnaire which can be used as an initial assessment tool for children with feeding problems.

Stevenson R D, Allaire J H 1996 The development of eating skills in infants and young children. In: Sullivan P B, Rosenbloom L (eds) Feeding the disabled child. Mac Keith Press, London

Although this book is devoted to feeding problems in the neurologically handicapped child, this opening chapter provides an account of the normal development of eating skills in early life.

REFERENCES

Barr R G 1996 Colic. In: Walker W A, Durie P R, Hamilton J R, Walker-Smith J A, Watkins J B, (eds) Pediatric gastrointestinal disease: pathophysiology, diagnosis and management. Mosby, St. Louis

Berkowitz D, Naveh Y, Berant M 1997 'Infantile colic' as the sole manifestation of gastroesophageal reflux. Journal of Pediatric Gastroenterology and Nutrition 24:231–233

Bock S A 1987 Prospective appraisal of complaints of adverse reactions to foods in children during the first 3 years of life. Pediatrics 79:683–688

Brown K H, Peerson J M, Fontaine O 1994 Use of non-human milks in the dietary management of young children with acute diarrhoea: a meta-analysis of clinical trials. Pediatrics 93:17–27

Cavataio F, Iacono G, Montalto G, Soresis M, Tumminello M, Carroccio A 1996 Clinical and pH-metric characteristics of gastro-oesophageal reflux secondary to cow's milk protein allergy. Archives of Disease in Childhood 74:51–56

Chandra R K, Puri A, Hamed A 1989 Influence of maternal diet during lactation and use of formula feeds on development of atopic eczema in high risk infants. British Medical Journal 229:228–230

Clayden G S 1994 Paediatric practice guidelines: childhood constipation. British Paediatric Association, London

Conway S P, Phillips R R, Panday S 1990 Admission to hospital with gastroenteritis. Archives of Disease in Childhood 65:579–584

Current Problems in Pharmacovigilance 1998 Cisapride (prepulsid): risk of arrhythmias. Current Problems in Pharmacovigilance 24:11

David T J 1998 Infant feeding causes all cases of asthma, eczema, and hay fever. Or does it? Archives of Disease in Childhood 79:97–98

de Jong M H, Scharp-van der Linden V T M, Aalberse R C, Oosting J, Tijssen J G P, de Groot C J 1998 Randomised controlled trial of brief neonatal exposure to cows' milk on the development of atopy. Archives of Disease in Childhood 79:126–130

Dellert S F, Hyams J S, Treem W, Geertsma A 1993 Feeding resistance and gastroesophageal reflux in infancy. Journal of Pediatric Gastroenterology and Nutrition 17:66–71

Drug and Therapeutics Bulletin 1997 Managing childhood gastro-oesophageal reflux. Drug and Therapeutics Bulletin 35:77–80

Edwards A G K, Halse P C, Parkin J M, Waterston A J R 1990 Recognising failure to thrive in early childhood. Archives of Disease in Childhood 65:1263–1265

Ferguson A 1992 Definitions and diagnosis of food intolerance and food allergy: consensus and controversy. Journal of Pediatrics 121:S7–S11

Fleisher D 1994 Functional vomiting disorders in infancy: innocent vomiting, nervous vomiting, and infant rumination syndrome. Journal of Pediatrics 125:S84–94

Gallagher B, West D, Puntis J W L, Stringer M D 1998 Characteristics of children under five referred to hospital with constipation: a one year prospective study. International Journal of Clinical Practice 52:165–167

Hamilton A B, Zeltzer L K 1994 Visceral pain in infants. Journal of Pediatrics 125:S95–102

Harris G, Booth I W 1992 The nature and management of eating problems in pre-school children. In: Cooper P J, Stein A (eds) Feeding problems and eating disorders in children and adolsecents. Harwood Academic Publishers, Reading

Høst A (ed) 1995 Cow's milk protein allergy and intolerance in infancy. Pediatric Allergy and Immunology 5(Supplement 5)

Hyman P E 1994 Gastro-oesophageal reflux: one reason why baby won't eat. Journal of Pediatrics 125:S103–109

Hyman P E 1995 Chronic intestinal pseudo-obstruction in childhood: progress in diagnosis and treatment. Scandinavian Journal of Gastroenterology 30 Suppl. 213:39–46

Jakobsson I, Lindeberg T A 1979 A prospective study of cow's milk protein intolerance in Swedish infants. Acta Paediatrica Scandinavica 68:853–859

Jones C A, Warner J A, Warner J O 1998 Fetal swallowing of IgE. Lancet 351:1859

Kiely E 1990 Surgery for gastro-oesophageal reflux. Archives of Disease in Childhood 65:1291–1292

Loening-Baucke V 1993 Constipation in early childhood: patient characteristics, treatment, and long-term follow up. Gut 34:1400–1404

Lucassen P L B, Assendelft W J J, Gubbels J W, van Eijk J T M, van Geldrop W J, Knuistingh Neven A 1998 Effectiveness of treatments for infantile colic: systematic review. British Medical Journal 316:1563–1569

Mackenzie A, Barnes G, Shann F 1989 Clinical signs of dehydration in children. Lancet 2(8663):605–607

Murphy M S 1998 Guidelines for managing acute gastroenteritis based on a systematic review of published research. Archives of Disease in Childhood 79:279–284

Odze R D, Wershil B K, Leichtner A M, Antonioli A 1995 Allergic colitis in infants. Journal of Pediatrics 126:163–170

Oldham K T, Massey M 1998 Antireflux surgery. In: Stringer M D, Mouriquand P D E, Oldham K T, Howard E R (eds) Pediatric surgery and urology: long term outcomes. W B Saunders, London

Rosenbaum M, Leibel R L 1988 Pathophysiology of childhood obesity. Advances in Pediatrics 35:73–137

Skuse D 1985 Non-organic failure to thrive: a reapraisal. Archives of Disease in Childhood 60:173–178

Tobin J M, McCloud P, Cameron D J S 1997 Posture and gastro-oesophageal reflux: a case for left lateral positioning. Archives of Disease in Childhood 76:254–258

Vanderhoof J A, Murray N D, Kaufman S S et al 1997 Intolerance to protein hydrolysate infant formulas: an under-recognised cause of gastrointestinal symptoms in infants. Journal of Pediatrics 131:741–744

Wilson A C, Forsyth J S, Greene S A, Irvine L, Hau C, Howie P W 1998 Relation of infant diet to childhood health: seven year follow up of cohort of children in Dundee infant feeding study. British Medical Journal 346:21–25

Wright C M, Waterston A, Matthews J N S, Aynsely-Green A 1994 What is the normal rate of weight gain in infancy? Acta Paediatrica 83:351–356

Wright C M, Callum J, Birks E, Jarvis S 1998 Effect of community based management in failure to thrive: randomised controlled trial. British Medical Journal 317:571–574

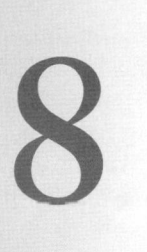

8 Disordered eating behaviours and therapeutic interventions

Malli Wadge   Peter Hodgkinson

INTRODUCTION

This chapter begins with the question, 'what is the importance of eating?'. Eating is a fundamental process, necessary for life, but it is also part of more complex psychosocial interactions. Due to the infant's dependence on its carers from birth, feeding is an inherently social process with the infant being cradled and given its first experience of social interaction. As the infant grows, these early interactions are built on and reinforced by socialization during family mealtimes: indeed, eating in groups would appear to be a cross-cultural phenomenon.

In many cultures the ritual of eating is indicative of stopping whatever one might be doing, joining as a group (family or social) and sharing the physical and sociological process of eating. Within our society, a walk down the high street in any town will bear testament to eating as a social phenomenon, with many multicultural dietary preferences being represented. The foods people choose to eat or reject can indicate cultural and belief systems, be they religious or moral. In Judaism, neither pork nor shellfish are eaten; the teachings of Islam also forbid the eating of pork; vegetarians choose not to eat meat; and vegans will refuse any products with a meat, fish or dairy content.

As the consumption of food has a strong social component, it also lends itself as a vehicle for expressing emotional upset or turmoil. Toddlers quickly learn the power of food refusal and can rapidly turn this to their advantage as they become aware of the concomitant increase in anxiety expressed by their care givers. It is easy, therefore, to understand how the process of eating can become a battleground, with the child not eating and the adult persuading and cajoling, each fuelling the position of the other. Indeed, carers can become anxious during a 'normal' toddler food fad if they consider that it has gone on too long. How many of us recognize that feeling of queasiness prior to an exam, the 'choc-attack' when under stress, or when feeling miserable suffering a loss of appetite or, alternatively, comfort eating to ease our distress? All of these are seen as common and acceptable experiences. The problems arise when these become more than fleeting symptoms – for example, the anxiety generated by a child who overeats and becomes obese, or the one who diets and manifests weight loss are easy to recognize.

ANOREXIA NERVOSA

Anorexia nervosa is not a modern phenomenon, and was first named by two physicians in 1873, one English – Sir William Withey Gull – the other French – Dr E C Lasegue. However, Richard Morton in 1689 seemed to be describing the same clinical picture when he described 'a skeleton only clad with skin'.

Definitions

The name anorexia literally means lack of appetite. However, this does not accurately describe the experiences of the young person suffering with anorexia nervosa. Anorexics do not suffer a lack of appetite, yet do have an unhealthy preoccupation with food and eating and try to stay in rigid control of food taken into their bodies and make great efforts to rid themselves of the calories that could result in weight gain.

Anorexia nervosa is a complex disorder, with many writers taking different perspectives when trying to understand it as a clinical entity. However, the clinical picture has been described in different yet similar ways. Dixon (1990) describes a voluntary semi-starvation in relentless pursuit of thinness, Crisp (1977) describes anorexia nervosa as a weight phobia with the anorexic demonst-

rating a preoccupation with maintaining a low sub-pubertal weight and avoiding any weight gain. Lask & Bryant-Waugh (1993) present a more comprehensive view, describing food avoidance, weight loss or failure to gain weight during the adolescent period with a preoccupation with body weight, calorie intake, a distorted body image, fear of fatness, self-induced vomiting, excessive exercise and laxative abuse.

Incidence and diagnostic criteria

Anorexia nervosa is frequently perceived as an illness associated with adolescence. Indeed, peak age of onset is in the mid-teens, with a female to male ratio of 10 to 1 (although, in some child studies a ratio of 10 to 3 has been reported). Onset before puberty is uncommon, although we have experience of children being diagnosed as young as 10. Other clinicians, including the authors, have experience of younger children (Fosson et al 1987) but these cases remain rare. Rates of prevalence vary slightly, but most researchers concur that in 11 to 15-year-old girls it is 0.1% and in 16 to 18-year-olds about 1%. Anorexia nervosa occurs in all social classes, although there is reported to be a bias towards girls from middle to upper-class backgrounds. Historically, anorexia nervosa has also been considered to be an illness that only occurred in people of white ethnic origin; however, modern studies report an increase in the incidence of anorexia nervosa in other communities (Timinn & Adams 1996, Holden & Robinson 1988).

The main diagnostic criteria used are derived from the ICD 10 (International Classification of Diseases) (WHO 1992), a set of criteria developed and published by the World Health Organization and DSM IV (Diagnostic and Statistical Manual) (American Psychiatric Association 1994), the American equivalent. Both identify similar criteria:

◆ low weight: being below 85% of expected weight for age and height, due to weight loss or failure to gain weight during the adolescent growth period
◆ due to deliberate dietary restriction, sometimes associated with the use of appetite

suppressants, deliberate vomiting or misuse of laxatives (or diuretics in the older age group) and excessive exercising
◆ associated with an intense fear of fatness, feeling fat even when underweight or only feeling happy when very underweight
◆ resulting in amenorrheoa in females past menarche, delayed puberty in early onset cases, and loss of sexual interest in males.

Features of anorexia nervosa

In general, self-starvation brings about a conformity and sameness both physiologically and psychologically within sufferers. These can be summarized as follows:

◆ starts in early adolescence
◆ severe weight loss or failure to gain weight during growth period
◆ morbid fear of fatness
◆ hyperactivity
◆ amenorrhoea
◆ feeling asexual
◆ binge eating
◆ preoccupation with appearance and body
◆ disturbed body image
◆ sense of ineffectiveness and/or low self-esteem
◆ denial of illness
◆ misjudgement regarding food needs
◆ obsessional behaviour
◆ rigid, 'dichotomous' thinking
◆ 'bird-like' eating with associated eating rituals
◆ hypotension
◆ bradycardia
◆ cyanosis of extremities
◆ increased hair growth (lanugo)
◆ electrolyte imbalance in severe cases
◆ high achievement in school.

BULIMIA NERVOSA

Bulimia nervosa (bulimia in Greek meaning 'ox hunger' or appetite) was historically seen as a feature of anorexia nervosa or, within the context of obesity, described as 'stuffing syndrome'. In 1980 the DSM III (American Psychiatric Association 1980) identified bulimia as a distinct syndrome from anorexia nervosa and in 1987 the DSM IIIR (American Psychiatric Association 1987) changed the term to bulimia nervosa.

Definitions

Bulimia nervosa is the term given to the eating disorder characterized by binge eating. Compared to anorexia nervosa, the disorder starts at a similar if not slightly later age, first being seen in later adolescence. Binges consist of secretive, frenzied consumption of large amounts of high-calorie food within a short period of time, an excess of 10 000 calories being consumed within 2 hours is not uncommon. This binge intake of calories is then counteracted by a variety of weight control methods, which may range from self-induced vomiting, to diuretic and laxative abuse, to fasting and excessive exercise.

These bingeing and purging cycles are followed by self-deprecating thoughts, depression and, unlike the anorexic, an awareness that there is a problem. Mood disorders associated with bulimia nervosa may also be accompanied by impulsive and self-harming behaviour, such as substance misuse, abuse and overdose and cutting or other self-mutilating behaviour.

Bulimia nervosa is not associated with dramatic weight loss, with weight usually being maintained within normal range. Complications observed may include menstrual irregularity, fluid and electrolyte imbalance, gastrointestinal upset and bleeding, dental caries and enamel erosion, muscle weakness and swollen salivary glands.

Incidence and diagnostic criteria

Hoek (1991) estimates the incidence of bulimia nervosa at approximately 10 per 100 000 of the general population, prevalence being predominantly female with only 4% of sufferers being male. Fairburn & Beglin (1990) report an incidence of 1 to 2% amongst young females. Prevalence among the student population has been reported as high as 4 to 19% (Hoek 1991).

As with anorexia nervosa, both ICD 10 (WHO 1992) and DSM IV (American Psychiatric Association 1994) diagnostic criteria converge greatly with regards to bulimia nervosa:

◆ The patient has a persistent preoccupation with eating and irresistible craving for food. The patient succumbing to binge eating:
  – eating in a discrete period of time, for example 2 hours, an amount of food that is definitely larger than the norm
  – a sense of lack of control during the binge.
◆ In order to avoid weight gain the patient engages in compensatory behaviours such as self-induced vomiting, purgative or other drug abuse, periods of starvation and excessive exercise.
◆ The binge–purge cycle occurs on average at least twice a week for 3 months.
◆ The patient has a morbid dread of fatness, patients setting themselves a sharply defined weight threshold, well below the pre-morbid weight that constitutes the optimum or healthy weight in the opinion of the physician.

DSM IV (American Psychiatric Association 1994) specifies:

◆ a purging type – during the current episode of bulimia nervosa, the person has regularly engaged in self-induced vomiting or the misuse of laxatives, diuretics or enemas
◆ non-purging type – during the current episode of bulimia nervosa, the person has used other inappropriate compensatory behaviours, such as fasting or excessive exercise, but has not regularly engaged in self-induced vomiting or the misuse of laxatives, diuretics or enemas.

Features of bulimia nervosa

Bulimia nervosa has the following features:

◆ starts in later adolescence
◆ weight is generally normal or within 10% of normal
◆ fear of fatness
◆ less frequent body image distortion
◆ irregular periods
◆ turns to food to cope
◆ binge eating – can consume in excess of four times the daily requirement in one binge
◆ binge associated with loss of control, self-loathing, purging, vomiting and use of laxatives
◆ has variable school performance

◆ recognizes illness
◆ often associated with mood disorders.

OBESITY

In the early nineteenth century, it was considered to be far more healthy to be overweight; indeed, to be overweight was to be beautiful, as thinness was a sign of malnutrition. As times and thinking have changed, however, it is now known that obesity has many associated health issues and often overweight people exhibit or hide concomitant psychological problems. Childhood obesity is on the increase, a trend which Schmidt (1998) attributes to an increasingly sedentary lifestyle and the widespread availability of high calorie snack foods.

Definitions

Ponto (1995) defines obesity as an excess of body fat stores by 20% as calculated by weight-for-height measures, although she does acknowledge the limitations of this definition.

Incidence and diagnostic criteria

It is stated by Lask & Fosson (1989) that obesity occurs in 10% of children of both sexes and all social classes. However, Groom (1995) suggests that the incidence is as high as 25 to 30% of pre-pubertal children, and 18 to 25% of adolescents. It is felt to be the most common disturbance of nutrition in children.

Obesity is not a recognized psychiatric illness and is therefore excluded from DSM IV, but when the psychological symptoms create major problems for a young person, it could be classed as 'eating disorders otherwise noted' (American Psychiatric Association 1994).

Features of obesity

Obesity can be diagnosed by eye alone, but examination and assessment need to include:

◆ weight and height for age
◆ skin fold thickness

- calculated body mass index
- family and personal history
- family and personal eating habits
- amount of exercise.

It is also important to exclude:

- endocrine disorders
- thyroid dysfunction
- altered metabolism.

AETIOLOGY OF EATING DISORDERS

Most authors writing about eating disorders agree that the aetiology of eating disorders is complex and multi-factorial (Hsu 1990, Bryant-Waugh & Lask 1995). When thinking about eating disorders from the perspective of assessment and treatment, it is important to consider a range of causative factors. Not only is it important to consider each causative factor, but also the interrelationship between these factors and their role in the genesis of eating disorders; this provides an important holistic perspective. Bryant-Waugh & Lask (1995) categorize these factors as predisposing, precipitating and perpetuating. They explain these as follows:

- *Predisposing factors* – the context and setting conditions in which the illness occurs, one of which needs to be present for the disorder to occur. This could be physiological, psychological or environmental.
- *Precipitating factors* – initiate the disorder and can be seen as the triggers within the pre-existing setting.
- *Perpetuating factors* – maintain the illness.

Cultural considerations

For many years writers have hypothesized about the importance of cultural issues. Certainly, with regards to anorexia and bulimia these disorders occur predominantly in young western females who live in societies where food is plentiful and thinness is valued. A quick perusal of magazines

 CASE STUDY

Josiah, a 13-year-old boy, was admitted with extreme obesity after all interventions by the community team had failed to help. His predisposing factor was his family's eating pattern and chaotic lifestyle, his obesity was precipitated by unhappiness and bullying at school, and perpetuated by the comfort and attention he gained by eating. There appeared to be a direct correlation between his level of unhappiness and eating – after a bad day at school he would admit to eating on his way home six Cornish pasties, four vanilla slices, jam doughnuts, chocolate bars and a litre of cola. Then he would arrive home in time for tea.

for both women and men provides a wealth of evidence as to the importance placed on body shape, weight and diet. Dieting is a multibillion-pound industry that offers participants opportunities of happiness, increased self-confidence and attractiveness. Is it therefore surprising that those people who are psychologically vulnerable fall into the dieting trap? Further, it is not surprising that Hsu (1990) hypothesizes that dieting – that is, a conscious restriction of food intake for whatever reason – provides the entrée into an eating disorder.

Feminist theorists would argue that, historically, the female form has been passive and depersonalized and held as an object of pleasure for men, to the extent that this role has been slowly integrated into every woman's experience of herself. These experiences have resulted in pressure exerted on teenage girls to conform to a fashion dictate that projects improbable shapes and weights, which is well documented. Although an important factor, culture is unlikely to be the sole issue in the development of eating disorders. Some men and many women are unhappy about their body shape and size and diet frequently and unsuccessfully to improve their perceptions of themselves, yet do not go on to develop an eating disorder (Wren & Lask 1993).

Groom (1995) suggests in relation to the effects of culture on obesity, that many food preferences and eating patterns are culturally determined and contributory to an increase in body weight. The increasing preponderance and acceptance into mainstream culture of fast foods, most of which are high in calories and often high in saturated fats, can be seen to be important in social eating. Many writers report a link between this trend and an increase in the incidence of childhood obesity, with some reporting that 25 to 30% of school age children are obese.

Psychodynamic theories

Within psychodynamic theory, anorexia nervosa is seen as a problem of the oral stage of development. It is believed that a domineering mother imposes a rigid care-taking schedule at her convenience. She does not respond well to the child's needs and, as a result, in later life the child is unaware of hunger and other needful bodily sensations (Bruch 1973, Lerner 1986). Bruch attributes the cause of anorexia nervosa to real rather than fantasized deprivation. She explains anorexic symptoms of delusional body image, altered perception of bodily need and overwhelming feelings of ineffectiveness as a product of real failure of the mother to respond to her daughter's infant needs. Bruch implies that instead of tending the child's needs she substitutes her own, her daughter therefore being conditioned to seek out what others want rather than recognizing her own needs. Orbach (1986) places the emphasis on the deprivation women suffer generally in our sexually unequal society. She argues that the failure of the mother to meet her daughter's needs is due to the mother's internalization of society's injunction to women to put the needs of others before their own. Women thereby become alienated from and fearful of their own needs, unable to respond to them within themselves or as projected by their daughters. Their daughters grow up equally cut off from the 'needy little girl' within themselves.

Edelstein (1989) has proposed an alternative mechanism in the development of eating disorders: the individual expressing and experiencing emotions in terms of physical sensations. Sadness or loneliness may be experienced as hunger, which is resolved by eating. This idea has been taken further by Magagna (1993), who has suggested that distorted body image arises from intense, suppressed negative feelings; these feelings are experienced by the sufferer as physical sensations, such as feeling full, bloated and heavy.

Family theories

The family model seeks to view the 'gestalt' – that is, the context in which an emotional problem is generated between family members – rather than viewing one member as being sick. The family theorists focus on the process between family members that perpetuates and enables the 'sick' behaviour of one identified member; all family members are seen as equally involved. For example, in the case of the anorexic, conflict between mother and daughter can serve the purpose of diverting parental attention away from facing conflicts within the marriage. The sick role behaviour thereby serves the purpose of keeping the family together. Though simplistic, this demonstrates that there is no one family member to be held responsible, but a set of circumstances which have given rise to an eating disorder. Common characteristics which have been identified by therapists working with the families of children with eating disorders include overly close, enmeshed relationships, avoidance of overt conflict and rigidity in interactional patterns (Minuchin et al 1978). These families have been described as psychosomatic and present as not needing or wanting change, preferring to use a limited range of ineffective coping strategies to cope with problems and avoiding altogether any problems that would lead to open conflict. Autonomy and independence are restricted, growing up and separating from the family discouraged, with this kind of environment leading to passive methods of defiance making it difficult for family members to assert their individuality.

By way of highlighting the complexities of these cases, it is also important to remember the contribution of other writers who question the role of family dysfunction. Hsu (1990) and Kog & Vandereycken (1988) agree that family dysfunction is more common in families where there is a young person with an eating disorder, yet there is no evidence that disturbed family interaction causes eating disorders and in opposition to Minuchin et al (1978) there is no empirical evidence to support any particular model of family interaction. This parallels our clinical experience where we have observed families where there is no sign of family dysfunction other than the stress and anxiety caused by having a young person with an eating disorder as a family member. Conversely, families have been observed where dysfunction is obvious and the patterns of behaviour fit those previously described by Minuchin et al.

In contrast to anorexia nervosa, the literature on bulimia nervosa and obesity in the family is minimal. However, literature regarding obesity shows that there is some evidence of the importance of family issues playing a role. Lissau & Sørensen (1994) propose that parental neglect increases the risk of obesity sevenfold. There is recognition that both genetic and environmental issues are significant contributors, but there is a need for further research in these areas (Flodmark 1997).

With regard to bulimia nervosa, there is as yet no empirical research and the reports that are in existence are based on very low numbers. To date there is little evidence that family interaction patterns play a significant role in the causation of bulimia nervosa.

Childhood sexual abuse

The role of child sexual abuse is becoming increasingly evident as an important factor in the genesis of eating disorders. A study by the NSPCC (1989) showed that of 411 children who had been abused, 5% showed symptoms of eating problems or disorders. Palmer et al (1990) found that out of 158 women attending an eating disorder clinic, one third reported an adverse sexual experience before the age of 16. In a study of abused women, Meiselman (1993) noted that a third of them were significantly overweight. Root (1991) expressed

the view that eating disorders are a gender-specific post-traumatic stress response to sexual assault.

When considering the experiences of bulimic young women, Pope & Hudson (1992) and Welch & Fairburn (1994) conclude that there is little evidence that sexual abuse is a particular risk factor for bulimia nervosa, rather that sexual abuse appears to be a risk factor for psychiatric disorder in general for young women. These findings concur with and support the earlier findings of Sloan & Leichner (1986) that sexual abuse is neither necessary nor significant for the development of eating disorders.

Renvoize (1993) states that eating problems are a symptom that many victims of child sexual abuse suffer. These may be present from early childhood, but many become more noticeable in adolescence when, sometimes, the young girl does not reach menarche at the expected time. Anorexia nervosa, bulimia nervosa or obesity can be ways in which the young girl punishes herself because of her perceived guilt or attempts to make herself so unattractive that she will be safe from further sexual abuse. The frequent purging of those with bulimia nervosa is not only a way of cleansing the body but also allows the victim to feel a sense of power over how their body is treated.

There is a paucity of literature surrounding male sexual abuse and the co-morbidity of eating disorders. However, we have experience of boys who have been admitted for treatment of anorexia nervosa who were all victims of child sexual abuse and who directly linked their eating disorders to their traumatic sexual experiences. This is also an experience reflected by approximately half of the young girls treated in our unit for eating disorders, who disclose sexual abuse during therapy. They again often draw a causal link between their abuse and their eating problems.

Biological theories

Research has indicated that there is a genetic susceptibility which plays a major role in the development of anorexia nervosa in particular (Holland et al 1988, Strober et al 1990). Little is known as to what the genetic contribution might be, but the evidence suggests some inherited predisposition. Gelazis & Kempe (1993) state that obesity often begins in early life and that genetic studies indicate that 60% of obese children have one or both obese parents. However, they feel that obesity is more a symptom of a calorific input/energy output imbalance.

It is important to remember that biological factors such as hypothalamic dysfunction, and gastrointestinal problems (for example, delayed gastric emptying) all need to be excluded by use of a complete medical investigation before psychological formulations and treatments are considered. Genetic influences also need to be taken into account. Twin studies indicate that genetics may play a large part in eating disorders, particularly in anorexia nervosa (Strober et al 1990). It is important that such biological factors are fully investigated to prevent misdiagnosis and therefore incorrect treatment.

Both of the case studies below are extreme, but emphasize the need to exclude organic causes prior to diagnoses being made. They also underline the necessity of assessing the young person holistically and not just concentrating on either biological or psychological factors to the exclusion of the other.

CASE STUDIES

Angela

Angela, a 14-year-old girl, was transferred to the unit for eating disorders with a diagnosis of chronic and intractable anorexia nervosa. On admission to the ward paediatric trained nurses questioned the diagnosis when they observed pigmentation changes of previous body scars during the assessment. This was brought to the attention of the medical team who then, after blood and urine tests, diagnosed Addison's disease. Angela then received appropriate treatment and was quickly discharged.

Brian

Brian, a 10-year-old boy, was transferred to the unit with a diagnosis of anorexia nervosa. Paediatric nurses noted his very unstable gait as he walked down the ward and pointed this out to their medical colleagues. A brain scan confirmed the existence of a brain tumour.

It can be seen that eating disorders have a complex and multi-factorial basis. There has been a wealth of research undertaken which has been unable to develop a clear understanding of the causation of eating disorders. Perhaps the most salient point after reading the research is not the importance of individual factors, but rather the importance of the interaction of many factors which can help develop a holistic understanding and, therefore, treatment of young people and families suffering from eating disorders.

NURSING CARE ISSUES

Assessment

As with all specialities of nursing care, assessment must include physical, psychological, familial, environmental and cultural, developmental, educational and spiritual elements within the individual young person's history. Assessment is seen as a dynamic process during the young person and family's therapeutic growth, and not an activity which is undertaken once and then forgotten. The following is by no means an exhaustive discussion of the assessment of the young person with a disorder, but covers some of the main areas which might be useful to address during an assessment interview. All discussion with the young person throughout the initial and subsequent assessments must be appropriate to their age and development.

Initial assessment

This is by far the most comprehensive assessment which takes place, providing nursing staff with a broad picture of the young person and the family's perception of the illness process and related problems and issues. (Further assessments within the boundaries of a deepening therapeutic relationship will provide further detail and insight that will help to clarify this broad picture.)

Physical assessment

◆ Height and weight – When plotted on a percentile chart, this gives an indication of what the young person's growth velocity should be and the present deviations from this.

◆ Temperature, pulse, respirations and blood pressure – Significant deviation from the 'norm' for age and development may indicate physiological disturbance such as fluid and electrolyte imbalances, or congestive cardiac failure.
◆ General appearance:
  – the presence of lanugo hair in anorexia nervosa
  – peripheral cyanosis associated with weight loss
  – skin condition – lack of subcutaneous fat leads to an increased risk of ulceration and skin breakdown, particularly over pressure points; in obesity there may be fungal infections in the skin folds
  – dryness, roughness or scaling of skin
  – increased sensitivity to cold or hypothermia
  – peripheral oedema
  – dehydration
  – restlessness
  – bruises or petechiae
  – finger clubbing
  – ulcers
  – hoarse voice
  – enlargement of salivary glands (parotid)
  – evidence of self-harm – scars, burn marks.
◆ Mouth – A torn fraenum linguae and eroded tooth enamel due to gastric acids, are both signs of repeated vomiting.
◆ Abdomen – Distension due to dilatation of stomach.
◆ Urine – Dip test to exclude diabetes.
◆ Bowels – To establish habits and investigate the inappropriate use of laxatives.
◆ Hygiene – Are there changes in levels of personal hygiene? Has the patient lost interest in personal appearance?
◆ Sleep – Are there any changes in the sleep patterns? Does he or she wake through the night? Does he or she sleep in the daytime? Is he or she troubled by dreams?
◆ Secondary symptoms – Is there evidence of psychosis? Is there evidence of memory impairment?

◆ Medical examination:
  – cardiovascular system for arrhythmias, cardiac failure, bradycardia, hypotension
  – respiratory system for increased respiratory rate, wheezing
  – neurological system for peripheral paraesthesia, muscle weakness, tetany, neuropathy.
◆ Haematology tests – Full blood count to include red blood cell indices, white blood cell indices and platelets.
◆ Biochemistry tests – Urea and electrolytes, serum magnesium, phosphate levels, serum bicarbonate levels, liver function tests, blood glucose, cholesterol, free fatty acids, serum carotene.
◆ Endocrinology – Thyroid function tests (especially T3 levels), prolactin levels, cortisol, growth hormone level, testosterone (in males), LH, FSH.
◆ Special investigations:
  – pelvic ultrasound examination (useful to assess improvement)
  – MRI of pituitary and hypothalamic regions
  – assessing bone density.

Psychological assessment
◆ Interaction:
  – Does patient have good eye contact?
  – Does patient have a distorted sense of body space, for example standing away from others?
  – Does patient stare?
  – Is patient self-centred?
  – What is patient's posture like?
  – Does patient fidget?
  – Does patient think in a polarized, 'all or nothing' way?
  – Does patient converse appropriately?
  – Does patient speak at the normal volume, rate and tone?
  – Does patient walk away while in conversation?
  – Does patient behave in the same way with friends as he or she does with family members?

◆ Assertiveness:
  – Is patient quiet or shy?
  – Does patient behave in an assertive manner?
  – Does patient behave aggressively?
  – Does patient seem suspicious of others?
  – Does patient show tactless behaviour?
◆ Body image – How does patient feel with regard to body size and weight? How would patient like to look? Get patient to draw a 'picture' of how they are and how they would like to be.
◆ Mood – Is the young person depressed, euphoric or euthymic? Is their mood perceived as a problem by themselves or the family? (There is a recognized co-morbidity between eating disorders and depression.)
◆ Illness perception – Does the young person acknowledge that he or she has an illness? Does the family acknowledge a problem?
◆ Stress and anxiety:
  – How does the patient cope with stress?
  – How does the patient perceive stress?
  – Is stress recognized in the family?
  – Are there any maladaptive behaviours with stress, for example substance misuse and abuse?
  – Are there any obsessional compulsive behaviours, such as frequent hand-washing or excessive exercising?
◆ Habits:
  – Has patient increased exercising?
  – Does patient steal food or money?
  – Has patient begun thumb-sucking or nailbiting?
◆ Eating behaviour:
  – What are mealtimes like?
  – Does the family snack?
  – What foods are eaten?
  – Is there evidence of dieting or bingeing?
  – Are there any food rituals or fads?
  – Is there evidence of food disposal?
  – Who eats where and with whom?
  – Has patient recently become a vegetarian?
◆ Self-esteem:
  – What is patient's self-worth?
  – How does patient feel about him or herself?
  – How does patient perceive his or her self-worth in the context of family and peers?

  – Are there fluctuations in patient's self-esteem in relation to his or her mood?
◆ Self-harm:
  – Is there any evidence of self-harm or suicide attempts?
  – How long has this been happening?
  – How does patient hurt him or herself?
  – Why does patient hurt him or herself?
  – Does this fluctuate with patient's mood?

It is very important to note that if there is evidence of self-harm or suicide attempts, a thorough risk assessment must be undertaken. Sullivan (1995) states that mortality in anorexia nervosa is twice as high as in any other psychiatric disorder.

Familial. This helps to set the context in which the problems arise and will help create a discussion which may elicit strengths, skills and resources for later use in treatment.

◆ Family relationships:
  – Use of a genogram (Figure 8.1) might be helpful to establish isolated or overly-close relationships.
  – Discussion of who talks to whom and who does not?
  – Who talks a lot and who speaks least?
  – Who are you like? Who are you least like?
  – Who do you like to be close to and who would you like to keep far away?
  – Would you like to change communication in your family? How?
  – Who sets boundaries and who keeps them?
  – Who helps who and who does not help?
◆ Family strengths and weaknesses – Who are the strong family members and who are the worriers?
◆ Impact of illness:
  – Does the family recognize the illness?
  – How does each family member see the illness?
  – Have relationships changed as a result of the illness?

Environmental, cultural and spiritual assessment. This provides a picture of the family's usual social and cultural context and investigates whether this has changed, and if so, how.

- ◆ Home environment:
  - How many rooms are there?
  - How many people share the house?
  - Who shares a room with whom?
- ◆ Social skills:
  - Who are patient's friends? Has this changed?
  - Has patient become more isolated?
  - Does patient try to 'buy' friends?
  - What are patient's hobbies?
  - Is patient worried in social situations?
  - Does patient partake in cultural family events?
- ◆ Religion:
  - Does patient still attend religious activities?
  - Has patient become more deeply involved in religion?
  - Does patient question religious beliefs?
- ◆ Spiritual:
  - Has patient's meaning of life changed?
  - Have patient's future aims changed?

Developmental assessment
- ◆ Maturational tasks:
  - Has patient reached expected maturation?
  - Has patient regressed in any way?

- ◆ Growth:
  - Is patient progressing along projected growth curve?
- ◆ Development:
  - Has patient reached menarche?
  - Have there been any changes in menstruation such as painful menstruation or cessation (check if there is a possibility of pregnancy)?
  - Are there age-appropriate signs of secondary sex characteristics?

Educational assessment (in conjunction with school teachers)
- ◆ School:
  - Have there been changes in grades at school?
  - Has patient become more conscientious with schoolwork?
  - Has patient's level of concentration changed?
  - Does patient strive for perfection or unrealistic goals?
  - Have school friendships changed?
  - Have attitudes to teachers changed?
  - Has patient become disinterested in work?
  - Does patient display 'acting out' behaviour?

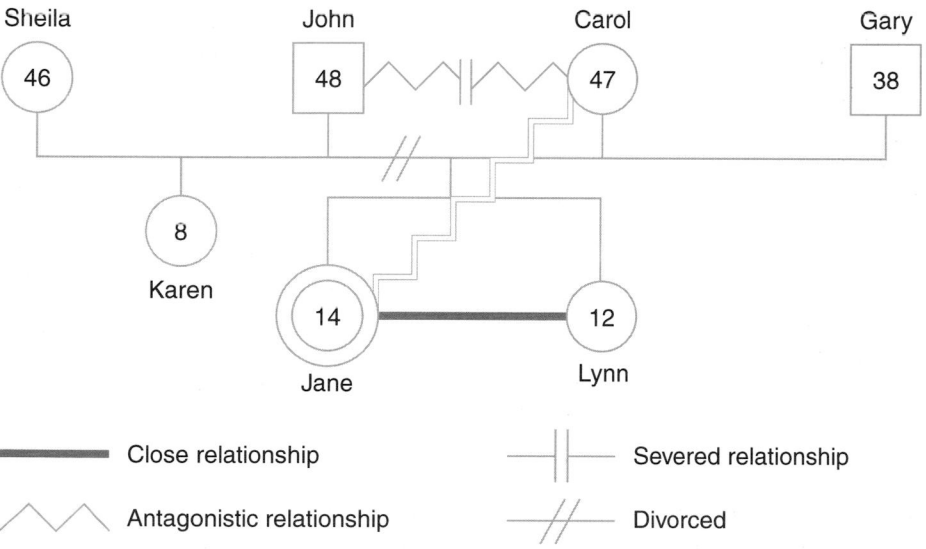

Figure 8.1   Example of a genogram

CARE IN CONTEXT

Tiers of provision

In 1995, the Health Advisory Service (HAS 1995) reviewed all the mental health services available to children and adolescents. From their findings they developed a four tier model of provision which has since been developed as government policy. The four tiers are described below.

Tier one

This is a provision of service from general practitioners, community-based social workers, education and health workers in schools, health visitors and workers in the voluntary sector. These professional groups are those to which patients often first turn for help. They provide basic advice and support but are also able to access help from the other tiers.

Tier two

This provision is by specialist child and adolescent mental health professionals when they work in a uni-professional manner, with no supporting team. These services may be based in a variety of settings, which might include clinics, schools, health centres or the home environment. This is the first specialist contact for families experiencing mental health problems. This group of professionals is also able to access other tiers.

Tier three

This tier provides more specialized services and treats problems of greater complexity. Care is provided by a multidisciplinary team which may comprise child and adolescent psychiatrists, psychologists, nurses and social workers. These services are offered on an outpatient basis and the professionals again may refer to other tiers.

Tier four

This tier provides treatment for highly complex problems which, within the context of the Health Service, includes inpatient psychiatric provision, secure provision and specialist provision for those with a sensory disability.

The theoretical basis for the tiered provision is that young people and their families receive the appropriate level of care related to the severity of their problem. In effect this means that they may pass through the different tiers, depending on the regression or recovery of their illness (see Figure 8.2)

Most young people with eating disorders are seen and treated at tiers one, two and three. Much of the following discussion of therapeutic intervention, from the nursing perspective, involves principles that may be applied in all settings. The authors manage a tier four inpatient setting where young people with eating disorders (and other mental health problems) receive treatment which is delivered in a multidisciplinary framework. The core professionals in this instance are child and adolescent psychiatrists, paediatricians, nurses, social workers, school teachers, physiotherapists and dietitians, with other specialist disciplines being co-opted as necessary.

A tier four perspective

All nursing interventions take place within a therapeutic milieu, in which the whole is

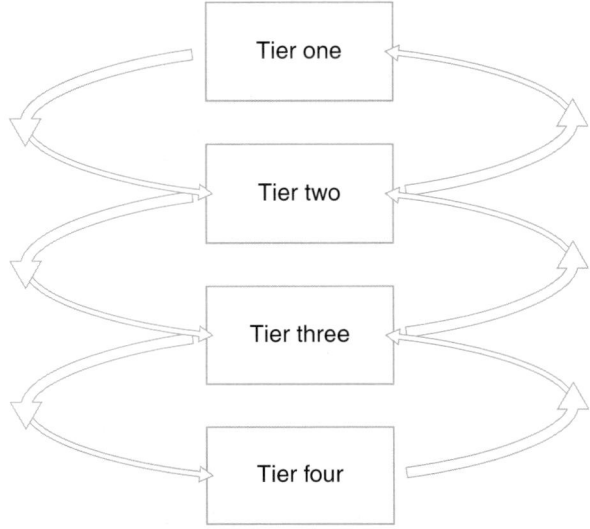

Figure 8.2 Possible flow chart for the tiered provision of child and adolescent mental health services

greater than the sum of the parts. As expressed by Keltner et al (1991) the milieu serves the purpose of reorganizing all interpersonal and environmental forces to develop an atmosphere that facilitates patient growth, rehabilitation and restoration. Benfer & Schroder (1990) include in the milieu the physical environment and the treaters who participate in that milieu as well as the interplay among the various components. From this it can be seen that the therapeutic milieu is a complex but important environment where all care takes place.

The theoretical underpinning of the authors' inpatient unit is that of the Developmental Framework of Peplau (1952). This framework highlights the parallel development of clients and nurses through the utilization and building of therapeutic relationships. Peplau views the use of therapeutic relationships as the cornerstone of all nursing care; this, in the authors' opinion, is the unique contribution of nursing. Within this framework, structure for assessment, planning and implementation of nursing care is provided by Roper et al's model of the Activities of Daily Living (1980). This is the format which will be utilized to describe nursing interactions. This will by no means be a comprehensive or exhaustive discussion, and it must be remembered that each young person's experience of an eating disorder will be individual.

NURSING CARE AND THERAPEUTIC INTERVENTIONS

Maintaining a therapeutic environment

Hospitalization is necessary for:

◆ prevention of suicide, self-harm or mutilation
◆ to correct electrolyte imbalances caused by starvation, vomiting or purging behaviours
◆ to help establish control of purging behaviours
◆ to establish appropriate dietary intake.

Communication

Individual communication

Individual therapy for young people with eating disorders can be from many different perspectives, depending on the training and interests of the therapist. All individual therapies seek to promote change, develop understanding, educate and motivate the individual to create solutions to the problems they are experiencing. Some of the approaches used which have been successful are:

◆ systemic therapy
◆ solution-focused therapy
◆ cognitive behaviour therapy
◆ client-centred therapy.

Issues that could be addressed during individual therapy are:

◆ feelings associated with food
◆ feelings associated with bingeing
◆ distorted body image
◆ feelings of low self-esteem
◆ feelings surrounding self-harm
◆ feelings associated with eating for comfort
◆ other interpersonal issues related to their perceived problems.

When considering psychotherapeutic intervention, it is important to note that cognitions associated with starvation need to be corrected before this can take place. This does not mean that the nurse who will provide the psychotherapy cannot begin to establish a therapeutic alliance during this time.

Individual psychotherapy, as with all interventions, has to relate to each young person's cultural background. Each therapist needs to be sensitive to and aware of all cultural issues affecting the illness process, and stereotyping must be avoided. The importance of assessing and treating each person as an individual and not as part of a cultural stereotype is paramount (Chang 1990).

Group communication

Group therapy

This can be an effective intervention for young people with disordered eating. The emotional support, reality testing and the hope from seeing others improve are important elements of group work. A number of major issues can be explored in the group experience. These may include:

◆ nutritional education
◆ social skills training (to help develop friendships)
◆ assertiveness training (to combat the passivity often associated with eating disorders)
◆ self-awareness
◆ exploration of limit setting and boundaries within community groups.

Group activities

Joint activities are useful, as many of the above skills can be practised in an environment that does not seem overly managed and is therefore more naturalistic. Examples of this are:

◆ art groups (both art therapy and therapeutic art)
◆ relaxation groups
◆ sailing
◆ rock climbing and other outdoor activities
◆ drama therapy
◆ music therapy
◆ dance
◆ puppetry
◆ storytelling.

There is much empirical evidence that activity groups have beneficial effects in terms of self-confidence, self-esteem and social skills, and the authors' experience strongly supports this.

Family communication

Therapeutic interventions with families seek to view problems within the context of the family and the wider social network. It is important to note that family therapy has moved away from 'pointing the finger of blame' at families to a position whereby family skills, strengths and resources are used to create change, solve problems and aid recovery.

Family communication can work on many levels, not only as formal therapy, but also as family counselling and parent support groups.

Together, this creates an environment that is both collaborative and cooperative. The development of therapeutic alliances with individuals and families in this way is the basis for all nursing interventions.

Breathing

If there is evidence of self-induced vomiting with the eating disordered young person, the nurse needs to be aware of the possibility of inhalation and secondary chest infections. Vomiting can also lead to metabolic alkalosis causing slow, shallow respirations which may lead to cyanosis and associated complications. Severely obese young people may experience shortness of breath limiting physical activity.

Eating and drinking

Table 8.1 identifies some potential problems and cognitive thoughts which are associated with anorexia nervosa, bulimia nervosa and obesity.

The role of the dietitian

The dietitian's role is of paramount importance in the treatment of all young people with disordered eating, as the provision of food by a person other than the nurse frees the nurse from the potential conflicts that can and do surround food. As and when conflicts arise, the nurse can refer the child back to the dietitian who can explore, discuss and educate the young person with regard to his or her dietary requirements. The dietitian is also in the ideal position to teach the young person about the merits of healthy eating, which can then be continued by nursing staff. The diets prescribed for individual children (which will include snacks and supplement drinks in the case of very low weight) are delivered ready prepared and individually named from the diet kitchen. The use of vitamin supplements is often advocated.

The role of the nurse

The input of the dietitian allows the nurse to build a therapeutic relationship which is free from the

Table 8.1 Potential problems and cognitive thoughts associated with eating disorders

	Anorexia nervosa	Bulimia nervosa	Obesity
Potential problems	Malnutrition with associated emaciation	Malnutrition from vomiting	Malnutrition from high sugar, high fat content foods
	Avoidance of high calorie foods Purging behaviours	Bingeing Purging behaviours	
	Delayed gastric emptying	Gastrointestinal manifestations such as bleeding or abdominal pain	
	Decreased intestinal motility leading to feelings of bloatedness and abdominal pain		
Cognitive thoughts	Distorted thoughts about food, weight, eating, body shape and size	Distorted thoughts about food, weight, eating, body shape and size	The use of food for comfort
	Manipulative behaviour with regard to food intake and weight	Manipulative behaviour with regard to food intake and weight	

traumas associated with food. The role of the nurse is to:

◆ explore food-related issues
◆ provide a supportive caring environment in relation to food
◆ establish boundaries for behaviour surrounding mealtimes, for example:
  – using the toilet before meals
  – not visiting the bathroom for an hour after meals
  – being available after meals to provide support and distracting from purging behaviours, treating these latter as a cry for help and not a behaviour to be condemned, but understood
◆ helping the young person to come to terms with feelings surrounding food
◆ eating with the young people and modelling appropriate eating behaviour.

Re-feeding the young person with anorexia nervosa

◆ It is sometimes necessary to rehydrate a youngster by use of an intravenous infusion, if there is a proven electrolyte imbalance.
◆ An initial assessment of dietary needs by the dietitian will indicate if oral or nasogastric feeding is required.
◆ If nasogastric feeding is to be undertaken then this should be by frequent bolus feeds which mirror the normal pattern of eating (four in a waking day). Some young people find continuous nasogastric feeding difficult as this acts as a constant reminder of the calories which they are fighting to avoid. This in turn adds to their psychological pain. The nurse begins reorientation of the social norm by talking throughout the feed. This also helps to decrease anxiety around nutrition.
◆ When bolus feeds are mirroring ordinary mealtimes (such as breakfast, lunch, tea and supper), and the emaciated young person is feeling stronger, an oral diet is offered. Any food eaten has its calorific value subtracted from the bolus feed and the remaining calories are given by nasogastric tube. This continues until a regular oral eating pattern is established.

◆ Initially, the anorexic young person may find it difficult to eat in a group situation and may not have eaten with their family for many months. In this case the meals are taken in a one-to-one situation with a nurse and the young person eating together. The nurse reinforces good social eating behaviour by engaging in conversation. The young person is gradually reintroduced to group eating as he or she feels able, beginning with the meals which he or she finds the easiest – usually snacks and tea (fruit and a drink).

◆ Rigid behavioural regimes appear not to be effective. What might be perceived as privileges in such a regime, such as access to television, games, visitors and peer group interaction, the young people in our unit have as a matter of course.

◆ Regular weekly monitoring of weight and height is necessary to establish progress, although the focus of improvement is not on weight but on eating behaviour. When weighing these young people it must be remembered that it is possible that the more manipulative might partake of behaviours to increase their weight; these might include drinking vast amounts of water, wearing extra clothes or hiding heavy objects in their clothes or hair. To decrease the possibility of such actions it is useful to ensure that the toilet is used immediately beforehand and that weighing takes place while only nightclothes or underwear are worn. Weighing should also be undertaken at the same time of day to avoid diurnal variations.

Elimination

Problems which may occur are:

◆ abnormal bowel pattern
◆ amenorrhoea
◆ menarche or recommencement of menstruation
◆ abuse of diuretics
◆ laxative abuse
◆ use of soap or toothpaste as laxatives
◆ inability to undertake own toilet hygiene in severely obese young people.

Many young people with disordered eating have misconceptions about normal bodily functions. Anxiety related to problems experienced in this area can be dealt with through a process of education to encourage understanding.

Cleansing/dressing

Possible problems in these areas are:

◆ obsessive compulsive self-cleaning
◆ self-neglect associated with mood disorders
◆ poor oral hygiene and dental caries due to excessive vomiting
◆ possible presence of fungal infections in the skinfolds of obese patients
◆ inappropriate clothing in low weight young people in an effort to burn off calories, such as wearing only a tee shirt in very cold weather
◆ inappropriate clothing to disguise excessive thinness
◆ excessive sweating in the very overweight.

Body temperature control

Young people with anorexia nervosa can exhibit abnormal thermoregulatory responses, including a lack of shivering when cold. These responses are controlled by the hypothalamus, and abnormalities are thought to be due to the effects of starvation. Other body temperature problems are related to poor circulation or the lack of subcutaneous fat.

All these problems will revert to normal once the anorexic has achieved a healthy weight. Until such time, nurses need to ensure a warm environment and encourage the wearing of appropriate clothing.

Mobilizing

Problems which might be present in this area are:

◆ excessive exercise in anorexic young people
◆ lack of mobility due to excessive weight in the more obese young person.

Regular exercise should be presented as necessary for cardiovascular, respiratory and general health. The anorexic can be assisted in developing an exercise programme that will help to attain these benefits. This is to replace the deficits caused by excessive exercise which interfere with the general health and activities of daily living. In overweight young people it is useful to produce a programme of increasing exercise to promote mobility.

Liaison with the physiotherapist is vital in creating programmes of exercise appropriate for the individual young person and his or her problem. The physiotherapist is also in an ideal position to encourage the underlying feelings of well-being associated with exercise, together with the improving fitness that will act as a reinforcement for weight loss.

Working and playing

The problems which might arise in these areas are:

◆ social isolation
◆ a desire to be liked
◆ boredom
◆ obsessional studying
◆ competitiveness
◆ bullying at school – either due to high or low standards or weight.

The child with an eating disorder will be helped by a relaxed ward atmosphere in which the nurses are approachable. Nursing staff should encourage the young person to join in group activities, while respecting the need for privacy. The eating disordered child may also be helped and feel supported in their studies if a mutually agreed study programme is designed.

Children who are inpatients on our unit should engage in a full school day. Our unit is fortunate as the local education authority provides a fully functional hospital school which is able to offer a full curriculum and liaison with each child's own school, providing a comprehensive educational package. In hospitals where this is not possible, the use of the Home Teaching Service is advocated.

Expressing sexuality

Problems here might include:

◆ avoidance of menstruation
◆ changes in body size and shape
◆ sexual activity – some adolescents may have had pleasurable or traumatic sexual experiences
◆ obese young people may feel sexually unattractive.

The nurse needs to be aware that there is a link between eating disorders and sexual abuse. There is a possibility that disclosure of such abuse will occur in the safety of the therapeutic relationship.

Nursing staff have an important role in emphasizing the importance of being happy with one's body shape and size, while underlining the importance of being a healthy weight.

The recommencement of menstruation or the reaching of menarche may be a cause for concern or anxiety, as this will be symbolic of the maturational process of puberty having been restored. This will have been associated with significant weight gain and possible feelings of bloatedness and depression as features of premenstrual syndrome. Young people with anorexia nervosa or bulimia nervosa may have feelings about being sexually mature and may need help in confronting the emotions associated with that sexual maturity.

Sleep

There are problems which may arise in this area, such as:

◆ decrease in the amount of sleep or fragmented sleep associated with starvation
◆ sleep disturbances associated with depression
◆ breathlessness in obese young people when lying down to sleep
◆ a feeling of poor sleep due to excessive and possibly distressing dreaming.

A physically active day – when the anorexic and bulimic patient's physical condition allows – will help with some of these sleep problems. A nurse being available at bedtime will often help, as this is when the rumination of problems occurs most. The use of relaxation tapes and teaching relaxation techniques can be helpful.

Dying

It is important to remember that eating disorders are potentially fatal, due to short or long-term physiological changes from starvation, purging or overeating. Death is also a possibility due to suicide, so the nurse must be aware of the mental state of the eating disordered young person and be open to the possibility of suicidal intent. Dealing with young people who exhibit self-harm and suicidal gestures is a feature of nursing these challenging children.

THE USE OF MEDICATION IN THE TREATMENT OF EATING DISORDERS

Anorexia nervosa

There is no research basis to underpin the use of medication for the treatment of anorexia nervosa. Many drugs, including amitriptyline, clonidine and opiate antagonists have been used to promote weight gain and food intake, but results of tests have been very disappointing. Depression is a common problem experienced by the anorexic; although this usually becomes less pronounced with weight gain, antidepressants can be a useful adjunct to treatment for those young people whose depression persists despite increasing weight. Care needs to be taken if a tricyclic antidepressant is to be used, since underweight patients may be vulnerable to hypotension and cardiac arrhythmia.

Bulimia nervosa

Medication seems to have a more useful role in the treatment of bulimia nervosa. The most encouraging evidence has been in relation to the use of antidepressant medication. These compounds have displayed consistent and reproducible antibulimic effects, such as reducing the frequency of bingeing and purging behaviours in both depressed and non-depressed bulimics (Walsh 1991, American Psychiatric Association 1994). However, the place of antidepressants in the overall treatment of bulimia nervosa remains unclear. Concerns centre around residual symptoms and long-term outcome.

Obesity

There is no indication for the use of medications such as appetite suppressants in the treatment of obesity in young people. Diet and lifestyle changes in conjunction with treating any underlying psychological issues should be the mainstays of treatment. Treatment of an associated depression may again be a useful adjunct to treatment.

Complementary medicine

Although this is an area which many medical establishments still treat with suspicion, health care workers should remain open-minded to all potential treatments. Hypnotherapy as a treatment strategy is regularly used in the authors' unit. The utilization of such alternative therapies and cultural treatments respects the beliefs of the children and their families. However, it is important that the families and the multidisciplinary team work equally and as collaboratively in this area as in any other.

ETHICAL ISSUES

This area mostly focuses around the issue of anorexia nervosa. Bulimic patients tend to look for help, do not usually have the cognition problems associated with starvation and, in our experience, always consent to treatment when supplied with all the necessary information (informed consent). The clinically obese young person also is cognitively able to consent and negotiate packages of care and, as with the bulimic, actively engage in the care process.

The problem with regard to anorexia nervosa can be described relatively straightforwardly. If the anorexic is not mentally competent due to the effects of starvation, then treatment – for example, re-feeding – without consent could be described as involuntary treatment. However, this may not be seen as a violation of autonomy for the young person's rational or true self would not have defied such a procedure. In other words, if the patient had been well, he or she would not have objected to such a procedure.

The ethical issues surrounding the treatment of young people with anorexia nervosa could be described as a minefield. Consent for any medical intervention has to be obtained from a person who is deemed competent. When discussing competent consent in young people under the age of 16, Gillick competence has to be established. (The young person is judged to be developmentally and psychologically able to make informed decisions regarding their treatment interventions.) In young people not deemed to be Gillick competent, consent for treatment can be given by the person who holds parental responsibility, as defined in the Children Act 1989. If this consent is still not forthcoming then, as a last resort, Section 3 of the Mental Health Act 1983 may be utilized. There have been cases where the courts have been called to intervene when consent has not been able to be obtained. The court has insisted, on occasion, that young people with anorexia nervosa should receive treatment against their wishes for their long-term benefit.

A further consideration in regard to treatment is that it is not uncommon in psychiatry that assessment automatically merges into treatment interventions, without express consent for treatment being obtained. With these young people it is particularly important that this does not happen as this can be experienced as abusive and may parallel previous abusive traumas for the young person.

Within a legal and health care framework which has a tendency to be paternalistic, professionals have a responsibility to frequently review the ethics of treatment packages. The focus should initially be on the individual, his or her rights, feelings, thoughts and concerns regarding treatment, with due consideration given to the family and also to the social and cultural environment that the young person comes from. Within a nursing framework, mechanisms should be established to foster ethical practice care, reflective practice, examination of critical incidents and clinical supervision.

Finally, the use of the Mental Health Act 1983 with these young people has huge ramifications for the rest of their lives. It is therefore more therapeutically beneficial that consent is gained in a collaborative and cooperative manner. The use of the Mental Health Act with young people with anorexia nervosa often brings with it emotional implications, not only for the person concerned but also for the team providing nursing care. It is the author's experience that when the Mental Health Act is utilized to enforce care, relationships frequently become fraught and traumatic. The use of the Act takes away young people's last area of control, leaving them feeling that their physiological and psychological being is controlled and at the behest of others.

In these difficult cases, the importance of clinical supervision is paramount. Despite this bleak picture, young people can emerge from this traumatic period better able to deal with the problems they find themselves confronted with. However, the establishment of therapeutic relationships based on trust is always coloured by these experiences.

THE DISCHARGE PROCESS

The discharge process begins during the initial assessment process, with aims and objectives brought into the discussion so that from the first day the young people and their families can see that we are all working to the common goal of discharge.

Depending on the young person's progress and negotiated care planning, usually when a regular eating pattern is established, the young person is encouraged to begin spending time at home during the weekends. This acts as a reinforcer for more appropriate eating behaviour, as well as allowing the recommencement of social relationships and structures. It is also a time for practising new and relearnt skills gained through varying therapeutic interactions.

This process begins with just an afternoon's visit and increases until the family feels able to manage a full weekend from Friday evening to Sunday evening. An important part of this is interviewing both the young person and the family to establish progress and identify any problems encountered, and to discuss the coping mechanisms used to overcome difficulties and mutually recognize and celebrate progress.

Often these families have been through significant traumas and do not feel that they have sufficient resources and coping strategies to manage the problems with which the family system is confronted. Therefore, acknowledgement and reinforcement of progress is essential to promote a climate in which change can happen with families feeling secure.

Once these periods at home are successfully established, a pre-discharge meeting is held. This includes the core multidisciplinary team, the parents and child (if he or she wishes), a representative from the child's own school and the local community services to whom the family will eventually be discharged. Issues raised at this meeting will include:

◆ acknowledgement and reinforcement of progress
◆ gradual reintegration back into the child's home school
◆ school issues – bullying, social isolation, dealing with difficult questions about the illness
◆ re-establishment and development of peer relationships
◆ management of eating behaviour.

The process, once established, continues with regular progress meetings until the young person is back at home and attending school full-time. Although the pace is determined by the multidisciplinary team, it tends to be set by the young person and their family.

SUMMARY

The eating disorders which have been discussed in this chapter are the three most commonly nursed. Other eating disorders are seen in child and adolescent psychiatry, but these tend to be unique and often of a purely psychological nature. Two examples of these cases include a little girl who stopped eating because a boy at her school said he had put a frog in her sandwich, and a young boy who would only eat green food. Obviously, each of these eating disorders was treated individually according to their unique presentation.

Eating disorders are extremely distressing for both young people and their families. It is hoped that wherever they are nursed, they are treated individually with the respect and understanding they deserve.

 ## FURTHER READING

Booth D A 1994 Psychology of nutrition. Taylor and Francis, London

Claude-Pierre P 1998 The secret language of eating disorders. Transworld, London

Craighead L W, Craighead W E, Kazdin A E, Mahaney M J (eds) 1993 Cognitive behavioural interventions: an empirical approach to mental health problems. Prentice Hall, Hemel Hempstead

Feltham C (ed) 1997 Which psychotherapy? Sage, London

Harbour A, Ayotte W (eds) 1994 Mental health handbook: a guide to the law affecting children and young people, 2nd edn. The Children's Legal Centre, London

Hudson O'Hanlon W, Weine-Davis M 1989 In search of solutions: a new direction in psychotherapy. W W Norton, New York

Lankton S L, Lankton C H 1983 The answer within: a clinical framework of Ericksonian hypnotherapy. Brunner/Mazel, New York

Levons M 1995 Eating disorders and magical control of the body: treatment through art therapy. Routledge, London

Rogers C R 1965 Client-centred therapy. Constable, London

Rowlands B 1997 The Which? guide to complementary medicine. Which?, London

Schaefer C E, Briesmeister J H, Fitton M E 1984 Family therapy techniques for problem behaviours of children and teenagers. Jossey-Bass, London

Shelley R (ed.) 1997 Anorexics on anorexia. Jessica Kingsley, London

REFERENCES

American Psychiatric Association 1980 Diagnostic and statistical manual of mental disorders, 3rd edn. APA, Washington DC

American Psychiatric Association 1987 Diagnostic and statistical manual of mental disorders, 3rd edn. (revised). APA, Washington DC

American Psychiatric Association 1994 Diagnostic and statistical manual of mental disorders, 4th edn. APA, Washington DC

Benfer B, Schroder P 1990 The eclectic approach: principles and general applications. In: Reynolds W, Cormack D (eds) Psychiatric and mental health nursing. Chapman and Hall, London

Bruch H 1973 Eating disorders, obesity, anorexia nervosa and the person within. Routledge and Kegan Paul, London

Bryant-Waugh R, Lask B 1995 Eating disorders: an overview. Journal of Family Therapy 17(1):13–30

Chang C 1990 Transcultural psychiatry. In: Guze B, Richeimer S, Siegel D (eds) The handbook of psychiatry. Yearbook Medical Publishers, Chicago

Crisp A H 1977 Diagnosis and outcomes of anorexia nervosa: the St George's view. Proceedings of the Royal Society of Medicine 70:464–470

Dixon K N 1990 Eating disorders: anorexia nervosa and bulimia. In: Coddington R D, Wallick M M (eds) Child psychiatry: a primer

for those who work closely with children. Warren H Green, Missouri

Edelstein E 1989 Anorexia and other dyscontrol syndromes. Springer, Berlin

Fairburn C, Beglin S 1990 Studies of the epidemiology of bulimia nervosa. American Journal of Psychiatry 147:401–408

Flodmark C E 1997 Childhood obesity. Clinical Child Psychology and Psychiatry 2:282–295

Fosson A, Knibbs J, Bryant-Waugh R, Lask B 1987 Early onset anorexia nervosa. Archives of Disease in Childhood 62:114–118

Gelazis R S, Kempe A R 1993 Therapy for clients with eating disorders. In: Rawlins R P, Williams S R, Beck C K (eds) Mental health – psychiatric nursing: a holistic life-cycle approach, 3rd edn. Mosby-Year Book, Missouri

Groom S 1995 Behavioural health problems of adolescents. In: Campbell S, Glasper E A (eds) Whalley and Wong's children's nursing. Mosby, Barcelona

Health Advisory Service 1995 Child and adolescent mental health services: together we stand. HMSO, London

Hoek H 1991 The incidence and prevalence of anorexia nervosa and bulimia nervosa in primary care. Psychological Medicine 21:445–460

Holden N I, Robinson P H 1988 Anorexia nervosa and bulimia in British blacks. British Journal of Psychiatry 152:544–549

Holland A, Sicotte N, Treasure J 1988 Anorexia nervosa – evidence for genetic basis. Journal of Psychosomatic Research 32:549–554

Hsu L K G 1990 Eating disorders. Guildford Press, London

Keltner W R, Schweke L H, Bostrum C E 1991 Introduction to milieu management. In: Keltner W R, Schweke L H, Bostrum C E (eds) Psychiatric nursing: a psychotherapeutic management approach. Mosby-Year Book, Missouri

Kog E, Vandereycken W 1988 The facts: a review of research data on eating disorders in families. In: Vandereycken W, Kog E, Vanderlinden J (eds) The family approach to eating disorders: assessment and treatment of anorexia nervosa and bulimia nervosa. PMA, New York

Lask B, Bryant-Waugh R 1993 Childhood anorexia nervosa and related disorders. Lawrence Erlbaum, Hove

Lask B, Fosson A 1989 Childhood illness: the psychosomatic approach. John Wiley, Chichester

Lerner H D 1986 Current developments in the psychoanalytic psychotherapy of anorexia nervosa and bulimia nervosa. Clinical Psychologist 39:39–43

Lissau I, Sørensen T 1994 Parental neglect during childhood and the increased risk of childhood obesity in young adulthood. Lancet 343:324–327

Magagna J 1993 Individual psychodynamic psychotherapy. In: Lask B, Bryant-Waugh R (eds) Childhood anorexia nervosa and related disorders. Lawrence Erlbaum, Hove

Meiselman K 1993 Incest: a psychological study of causes and effects with recommendations. In: Hall L, Lloyd S L (eds) Surviving childhood sexual abuse, 2nd edn. Falmer Press, London

Minuchin S, Bosman B L, Baker L 1978 Psychosomatic families: anorexia nervosa in context. Harvard University Press, Massachusetts

National Society for the Prevention of Cruelty to Children 1989 Child sexual abuse in Greater Manchester: a regional profile of child sexual abuse registrations. NSPCC, Manchester

Orbach S 1986 Hunger strike. Faber & Faber, London

Palmer R, Oppenheimer R, Dignon A, Chaloner D, Howells K 1990 Childhood sexual experiences with adults reported by women with eating disorders. British Journal of Psychiatry 156:699–703

Peplau H 1952 Interpersonal relations in nursing. In: Simpson H 1991 Peplau's model in action. Macmillan, Basingstoke

Ponto M 1995 The relationship between obesity, dieting and eating disorders. Professional Nurse 10(7):422–425

Pope H, Hudson J 1992 Is childhood sexual abuse a risk for bulimia nervosa? American Journal of Psychiatry 149:445–463

Renvoize J 1993 Innocence destroyed: a study of child sexual abuse. Routledge, London

Root M 1991 Persistent, disordered eating and gender specific post-traumatic stress response to sexual assault. Psychotherapy – Theory, Practice and Research 28:96–102

Roper N, Logan W W, Tierney A J 1980 Elements of nursing. Churchill Livingstone, London

Schmidt U 1998 Eating disorders and obesity. In: Graham G (ed.) Cognitive behaviour therapy for children and families. Cambridge University Press, Cambridge

Sloan G, Leichner P 1986 Is there a relationship between sexual abuse or incest and eating disorders? Canadian Journal of Psychiatry 31:656–660

Strober M, Lampert C, Morrell W, Burroughs J, Jacobs C 1990 A controlled family study of anorexia nervosa. International Journal of Eating Disorders 9:239–253

Sullivan P 1995 Mortality in anorexia nervosa. American Journal of Psychiatry 152:1073–1074

Timinn S, Adams R 1996 Eating disorders in British Asian children and adolescents. Clinical Child Psychology and Psychiatry 1(3):441–456

Walsh B T 1991 Psychopharmacologic treatment of bulimia nervosa. Journal of Clinical Psychiatry 52(suppl):34–38

Welch S, Fairburn C 1994 Sexual abuse and bulimia nervosa: three integrated case control comparisons. American Journal of Psychiatry 151:402–407

World Health Organization 1992 The ICD 10 classification of mental and behavioural disorders. Clinical descriptions and diagnostic guidelines. WHO, Geneva

Wren B, Lask B 1993 Aetiology. In: Lask B, Bryant-Waugh R (eds) Childhood onset anorexia nervosa and related eating disorders. Lawrence Erlbaum, Hove

9 Feeding children with special needs

Liz Allott

KEY ISSUES

- ◆ Prevalence
- ◆ Causes of feeding difficulties
- ◆ Nutritional assessment
- ◆ Normal and abnormal swallowing
- ◆ Failure to thrive
- ◆ Low body weight
- ◆ Poor growth
- ◆ Constipation
- ◆ Dental caries
- ◆ Vitamin and mineral deficiencies
- ◆ Management of feeding
- ◆ Texture
- ◆ Fluids
- ◆ Increased energy intake
- ◆ Role of enteral feeding
- ◆ Encouraging fibre
- ◆ Special equipment
- ◆ Positioning
- ◆ Nutrition in special schools
- ◆ Nutritional support
- ◆ Cultural issues

INTRODUCTION

The first part of this chapter looks at some of the problems faced by children with special needs, and considers such issues as the prevalence and causes of feeding difficulties, nutritional assessment and some of the problems which can arise from feeding difficulties. The chapter then goes on to give some practical guidance on overcoming these problems.

KEY POINTS

- ◆ Children with special needs should aim to achieve their optimal nutritional status, to give them the greatest chance of reaching their potential in life.
- ◆ Hungry children do not concentrate at school.
- ◆ Overweight children with mobility problems may be unable to walk.
- ◆ Underweight children who are wheelchair-bound are more likely to develop pressure sores.
- ◆ Parents are often the expert source of information, and should never be under-estimated in their ability to take on new ideas.
- ◆ Life should be enjoyed, not endured. Good nutrition is a vital step required to achieve this aim.

PREVALENCE

Children with special needs are usually referred to a local child development unit at an early age, for assessment by a multidisciplinary team. Educational recommendations are made for the most appropriate school for the child. However, due to inequalities of service provision and standards throughout Britain, nutritional services to these children are not consistent.

There is a prevalence of feeding difficulties and nutritional problems are common (Stevenson 1995). In 1989 it was found that 40% of children with special needs had feeding problems (Bax

Table 9.1 Common causes of feeding problems

Problem	Result
Neurological problems	
Inability to move food around the mouth with the tongue.	Bolus of food is not formed. If a bolus of food is formed, it may not be moved efficiently to the back of the mouth to trigger the swallow reflex. Food may be stored in the cheeks or roof of the mouth.
Uncoordinated swallow.	Choking on food or fluids. Swallowing of air.
Delayed feeding developed as part of global developmental delay.	Feeding development may be following the normal progression, but at a much slower rate.
Anatomical problems	
High roof of the mouth.	Food storage in the roof of the mouth. This can then 'fall down' when the child is not expecting it and cause the child to choke.
Unusual dentition.	Absence of normal bite, making chewing more difficult.
Large tongue.	Difficulty in moving food around the mouth. Where tongue thrust is present, there is also difficulty keeping food in the mouth.
Poor lip closure.	Difficulty in swallowing food. Fluid loss from the mouth. Difficulty in using a cup. Difficulty in removing food from a fork or spoon.
Physiological problems	
Fatigue, e.g. due to congenital heart problems, anaemia, chronic undernutrition or medication.	The child is too tired to continue eating a meal, so stops eating before satisfying nutritional requirements.
Taste alterations, e.g. due to trace element deficiency or medication.	Food may not taste as the carer expects, so more or less seasoning may be required.
Lack of appetite due to illness or constipation.	Poor nutritional intake.
Communication problems	Inability to express food preferences, hunger or satiety until a simple communication method has been developed to suit the child.
Prolonged enteral/parenteral feeding in the early months of life due to prematurity, medical or physical problems.	Feeding development may be significantly delayed. Oral stimulation techniques can reduce this effect.
Behavioural problems	
Fear of choking or vomiting from previous experience.	The child may refuse to open mouth, or may store food in the cheeks rather than swallowing it. Behavioural problems may also develop due to other areas covered in this table.
Hypersensitivity of the mouth or area around the mouth.	The child may startle or gag or appear to be in discomfort when these areas are touched.

1995). A validated nutrition risk screening tool specially designed for these children will be available in the future. This will enable nursing and medical staff to identify children with nutritional or feeding problems quickly and reliably.

CAUSES OF FEEDING DIFFICULTIES

It is important that the causes of feeding difficulties are identified so that the most appropriate medical and nutritional treatment can be offered. Increasing a child's nutritional intake without knowing if the child can swallow safely is dangerous (Sullivan 1997).

Essential first steps for a child with feeding difficulties

◆ If the child has a named syndrome, ask the experts or find out more.
◆ Obtain a recent neurological assessment.
◆ Obtain a recent assessment by a speech and language therapist with special feeding assessment skills.
◆ Obtain a recent assessment by a dietitian.
◆ Review the recommendations for feeding by the speech and language therapist and dietitian, based on the above information.

Table 9.1 shows some common causes of feeding difficulties. The action needed to help the child optimally manage their feeding difficulties is discussed in the second half of this chapter.

NUTRITIONAL ASSESSMENT

KEY POINT

Nutritional assessment aims to determine the child's food and fluid requirement to achieve optimal growth and nutritional status.

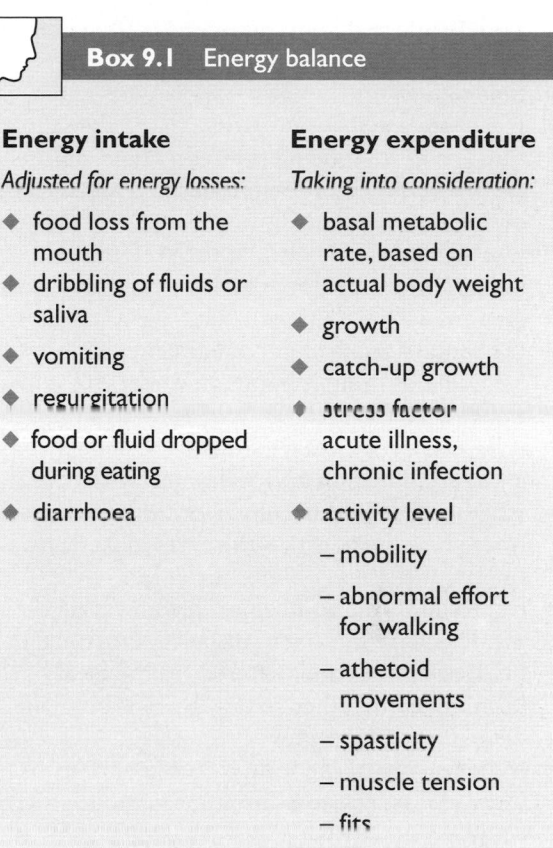

Box 9.1 Energy balance

Energy intake	**Energy expenditure**
Adjusted for energy losses:	*Taking into consideration:*

Energy intake — *Adjusted for energy losses:*
◆ food loss from the mouth
◆ dribbling of fluids or saliva
◆ vomiting
◆ regurgitation
◆ food or fluid dropped during eating
◆ diarrhoea

Energy expenditure — *Taking into consideration:*
◆ basal metabolic rate, based on actual body weight
◆ growth
◆ catch-up growth
◆ stress factor acute illness, chronic infection
◆ activity level
  – mobility
  – abnormal effort for walking
  – athetoid movements
  – spasticity
  – muscle tension
  – fits

All nutrients must be available to the child in the correct quantities if the child is to thrive. Energy requirements will be discussed as these are the most difficult to assess. If nutritional energy intake equals expenditure then the child is in energy balance and will achieve optimal growth. Box 9.1 shows some important considerations when calculating energy balance.

Food and fluid intake

It is easy to quantify the amount of food or fluid contained in a plate, bowl or cup. It is much more difficult to assess the amount that the child successfully retains. The quantities lost will vary according to the following factors:

◆ whether the child is well or ill

- an epileptic child will often refuse food before a fit
- time of day
- size of the meal
- the type of food being offered – some children are very clever at allowing disliked foods to fall out of their mouth!
- whether the food is still at the preferred temperature – prolonged meals can easily mean cold food
- the venue – some children eat better at McDonalds than at home, or prefer to eat in a quiet place
- if the child requires feeding, he or she may have a preferred person and technique for feeding
- whether the child is hungry or thirsty when offered food or drink – the carer must be aware of how the child communicates this
- if the child has become bored with eating the meal because it has taken such a long time, or because all the foods offered for the meal have been mixed together so that there is only one taste to enjoy
- if the texture of the food is inappropriate
- if the child has a sore mouth, e.g. mouth ulcers or thrush
- if the child has tooth decay or is losing a tooth.

Energy expenditure

Both recommended daily allowances and growth charts are based on active children with normal growth. These may not be appropriate for many children with special needs. Without knowledge of the expected growth pattern for an individual child, it is impossible to accurately predict their nutritional requirements. Some growth charts for children with specific diagnoses have been developed:

- Down's syndrome (Cronk et al 1998)
- Williams syndrome (Nardella 1996)
- Prader-Willi syndrome (available from the Prader-Willi Syndrome Association UK)
- cerebral palsy – charts being researched (C Fairhurst, personal communication, 1997).

Data plotted on any growth chart need careful interpretation, as factors such as associated breath-ing problems, renal disease or cardiac problems will also affect growth. However, energy requirements still have to be assessed to meet the individual child's expenditure. Krick et al (1992) have proposed a formula for calculating energy needs for children with cerebral palsy which includes:

- basal metabolic rate
- muscle tone
- movement/activity
- energy for growth
- energy for catch-up growth.

A similar approach may be possible with other groups of children.

Measuring growth

Weight

A variety of types of weighing scales are available:

- standing scales
- sitting scales
- hoist scales, as a freestanding hoist or as part of a bath hoist
- wheelchair scales.

The same method should ideally be used on each occasion for the child. Some small children can be weighed most reliably on the lap of an adult, where they feel safe and will stay still. Note should be made if the child is weighed wearing callipers, splints, etc., and the weight of these should be deducted.

Height

Measuring children's height is not easy. Errors in measuring children's standing height have been established (Voss et al 1990). Reliable height and length measures in children with disabilities have been considered in a number of studies. Spender (1989) has discussed the use of upper arm and tibial length measurement in children with cerebral palsy, and has produced growth charts for these measurements. Stevenson (1996) recommends the use of upper and lower limb anthropometry for length evaluation. The easiest measurement is probably tibial length, using a tape measure. A formula can then be used with the child's age to estimate total height (C Fairhurst, personal communication, 1997). Growth charts of tibial length for age would be even more accurate, as any errors in conversion would be eliminated.

In summary, the dietitian must:

◆ weigh and measure the child using appropriate methods
◆ assess the child's present nutritional intake
◆ assess the child's likely requirements
◆ advise the child and their carers how to meet their requirements
◆ reassess after a period of time to find out if optimal growth is being achieved
◆ if optimal growth is not being achieved, the requirements must be revised accordingly.

NORMAL AND ABNORMAL SWALLOWING

The normal swallow has four stages (Winstock 1994).

1. *Anticipation* – by all the senses. If one of the senses is lacking (e.g., due to visual

> **KEY POINT**
>
> Children with swallowing problems should be assessed by a speech and language therapist who can recommend safe feeding methods. They may also be able to prescribe treatment techniques to allow the child to further develop his or her feeding skills.

impairment) then extra cues should be given verbally, and by familiar cooking noises and smells.

2. *Oral stage* – food enters the mouth and is moved around to form a bolus. The bolus is moved to the back of the mouth by the tongue to trigger a swallow. As the swallow reflex is triggered, breathing stops.

3. *Pharyngeal stage* – the larynx is closed by a sequence of events, to protect the airway and prevent aspiration of food or fluid. The food bolus moves into the oesophagus.

4. *Oesophageal phase* – food travels by reflex action down the oesophagus to the stomach.

Table 9.2 Ages at which new feeding skills are developed. (Adapted from Winstock 1994, with permission.)

Age	Lips	Tongue	Jaw	Gag reflex
Birth–3 months	Sucking, lip seal around breast or teat – some fluid loss normal	Forward and backward tongue movement	Up–down jaw movement	Very sensitive gag reflex
3–6 months	Sucks food from a spoon using forward–backward tongue movement			
6–9 months		Sucks food placed on tongue	Learns to bite food placed at side of mouth	
9–12 months	Upper lip removes food from spoon	Tongue able to move food from side to side of the mouth, i.e. chewing developing		Gag reflex less sensitive
12–18 months	Lip closure some of the time during chewing	Chews efficiently with lateral and rotatory movements	Jaw movement 'mirrors' tongue movement	
18–24 months	Can chew with lips closed	Able to chew firmer foods		
24–36 months	Eating and drinking well with little spillage			

CASE STUDY

Jo is 6 years old. His feeding development is that of a 3-month-old child. He cannot be expected to manage lumpy food as this will trigger his gag reflex, and may eventually make him frightened to eat. Puréed food will be managed. The thickness of the purée can very gradually be increased so that he learns to manage the texture in his mouth. Careful observation will be required to assess when he is ready to start lumpy foods.

Once this reflex is triggered, breathing starts again.

A child can have problems with one or more of these stages. It is important to work out what stages are normal, abnormal or malfunctioning. Feeding must be appropriate to the child's stage of feeding development.

A multidisciplinary approach to the assessment of a child's feeding development and swallowing ability is ideal, but is not always possible. Video recording can be a useful method of assessing progress. Some children may develop abnormal feeding habits that need to be identified in order to progress further.

FAILURE TO THRIVE

Children with special needs are at risk of failing to thrive due to:

◆ underlying chronic disease
◆ acute illness
◆ feeding difficulties
◆ malabsorption
◆ decreased intake in a child with a degenerative condition
◆ increased requirements due to cardiac problems, chronic infection or malignancy
◆ presence of a syndrome where the growth pattern is not understood
◆ exhausted carers trying to manage a very demanding child.

The cause of the weight loss or poor weight gain must be sought. This must be treated appropriately, whether by medical or surgical intervention or through the identification of suitable respite facilities. A detailed nutritional assessment should form part of the investigation, and should precede any invasive medical tests.

The most common cause of non-organic failure to thrive (where the cause is primarily external to the child) is inadequate nutrition (Maggioni & Lifshitz 1995). This can occur unintentionally

CASE STUDY

Ben was 8 years old, weighed 14 kg, and had a height of 104 cm. His height had not increased for a year. His weight had fallen by 1 kg over the preceding 6 months. He had had no significant illnesses during this period. He had severe feeding problems, managing a thick puréed consistency of food and small quantities of fluid. His carers spent at least an hour feeding him at each of three meals a day, and a further hour preparing the food, cleaning him afterwards, cleaning themselves and the area where he has been fed. Drinks were given between meals, but this was also a slow and messy business. Ben showed no enjoyment from eating after the first few mouthfuls and was exhausted at the end of a meal. On assessment he was only managing 70% of his nutritional requirements, despite advice from the dietitian to increase the energy content of his meals having been followed. Ben's actual food intake had not altered significantly for 3 years. Until then his growth was following a course below the third centile, but parallel to it. At age 6 his growth was noted to be slower than before, and had now stopped. His nutritional intake had been sufficient for him at 5 years old, but his eating ability had prevented him from achieving normal growth since then.

Ben is now a happy and thriving 10-year-old. He has the majority of his nutritional needs satisfied by gastrostomy feeding, and eats for pleasure. His drinking ability has improved now that less time is spent on feeding. His family are also enjoying their meals again.

with special needs children who are difficult and slow to feed.

Catch-up growth

Catch-up growth is defined as the acceleration in growth that occurs when a period of growth retardation ends and favourable conditions are restored (Maggioni & Lifshitz 1995). This can occur if:

◆ high nutritional requirements return to normal levels, e.g. after correction of congenital heart defects in a child with Down's syndrome
◆ energy and protein intake is increased
◆ a combination of these conditions occurs.

The formula commonly used to determine energy requirements for catch-up growth is as follows (MacLean et al 1990):

$$\frac{\text{kcal/body weight}}{\text{(in kg)}} = 120 \times \frac{\text{ideal body weight for height}}{\text{actual body weight}}$$

Protein intake should also be increased to provide at least 9% of energy intake to support rapid growth (Jackson 1990).

Carers often become concerned during catch-up growth, as the child at first appears to be gaining body weight rapidly before growth in height is restored. This can cause problems with lifting the child, and should always be discussed when the new regimen is developed so that appropriate equipment can be made available through occupational therapy or physiotherapy services.

Monitoring by the multidisciplinary team and carers should be carried out during catch-up growth, and adjustments made where necessary – to the diet, size of the wheelchair, standing frame and so on.

LOW BODY WEIGHT

Many features seen in a child with low body weight are common with those in children with failure to thrive. Information from the child's growth chart should be used to establish whether the child has always had a low body weight in proportion to his or her height, or if the child is failing to thrive. There may be a number of reasons for low body weight:

◆ weight may be normal for a child with their syndrome, although this may appear to be a low weight on normal growth charts
◆ feeding problems
◆ food refusal for social, psychological or behavioural reasons, e.g. expressing unhappiness when parents' marriage breaks down
◆ appetite changes due to medication
◆ adolescent growth spurt when the child may find it difficult to eat enough to meet requirements
◆ inappropriate food intake for the child's age – a small teenager with learning difficulties who is developmentally functioning at a 5-year-old level can all too easily be given food portions suitable for a much younger child.

Low body weight is often due to lack of sufficient energy intake rather than lack of a wider range of nutrients. Nutritional assessment will help identify this. Energy intake should be increased gradually using three meals with snacks between meals for most children. Fun, enjoyable food can be used to encourage the child to eat, although extra dental care may be needed if many sweet foods are used. If a child is on any medication this will need to be monitored if the dosage is dependent on body weight. Epileptic children have been observed to have more fits during a period of rapid weight gain.

The psychological and practical aspects for the family of a child's low body weight should be considered:

◆ a small child in a buggy may be easier to take on outings than a larger child in a wheelchair
◆ a child weighing more than about 17 kg becomes too heavy to lift easily and carry upstairs.

Any weight gain planned at this stage needs to be carefully discussed with the family. The occupational therapist should be involved to discuss plans for hoists, house adaptations and so on. There are no clear guidelines about the provision of hoisting equipment for children.

POOR GROWTH

Poor growth, failure to thrive and poor weight gain have features in common. Where there appears to be a problem with poor growth, the following steps should be taken:

◆ nutritional assessment should always be carried out
◆ growth of other individuals with the same syndrome should be examined
◆ techniques for catch-up growth can be applied
◆ poor growth during puberty is common in children with feeding problems, due to the high requirement for food during this period
◆ carers may need to be encouraged to increase food intake in readiness for the child's pubertal growth spurt when other signs of early puberty become evident
◆ growth during puberty may also be compromised if the adolescent child is unable to express his or her emotions at this stage – food refusal may be one of the child's only means of rebelling.

CONSTIPATION

Chronic constipation can be a major problem in children with special needs. It may be exacerbated by:

◆ immobility
◆ poor gut motility – e.g. in cerebral palsy
◆ medication – e.g. some anticonvulsants, iron preparations
◆ poor fluid intake due to feeding problems, spillage or hypersalivation
◆ low fibre content of foods in some poor eaters or fussy eaters
◆ reliance on milk for a large part of the child's nutritional needs
◆ toilet training, if the child is worried about having an 'accident'.

Prevention, by eating a healthy diet with an adequate fluid intake, should always be the first line of action in susceptible individuals. Guidelines for avoiding constipation should be made easily available to the carers of special needs children at an early age, through child development units, health visitors, community nurses and dietitians. A child who is already constipated should gradually have his or her diet improved to include fibre, in the form of fruit and vegetables, at each meal. Children should be encouraged to have fruit as a snack, and to drink plenty of fluids.

Chronic constipation that is not successfully treated can cause pain, discomfort, loss of appetite, lethargy and taste abnormalities. Some children will still be constipated despite an excellent diet. These children will require medication.

DENTAL CARIES

Preventive treatment by a dentist and dental hygienist should be introduced from an early age. Dietitians should avoid recommending sugary snacks and drinks between meals or at bedtime, except where this is the only way to satisfy energy requirements. Dental caries and gum disease can be a problem for children with special needs due to:

◆ difficulty in cleaning the teeth because of oral hypersensitivity or lack of cooperation
◆ poor enamel formation
◆ medication
◆ lack of normal chewing and tongue movements to move food around the mouth and clear food away from the teeth
◆ lack of ability of the child to indicate that a tooth is sensitive to temperature or sweet tastes, causing decay to develop further before treatment – this may be shown by a reluctance to eat
◆ snacks with a high sugar content used to increase a child's weight

◆ excessive toothwear due to acidic drinks or tooth grinding
◆ difficulty in giving dental treatment, as this can be frightening to the child – some children require sedation for treatment.

Box 9.2 shows some ways of preventing dental disease (Harris & Harris 1998).

VITAMIN AND MINERAL DEFICIENCIES

For normal growth and development to occur it is important that the child's diet is sufficient in every respect, including vitamins and minerals. Intakes of the water-soluble vitamins B and C from food may be reduced if food is:

◆ cut up, mashed or puréed
◆ cooked for a long time to make the texture suitable

◆ kept warm for a long time due to slow eating
◆ reheated during a meal or for another meal.

Most of the above are unavoidable for a child with feeding difficulties. Dietary assessment will not take full account of these vitamin losses, but the dietitian's recommendations should allow for losses.

Fat-soluble vitamins will not be absorbed well if mineral oil preparations are used to ease constipation. These laxatives are not normally prescribed, but are purchased by some individuals.

Minerals such as iron and zinc are often found to be lacking on dietary assessment, as rich sources of these minerals are not found in 'easy to eat' foods.

MANAGEMENT OF FEEDING

A consistent approach should be used by all the carers who feed a child. This should be formulated by the parents with the multidisciplinary team (Taylor et al 1996). If a team approach is not available or appropriate then the parents, the child and the dietitian should work together with the speech and language therapist, calling in other experts as and when necessary. A feeding programme or nutrition care plan should be written, to be followed by anyone who feeds the child.

Box 9.2 Prevention of dental disease

Dietary measures

Avoid sugary snacks and drinks between meals or at bedtime.

Use 'tooth friendly' drinks. Discourage use of bottles and feeder cups for sweet drinks.

Long-term medication should be sugar-free whenever possible.

Discourage acidic drinks and foods, especially between meals.

Brushing teeth after drinking acidic drinks may exacerbate toothwear.

Preventive dentistry

Good oral hygiene through regular brushing of teeth.

Electric toothbrushes may be recommended by some dentists.

Fluoride use – in toothpaste, fluoride mouth rinses or brush-on gels, drops or tablets, as recommended by the dentist.

Fissure sealing.

Prevention of trauma.

Prevention of toothwear, including effective treatment of gastric reflux and vomiting.

KEY POINTS

A very positive approach should be taken to feeding with praise given freely. Meals should:

◆ be enjoyable
◆ be relaxed
◆ be fun
◆ be a happy time
◆ fulfil nutritional needs.

The feeding programme should aim to allow the child to achieve safe feeding practices and to eventually develop as much independence in feeding as possible. Every child will need an individual approach. Some children will achieve this if they are not pressurized at all, while others need to have clear expectations set. Incentive schemes for achieving small goals may be useful: e.g. sticker charts, a certificate from the class teacher after a week of reaching a goal, a certificate from the head teacher presented in assembly for 4 weeks of achieving a goal. Children with visual problems should have agreed prompts to let them know that food or drink is coming: e.g. shaking the cup before offering a drink. They should have food described to them before it is eaten so they know what to expect. A mouthful of rice pudding will never taste good if you were imagining it to be chocolate mousse!

TEXTURE

Speech and language therapy assessment will determine the texture of food suited to the individual child. This will be based on safety and on the child's stage of feeding development. The most difficult texture that a child can manage safely will encourage further development, but

CASE STUDY

Helen is 7 years old, has cerebral palsy and has always had feeding problems. As a toddler she used to become distressed and scream at mealtimes. She has needed a gastrostomy to fulfil the majority of her requirements since she was 2 years old. After detailed assessment it was found that her swallow appeared to be safe and therefore she could be encouraged to eat more than the two to three teaspoons of puréed food that she had been having for a long time. She learnt how to indicate 'yes' and 'no'. She was told that she was expected to eat five teaspoons of lunch at school and could then indicate to say if she wanted more. After five teaspoons of food she was praised at whatever stage she decided to stop eating. This approach has been developed further over many months. She can now choose to select the food that she has for her lunch, but she has to eat it.

may sometimes decrease the child's total intake, due to the effort involved. During periods of illness or if the child is very tired, the texture may be made easier to ensure that enough is eaten. Texture is very difficult to describe. Using a blender with different foods gives a different effect. For example, whilst blended pasta on its own resembles glue, blended mashed potato is smooth and manageable.

The following texture classification is useful (Martin & Backhouse 1993):

◆ bite size
◆ easy chew
◆ smooth and thick
◆ thick fluids.

Each of these textures can contain a number of components:

◆ hardness
◆ crunchiness
◆ adhesiveness
◆ cohesiveness
◆ chewiness/gumminess
◆ particle size
◆ rate of breakdown.

These textures are self-explanatory, but experience will help to find the combinations that suit the individual child. If the texture of a food is being modified, attention must always be paid to the presentation, taste, smell and temperature of the final product.

Bite size

◆ Foods to be cut up with knife and fork into pieces of a manageable size.
◆ Gravy or sauces may be used to provide moisture and to stop food falling off the fork or spoon.

Easy chew

◆ Foods may be finely chopped or mashed lightly with a fork.
◆ Gravy or sauce will be needed to keep the food moist and to form a bolus easily in the mouth.

Smooth and thick

- Foods will need to be blended with added liquid.
- Care must be taken to ensure that the food does not become runny.
- Adding fluid increases the volume of food, so a normal portion for a child may be far too much once it is blended.
- Nutritious fluids should be used whenever possible to ensure an adequate intake.
- Foods should be blended separately and presented separately on the plate. This improves the appearance of the meal and offers a variety of tastes. A divided plate can be useful.
- Commercially available moulds can be used to shape puréed food to resemble the original product.

Here are some practical suggestions to achieve the desired consistency of food:

- to thicken savoury food – instant mashed potato, tomato purée, fromage frais, baby rice, instant sauce mix, stuffing mix, breadcrumbs, commercial thickeners
- to thicken sweet food – fromage frais, thick and creamy yoghurt, instant whip powder, instant cheesecake mix powder, baby rice, instant oat cereal, commercial thickeners
- energy-containing liquids to add to dry savoury food – yoghurt, cream, ready-made tins or jars of sauce, curry sauces, cheese sauce, condensed soup, salad cream, mayonnaise
- energy-containing liquids to add to dry sweet food – custard, cream, fromage frais, evaporated milk, sweetened condensed milk, ice cream, creamy yoghurt, ice cream sauces, melted chocolate.

FLUIDS

Many children with special needs struggle to drink sufficient fluids. This can cause:

- dehydration
- problems with temperature control
- constipation
- urine infections.

Fluid requirements are difficult to assess. In practice, if a child's fluid intake is thought to be borderline, then the volume and appearance of their urine is used as a guideline.

Many special needs children who find it difficult to drink enough fluid are also underweight. They may be eating enriched foods and having some nutritional drinks to satisfy their energy needs. It is important that these children also drink non-nutritious fluids, such as water or squash.

 CASE STUDY

Sam is 15 years old and has profound and multiple learning disabilities. His first assessment was carried out recently. He weighed 25 kg and was 140 cm tall. He was very thin. The fluid requirement for a 15-year-old boy is 50 ml per kilogram of body weight per day. This would suggest that Sam needs 1250 ml of fluid per day. Sam sweats profusely, like many 15 year old boys. As he is thin he has a large surface area, so the suggested fluid intake is unlikely to be sufficient. With a body weight of 25 kg Sam might be expected to be about 6 years old, with a fluid requirement of about 80 ml per kilogram of body weight per day. This would give Sam a daily intake of 2000 ml. Sam's actual fluid requirement is probably somewhere between 1250 and 2000 ml/day. His present intake was assessed, and he was asked to gradually increase his intake to a level he could manage, probably about 1800 ml/day.

Children with feeding problems may lose fluids during drinking due to poor lip closure. This can be minimized by speech and language therapy programmes and the use of adapted cups. Fluid losses must always be taken into account when working out how many cups of fluid to offer a child each day.

Children who can use a cup themselves may find it difficult to control the amount of fluid entering the mouth at once. Fluid is quite difficult to handle in the mouth as it does not form a distinct bolus for swallowing, and too much fluid at once can easily cause choking. These children may manage better if a small amount of fluid is put in the cup, with the cup being refilled repeatedly.

Fluids that have a natural diuretic effect (e.g. tea, coffee and coke) should not be used as the sole source of fluid intake.

Thickened fluids

Thickened fluids are used if the child has difficulty safely swallowing thin fluids. This is to allow the fluid to be more easily controlled within the mouth, ready for swallowing.

The speech and language therapist will recommend the thickness required. Prescribable thickening powders are used to produce the right 'grade' of thickness:

> Grade 1 – slightly thickened, syrup consistency
> Grade 2 – thickened but still drinkable: e.g. pourable yoghurt
> Grade 3 – thickened to a spoonable consistency: e.g. mousse.

Thickening powders can be used for both hot and cold drinks. Different fluids require different amounts of powder to achieve the same grade of thickness. Other thick drinks include:

◆ thick milkshakes
◆ some yoghurt drinks
◆ milkshake made using instant whip powder or ice cream.

INCREASED ENERGY INTAKE

Children with low body weight often only need their energy intake to be increased. This is done by increasing fat and carbohydrate eaten in foods, or by the use of special products. Ideas for increasing the energy content of normal foods include the following:

◆ fry foods
◆ add butter or margarine to mashed potato, vegetables, pasta or rice
◆ spread butter or margarine generously on bread or toast

◆ use thick yoghurt and fromage frais, clotted cream, tinned rice pudding or custard
◆ add double cream to puddings, in porridge or on breakfast cereal
◆ make sauces for savoury dishes, or use ready-made sauces
◆ add mayonnaise or cream to pasta dishes
◆ spread butter icing or a melted Mars bar on cakes
◆ enjoy trifle, ice cream desserts or gateau
◆ add grated cheese or cream cheese to sauces, baked beans or mashed potato
◆ add jam or honey to milk puddings, yoghurt and porridge
◆ use pots of pudding: e.g. chocolate mousse, individual cheesecakes, crème caramel.

Snacks between meals can also be encouraged, as long as the child's appetite for the next meal is not spoilt. Some snack ideas include:

◆ cake
◆ savoury scones with cream cheese
◆ a pot of yoghurt, fromage frais or pudding
◆ ice cream
◆ milk shake with cream or ice cream added
◆ hot chocolate or malted milk drinks
◆ biscuits or Jaffa cakes
◆ savoury crisp snacks
◆ cheese sandwich biscuits.

ROLE OF ENTERAL FEEDING

Children with feeding problems may not be able to meet their nutritional requirements, despite every effort being made by the child and his or her carers. Children with a degenerative condition (e.g. Batten's disease) may reach a stage at which their swallow is unsafe. Enteral nutrition may then be considered. This must be discussed fully with the family before any decision is made. Some families find enteral feeding very difficult to accept, and it may not be the best solution for every child. The following recommendations have been made (Townsley & Robinson 1997).

Before enteral feeding is established:

◆ All parents should receive verbal and written information about not only the practical aspects of tube feeding, but also the social and emotional impact it may have. A succinct checklist of 'issues to consider' should be available to all parents.
◆ Whenever possible, families should have an opportunity to talk to other parents who have direct experience of enterally feeding a child.

If enteral feeding is started, children with a safe swallow can eat and drink for pleasure, whilst receiving the majority of their nutritional intake without effort. Once feeding is established, children can expect to return to their normal growth pattern, and become nutritionally fit, without problems from constipation. Regular assessment of feeding should be carried out by the dietitian and support should be readily available.

The time during the day spent feeding the child is much reduced, and the family may find that this is a welcome relief. Feeding can be carried out discreetly during the day using a portable battery-operated pump and feeding bag in a cover. Feeding can then procede anywhere – in the pub, during car journeys, while shopping, at football matches, during days out. The child is often very contented when being fed, which improves everybody's enjoyment of the day. The child with a safe swallow can still enjoy some food orally while the feed is in progress, but will not have to be pressured into eating. The feeding regimen will have to be slightly flexible to fit in with other activities: e.g., swimming.

There is concern about the coordination of services, provision of training, support and assessment for children on home enteral feeding (Townsley & Robinson 1997).

ENCOURAGING FIBRE

Children who are poor eaters and require a modified texture of food often have a low fibre intake. Carers are encouraged to enrich the child's food. This can sometimes reduce the child's intake of fruit and vegetables, which are bulky but have a low energy content. Great care must be taken when advising carers to ensure that fibre is included. Children who have used baby foods for a prolonged period are particularly at risk.

Soluble fibre in the form of fruit, vegetables and oats is easily included and has the benefit of tasting good and offering other nutrients too. Increasing the soluble fibre content of the child's diet does not require extra fluid to be consumed. However, cereal fibre and foods containing bran do require extra fluid, and natural bran should not be added to foods.

Fruit purées are an excellent way of improving the fruit intake of a child needing a smooth and thick texture of food. These can be made from:

◆ tinned fruit compote
◆ tinned or dried apricots
◆ peaches
◆ mixtures of fruit including prunes and figures
◆ stewed apples
◆ tinned apple sauce.

The fruit purée could be added to:

◆ instant oat cereal
◆ porridge
◆ milk puddings
◆ custard
◆ yoghurt
◆ fromage frais.

To be effective for combating constipation, fibre should be included at each of the three meals, and preferably in snacks, too. Fruit juices, especially orange, prune and grape juice, can also help some children. Increasing the fibre and fruit juice intake of any child's diet should be done gradually, if abdominal pain and wind are to be avoided. An adequate fluid intake must also be consumed.

SPECIAL EQUIPMENT

Special feeding equipment can allow a child to gain as much independence as possible in feeding. Assessment and advice should be given by the occupational therapist and speech and language therapist.

Cutlery:
◆ small, flat soft plastic spoons
◆ use of a 'splade' instead of a fork

- cutlery with a large soft handle for easier grip
- angled cutlery for children with limited arm or wrist movement
- handles with straps to attach round the hand.

Plates:
- high-sided
- angled side to aid spoon loading
- sloped and angled for easy spoon loading
- guards to fix to ordinary plates
- divided plates to keep different tastes separate.

Cups:
- angled cups
- cups with an inset lid with holes for drinking
- spouted beakers with various sized holes
- straws
- valved straws
- fun cups and glasses
- cups with large handles.

Eating aids:
- counterbalanced arm supports, for those with limited arm movement and power – allows food to be collected from the plate and lifted up to the mouth
- rotating plate, controlled by a lever to put a new area of food in reach
- non-slip mats
- mirror on the table in front of the child.

New equipment should be introduced when the child is alert, not at the end of the day when the child may be tired. When a child is learning to use new equipment for independent feeding, a lot of effort is required and total food and fluid intake may be reduced. When the child is successful, great excitement can mean more spillage! Small goals should be set and plenty of praise given.

POSITIONING

The occupational therapist and physiotherapist should assess the child to recommend the best seating for feeding:

- the child must feel safe and secure to eat
- individual seating should be adjusted to achieve a well-supported upright position

- the head should be in the midline, not tilted back or dropping forward onto the chest
- if the child does not have good head control, the head may need to be supported in a suitable position
- if the child is feeding him or herself, the table must be at an appropriate height
- feeding in a standing frame can be appropriate for some children
- any straps must be quickly and easily removable in case the child chokes
- school dining rooms can be noisy places, so care must be taken with seating children who startle at loud noises or who are liable to fit.

NUTRITION IN SPECIAL SCHOOLS

A multidisciplinary approach with education and health is vital if children with special needs are to get optimum benefit from school. Health staff involvement in special schools is variable across the country, and many schools do not have regular contact with a specialist dietitian. Many people are involved in the nutritional care of a child.

The school nurse:

- provides valuable liaison between health professionals, the children and their parents, and will often identify children who need nutritional intervention – nutritional screening carried out at school would aid this process
- weighs and measures children and completes growth charts
- informally observes children during the school day – (eating, in the playground, in corridors, in lessons) – useful information is often gathered in this way
- liaises with families
- liaises with teaching and support staff
- liaises with paediatricians
- liaises with the dietitian and passes on concerns from children, families and staff
- reinforces nutrition care plans and individual targets.

The dietitian:

◆ should act as a resource to all the staff
◆ liaises with medical staff
◆ ensures that there is a local policy for enteral feeding at school
◆ organizes training for enteral feeding, with written back-up information
◆ assesses and monitors individual children with their parents
◆ provides written nutritional care plans for children with complex dietary needs
◆ provides targets for other children they have been working with – these can be incorporated into the child's individual education plan
◆ liaises with the school catering adviser and cook and advises about menu adaptation.

The speech and language therapist (with feeding assessment qualifications):

◆ assesses children
◆ carries out treatment programmes to develop the child's feeding skills
◆ recommends suitable textures of food for the child
◆ recommends the thickness of fluid required if thin fluids are not safe.

The occupational therapist:

◆ advises appropriate seating for feeding
◆ advises about special eating equipment
◆ may be able to advise about feeding techniques.

The physiotherapist:

◆ advises about seating.

The teaching staff:

◆ incorporate the child's targets from the nutritional care plan into lessons where appropriate
◆ may work with special school assistants feeding children and doing enteral feeding
◆ encourage certain children to have snacks and drinks between meals.

The special school assistant:

◆ feeds individual children

◆ carries out enteral feeding
◆ encourages certain children to have snacks and drinks between meals.

The school cook and catering adviser:

◆ adapt the school menus to provide suitable food for all the children
◆ provide food of the appropriate texture
◆ present the food attractively.

NUTRITIONAL SUPPORT

If a child cannot manage a sufficient intake using normal food, then prescribable supplements may be needed. These should be used in addition to food, not as a replacement for it. Children may need a nutritionally complete supplement, or one that provides extra energy. The protein content of some supplements is too high for children under 20 kg in weight or under 6 years old. The dietitian should advise the type and quantity of supplement to be used and should review the child regularly.

Table 9.3 shows examples of supplements suitable for children.

Care must be taken when giving any child a supplement containing more than 1 kcal/ml, to ensure an adequate fluid intake. Glucose polymers, calogen, liquigen and duocal must only be used in quantities advised by a dietitian. Duobar is a confectionary type bar containing 600 kcal in a 100 g bar. It is an extremely concentrated source of energy and should only be used on rare occasions with dietetic advice.

CULTURAL ISSUES

Children with special needs are found in all cultural groups. Some specific problems arise due to:

◆ religious dietary restrictions and customs
◆ cultural customs
◆ poverty.

The main implications for the diets of children with special needs are vegetarian and vegan diets, prolonged use of cow's milk as the main source of nutrition, and prolonged use of baby foods.

Table 9.3 Examples of supplements suitable for children (Russell et al 1988)

	Age 1–5 years (8–20 kg)	Age 6 years (over 20 kg)
Nutritionally complete sip feeds		
1 kcal/ml	Nutrini Frebini Paediasure	Fresubin Clinifeed Iso Ensure Nutrison standard
1.5 kcal/ml	Nutrini Extra *These can be flavoured with milkshake flavouring if necessary.*	Fortisip Entera Ensure plus
Sip feeds – not nutritionally complete		
1 kcal/ml	1/2 strength Scandiskake	
1.25 kcal/ml		Provide Xtra Enlive Fortijuice
2 kcal/ml		Scandishake
Energy supplements (energy from carbohydrate-glucose polymers)	caloreen polycal maxijul polycose vitajoule	caloreen polycal maxijul polycose vitajoule
energy from fat	calogen	calogen liquigen (MCT)
energy from carbohydrate and fat	duocal powder duocal liquid	duocal powder duocal liquid duobar

As with any child, schools should be made aware of any cultural dietary needs. Vegetarian and vegan children should be encouraged to eat a wide variety of suitable foods, including pulses, cereals and plenty of fruit and vegetables. Care must be taken when encouraging children to eat nuts, due to the danger of aspiration. Vegetarian and vegan diets can lack energy density, so fats and sugars may be needed to increase the energy content. Special care must also be taken to ensure an adequate iron intake in vegetarians. The vegan diet is at risk of being deficient in protein, energy, iron, fat-soluble vitamins, vitamin B_{12}, riboflavin, calcium and zinc. Dietary assessment will be needed for vegans in order to offer appropriate advice. Children depending on cow's milk and those on baby foods when they reach the nursery class at school are unlikely to be thriving. These children need to be encouraged to try new foods at school, and their progress should be reported to their family. The dietitian should be involved in helping the family to learn about healthy eating, and giving them guidance about feeding their child.

Questions

Answers are given in Appendix 2.

1. Anna is 4 years old and has just moved into the area. The move included spending 6 months living in temporary rented accommodation. She has cerebral palsy and visual problems. She weighs 11 kg and is 92 cm tall. Her mum and dad are 178 cm and 190 cm tall respectively. Until a year ago her height and weight were increasing along the third centile. She has some feeding difficulties but can reliably manage a smooth and thick texture of food. She has started school for the first time this week. She has eaten very little at school, and has become distressed very easily. Discuss her situation and make recommendations.

2. Claire is 15 years old. She has learning and physical disabilities as a result of a head injury 8 years ago. She can walk slowly but has coordination problems and falls easily. She can eat

independently and has some verbal communication skills. She enjoys television and using a computer. Her weight has been increasing faster than her height for the last 2 years. Her height is 168 cm and her weight is 82 kg. She can be very demanding at times, and has some behaviour problems. She enjoys food and often asks for food between meals. Her parents feel that eating is one of her pleasures in life. She is constipated. Her behaviour has been found to deteriorate when her constipation is severe. How can we help her?

FURTHER READING

Winstock A 1994 Eating and drinking difficulties in children. Winslow Press, Bicester

An excellent account of feeding development, assessment of eating and drinking, and its management from a speech and language therapist.

Martin J, Backhouse J 1993 Good looking, easy swallowing – creative catering for modified texture diets. JFC Foundation, Australia

Dysphagia and its practical management are discussed. Over 300 pages of recipes with colour photos and texture classification are included.

REFERENCES

Bax M 1995 Eating is important. Developmental Medicine and Child Neurology 31(3):285–286

Cronk C, Crocker A C, Peuschel S M et al 1998 Growth charts for children with Down's syndrome: 1 month to 18 years of age. Paediatrics 81:102

Harris J C, Harris I R 1998 An overview of dental care for the young patient: 1. Introduction, priorities and disease prevention. Dental Update March:65–72

Jackson A A 1990 Protein requirements for catch-up growth. Proceedings of the Nutrition Society 49:507–516

Krick J, Murphy P E, Markham J F B, Shapiro B K 1992 Proposed formula for calculating

energy needs of children with cerebral palsy. Developmental Medicine and Child Neurology 34:481–487

MacLean W C Jr, Lopez de Romana G, Massa E, Graham G G 1990 Nutritional management of chronic diarrhoea and malnutrition: primary reliance on oral feeding. Journal of Paediatrics 97(2):310–323

Maggioni A, Lifshitz F 1995 Nutritional management of failure to thrive. Pediatric Clinics of North America 42(4):791–810

Martin J, Backhouse J 1993 Good looking, easy swallowing – creative catering for modified texture diets. JFC Foundation, Australia

Nardella M 1996 Early nutrition intervention with Williams syndrome and hypercalcaemia. Nutrition Focus 11(5):1–8

Russell C, Micklewright A, Scott D et al 1988 Paediatric enteral feeding solutions and systems. A report by the joint working party of the paediatric group and parenteral and enteral group of the British Dietetic Association. BDA, Birmingham

Spender Q W, Cronk C E, Charney E B, Stallings V A 1989 Assessment of linear growth of children with cerebral palsy: use of alternative measures to height or length. Developmental Medicine and Child Neurology 31:206–214

Stevenson R D 1995 Feeding and nutrition in children with developmental disabilities. Paediatric Annals 24:255

Stevenson R D 1996 Measurement of children with developmental disabilities. Developmental Medicine and Child Neurology 38:861–866

Sullivan P B 1997 Gastrointestinal problems in the neurologically impaired child. Ballière's Clinical Gastroenterology 11(3):529–546

Taylor S, Wheeler L C, Taylor J R, Griffin H C 1996 Nutrition: an issue of concern for children with disabilities. Nurse Practitioner 21(10):17–18, 20

Townsley R, Robinson C 1997 Effective support services to disabled children who are tube fed – interim report to the NHS executive. Nora

Fry Research Centre, University of Bristol, Bristol

Voss L D, Bailey B J R, Cumming K, Wilkin J, Betts P R 1990 The reliability of height measurement (the Wessex growth study). Archives of Disease in Childhood 65:1340–1344

Winstock A 1994 The practical management of eating and drinking difficulties in children. Winslow Press, Bicester

10 Growth and nutritional assessment of children

Jeremy Kirk

KEY ISSUES

◆ The importance of growth and nutrition
◆ Measurement of growth and nutrition
◆ Growth charts
◆ Factors involved in growth
◆ Growth problems

INTRODUCTION

The investigation of growth and nutrition is for the most part a simple and inexpensive process, producing reproducible measurements that can be compared with data for normal children. Growth is a complex process, which does not only involve increase in height. A number of different factors, including nutrition, affect the ability of an individual to achieve his or her genetic potential, and these must be considered within the assessment process. The principles of measurement and charts and their part in the assessment of growth and nutrition will be described in this chapter.

THE IMPORTANCE OF GROWTH AND NUTRITION

Growth in children is not simply an increase in height and weight, but is instead a complex process involving increases in both the size and number of cells. It is influenced not only by genetic factors, but also by a number of other factors (including nutrition) which may act to prevent the individual achieving his or her genetic potential. Growth is a critical indicator of child health and is recognized by the World Health Organization, which identifies growth assessment as the best single measure for defining the nutritional status and health of children, as well as being an indicator for populations as a whole for quality of life. In the United Kingdom the NHS Executive publication 'Child health in the community: a guide to good practice' also recognizes the critical role of growth, and says:

Growth is a key indicator of normal health and development. Failure to grow at an appropriate rate may be associated with a primary growth disorder, but is more commonly due to a general failure to thrive which can be a pointer to chronic ill health eg. recurrent urinary tract infections, poor feeding practice, neglect or abuse. Early detection of an abnormal pattern of growth is a valuable pointer to many conditions which can cause avoidable disability. (Schilg & Hulse 1997, p.3)

Principles of growth

Figures 10.1a and 10.1b demonstrate the most famous and early of growth charts: that of the son of the Comte Philibert de Montbeillard, measured by his father every 6 months throughout childhood. This graphic plot demonstrates the characteristic pattern which is unique to humans and primates. Figure 10 shows the same data plotted in different ways: Figure 10a is a static chart which shows the data in terms of height achieved; Figure 10b is a dynamic chart which shows the data in terms of height increase over a period of time. If the process of growth is thought of as a journey, then Figure 10a is equivalent to the distance travelled (milometer), whilst Figure 10b is equivalent to the speed during the journey (speedometer). The same type of static and dynamic format of measurements is also commonly used for weight. Each type has its advantages and disadvantages.

Static chart

Advantages. The advantages of static charts are as follows:
◆ may only require a single measurement
◆ can be performed at any age using suitable charts
◆ repeated measurements can give an indication of rate of change (using centile crossing).

Disadvantages. The disadvantage is:
◆ a single measurement will not give any indication of the rate of change, whether past, present or future.

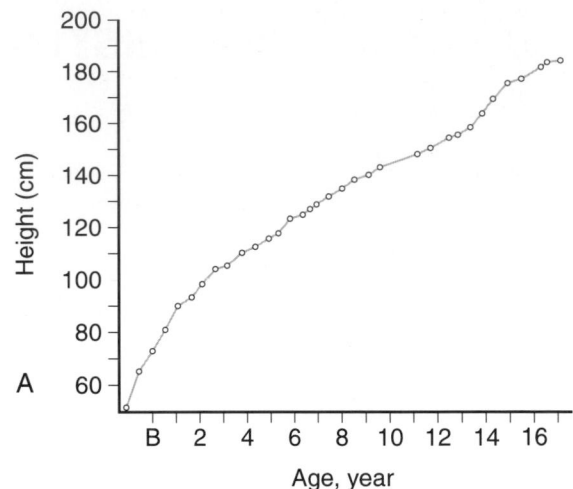

Figure 10.1a Distance chart of the growth of the son of Comte Philibert de Montbeillard

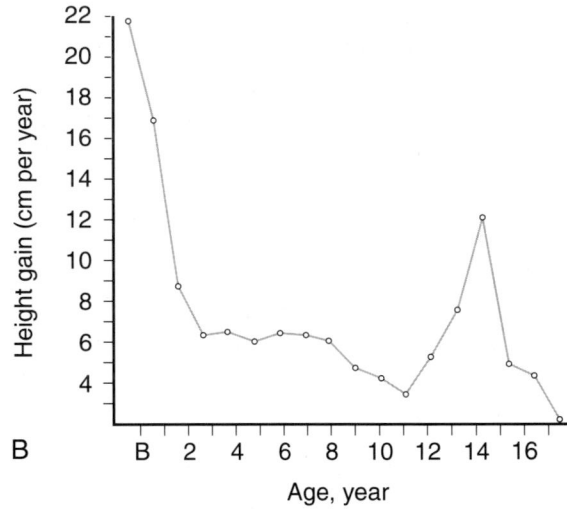

Figure 10.1b Velocity chart of the growth of the son of Comte Philibert de Montbeillard

Dynamic chart

Advantages. The advantages of dynamic charts are as follows:
◆ give an indication of rate of change, and therefore a dynamic measurement
◆ abnormal rate may indicate underlying pathology
◆ response to therapy can also be documented.

Disadvantages. The disadvantages are:
◆ at least two measurements are required
◆ need calculation of velocity from raw data
◆ several measurements increase potential for inaccuracy
◆ require measurements to be performed over at least a year to produce meaningful data.

In assessing growth, it is important to bear in mind that it consists of three phases superimposed upon each other. Each phase can be described mathematically, but more importantly each appears to be under different controls, both nutritional and hormonal.

Infantile phase

This is a continuation of the intrauterine growth curve, and is a rapid and rapidly decelerating growth curve lasting from birth to 3 years. During the first year of life an infant grows more rapidly than at any other period of his or her (extrauterine) life. Body length increases by 50% in the first year of life, and during the first months an infant can grow 2.5 cm a month. By 2 years of age a child is roughly half the adult height, indicating that 50% of growth has occurred by this time. This period of growth is predominantly under nutritional control, as children with congenital hormone deficiencies usually have relatively normal birthweights and lengths.

Childhood

This is a steady and slowly decelerating growth curve which starts at around 2 to 3 years and continues until puberty. By their eighth birthday most children will have achieved around three quarters of their final height. Although at this age there is little height difference between the sexes, boys tend to be slightly taller than girls. This phase of growth is under hormonal control (predominantly growth hormone), although nutritional factors do play a role.

Puberty

This is a phase of growth which lasts from adolescence onwards and has different timing and

Table 10.1 Percentage of final height achieved		
Age (years)	Boys (%)	Girls (%)
2	50	52
3	55	58
4	58	62
5	62	66
6	66	69
7	69	73
8	73	77
9	76	80
10	78	83
11	81	87
12	84	92
13	88	97
14	92	98
15	97	100
16	99	100
17	100	100

strength in the two sexes. It is this phase of growth which accounts for the major sex differences in final height of around 12.5 cm between males and females. Girls tend to enter their growth spurt earlier, although the amount of the growth spurt is not as great as that in boys (adding 20 to 25 cm in girls, and 25 to 30 cm in boys). This phase is under the control of growth hormone and sex hormones acting synergistically.

Table 10.1 shows the percentage of final height achieved by boys and girls aged from 2 to 17.

MEASUREMENT OF GROWTH AND NUTRITION

Measurements of growth, body dimensions and body composition (anthropometry) are easily and rapidly performed and are non-invasive. In addition to measuring growth they enable nutritional status (both short and long-term) to be assessed. However, it is important to ensure that measurements are performed consistently, using appropriate (though not necessarily expensive) equipment, and also using trained staff. Inconsistencies can occur at a number of stages, including in the setting up and calibration of equipment, measuring technique and recording of data. Most measurements are accurate to within several percentage points, which is significantly better than the accuracy seen in many biochemical investigations.

Measuring equipment and techniques

Standing height

Although traditionally recommended from 2 years of age onwards, this is commonly performed as soon as the child can stand. This measurement is on average 1 cm less than the corresponding supine length. This measurement should be performed without shoes, and wearing no more than thin socks. The head is held in the Frankfurt plane (an imaginary line drawn from the centre of the auditory meatus to the lower border of the eye), so that the child looks forward with heels and back in contact with an upright wall. As there is settling of the intervertebral discs during the day (an average of 7 to 8 mm) it is usually recommended that repeat height measurements are carried out at the same time of day, and that gentle but firm upward pressure be carried out by the measurer to the mastoid process to overcome this. Although this increases the unstretched height there is no evidence that the accuracy of measurements is improved by this manoeuvre. Whilst stadiometers are the measuring equipment of choice in hospital, the book and tape method can produce acceptable measurements over a 3-month period.

Height: supine length

Height is traditionally measured lying down until 2 to 3 years of age (with overlap with standing height from 2 years). This measurement requires two people: one to hold the head vertically against the headboard in the Frankfurt plane, and the other to straighten the knees and hold the feet flat against the footboard while the measurement is being made. There is no evidence that this manoeuvre causes hip dislocation. Various different pieces of measuring equipment are available, with accuracies of 1 to 5 mm. Reliable measurements can be produced in infants, with an accuracy comparable to that of older children.

Foot length in the infant is correlated with supine length, and this can be used as an indirect measure in sick premature infants.

Although in the past it was felt that expensive equipment was required to accurately measure height, it is now clear that much of the discrepancies arise from the observer. In a survey of 230 instruments it was discovered that one in seven was inaccurate by more than a centimetre. There is now a range of equipment costing from £20 to £1000 which, when properly set up and maintained, will produce accurate and consistent measurement in appropriately trained hands. It is expected that measurements of both supine and standing height should be accurate to within 3 mm.

Height velocity

Growth is not a continuous process, with short-term growth spurts and intervening growth arrest (saltation and stasis); seasonal variation in growth (growth is faster in spring and summer compared to autumn and winter); and longer term variation over a number of years. Repeated (longitudinal) measurements of growth enable an estimate of height velocity to be produced. The height velocity standards have been devised over a 1-year-period, and intervals of less than this will tend to emphasize measurement errors.

In the first 6 months of life a child grows around 14 cm. This growth rate slows, so that by the age of 2 years the growth rate is 9 cm per year. At 10 years of age the growth rate is 5 cm per year, and usually the slowest rate of growth is immediately prior to entering the pubertal growth spurt.

Weight

Weight is a variable that can be measured accurately without expensive equipment, and with minimal training. Electronic scales do not usually require regular calibration, although when using any type of scale it is worth having an object of known weight for calibration. Infants under 2 years of age are usually measured naked, and then after that in light clothing only, with nappies and shoes removed. If minimal clothing is used then its estimated weight (about 100 g) should be subtracted before weight is recorded. Recommended infant scales are usually graduated to 10 g, and for toddlers to 100 g. However, although easy to measure, weight gain alone is a poor guide to the health of a child, and other ways of assessing nutritional status are required.

Characteristically, an infant doubles its birthweight in the first 4 months of age (gaining 150 to 190 g in weight per week), and trebles it by 1 year. A child is approximately half the adult weight by 9 to 11 years of age.

Weight velocity

As with height velocity, this needs to be calculated over a year. This measurement is, however, rarely used.

Weight for height

Weight alone is not always a good way to assess nutritional status, as it goes without saying that a child who has a low weight is not necessarily thin, and one with a high weight is not necessarily fat! In order to make an assessment, comparison needs to be made with height. Weight for height can be used as an indication of the nutritional status of a child when expressed as percentage of ideal body weight (IBW). Box 10.1 shows the relationship between percentage IBW and nutritional status.

The ideal body weight can also be used to provide a weight goal for an individual child. Although weight for height is a simple way of assessing nutrition, it may be affected by a number of factors such as abnormal body proportions, variations in pubertal onset and also different body builds.

Body mass index

As weight for height is affected by a number of factors, an alternative way of assessing nutritional status is by using the body mass index (BMI), which is calculated by taking the weight (in kilograms) and dividing by the square of height (in metres) (w/h^2). The BMI has been used widely in adults to assess nutritional status, although there are problems using it in children as BMI varies throughout childhood. The BMI rises steeply in infancy, falls during the pre-school years, and then rises progressively into adulthood.

Measurements

There are a number of measurements which provide a non-invasive means of assessing nutrition. These involve measuring circumferences and skinfold thickness at sites which are sensitive to nutritional intake.

Skinfold thickness

Skinfold thickness gives an indication of subcutaneous fat, and hence nutritional status. These measurements are made by pinching the skin between two fingers and measuring the skinfold thickness using specialized skinfold callipers. These are expensive and require experience to produce accurate and reproducible measurements, although in trained hands an accuracy of 1.0 to 1.5 mm is possible. The two standard sites for skinfold measurement are the triceps and subscapular areas. Reduction in the triceps skinfold reflects depletion of fat store in chronically undernourished children. The subscapular skinfold is an indicator of truncal fat stores and reflects long-term rather than short-term nutritional status. With additional measurements of the skinfolds of the biceps and suprailiac regions, it is also possible to calculate fat mass (Brook 1971).

Box 10.1 Percentage IBW and nutritional status

>120%	Obese
110–120	Overweight
90–110	Normal
80–90	Mild wasting
70–80	Moderate wasting
<70	Severe wasting

Mid-arm circumference

This is a relatively easy measurement to perform using simple equipment, with an error of less than 0.5 cm. Using a non-stretchable tape, measurements should be taken in triplicate at the midpoint of the upper arm. The midpoint is reached by halving the distance between the acromion of the shoulder to the olecranon of the elbow. Despite measuring bone, muscle, fat and skin, the mid-arm circumference is a good reflection of current nutritional status. It can be used in all age groups for the assessment of nutritional status (both under- and overweight), and thus provides a rapid screen in childhood. The mid-arm circumference can be expressed as raw data, or as a percentage of expected circumference for age and sex.

Head circumference

The measurement of head circumference can be one of the most accurate and reproducible measurements if performed correctly. The maximum head circumference is usually taken; in practice, this is from the midpoint of the forehead to the occipital prominence (Figure. 10.2). The head grows rapidly in the first years of life, with a relative plateau period of growth in mid-

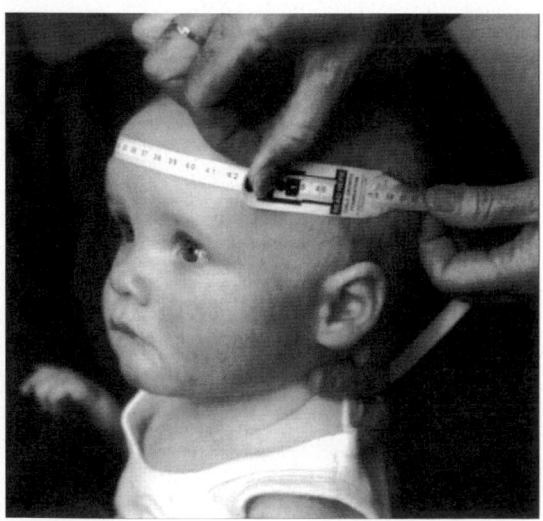

Figure 10.2 Taking a head circumference measurement. (Child Growth Foundation, reproduced with permission.)

childhood and a further increase from puberty onwards. In older children it is important to remember that a 1 mm depth of scalp will increase the head circumference by around 6 mm. Measurement should be made to the nearest millimetre, and ideally repeated. Head circumference is routinely measured up until the age of 2 years, but is only usually measured subsequently if there are clinical concerns regarding either disparity between head circumference and height, or abnormal head growth. It is important that a tape of non-stretchable material is used: the Lasso-o from the Child Growth Foundation is cheap and is designed specifically for head circumference measurement.

At birth the head circumference is approximately 75% of its adult size, with the majority of the postnatal growth occurring in the first year of life. During this period the head circumference increases by a mean of 13 cm, whereas between 3 and 14 years it only increases by a further mean of 7 cm.

The ratio of head circumference to mid-arm circumference is an easily performed and reproducible measurement in children aged 3 to 48 months. It is independent of age and sex, and can be used to assess both over- and undernutrition. The ratio of head to chest circumference is not as reproducible a measurement in the 1 to 2-year age group, but provides a crude indicator of undernutrition.

Sitting height

Determination of body proportions may be clinically relevant in forms of short stature with disproportion. This may be due to skeletal dysplasias (such as achondroplasia), where limb length is usually reduced, or alternatively to spinal irradiation in the treatment of malignant disease, where spinal growth is retarded. Prior to 2 years of age crown to rump length should be measured; after this, sitting height should be measured with appropriately constructed equipment. Sitting height measurements can be subtracted from the standing height to give the subischial leg length. The sitting height and subischial leg length are then plotted onto appropriate charts to see whether there is any discrepancy between the two measurements suggestive of disproportion. In the absence of a sitting height stadiometer, the relationship between standing height and arm span have also been used, and also upper and lower segment measurements (taken from the pubis). In addition, upper arm length and lower leg length are alternative measurements.

Body composition measurement

Measurements of body composition are important in nutritional assessment. Although in adults changes in weight are usually associated with changes in body fat, this is clearly not the case in children who are growing. Body fat rises in the fetus from 2.2% at 1 kg bodyweight to 12% at term, and by 6 months of age is 25%. Although it has been suggested that total fat mass can be calculated from the sum of four skinfold measurements (Brook 1971), this equation may not be as accurate as originally thought, as distribution of fat within the body may vary with sex, age and race.

Direct methods for measuring body composition in adults include densitometry, total body potassium and neutron activation. These techniques involve, respectively, immersion, isolation in a counting chamber, and radiation exposure, and for these reasons none is particularly useful, especially in younger children. As body weight equals fat mass plus fat free body mass (FFB), techniques which measure the FFB can be used by subtraction to produce the fat mass. However, this is based on an assumption that the components of the body maintain a relatively constant composition, and this assumption does not hold true for childhood.

Stable isotopes

As neutral fat does not bind water, measurement of the total body water can be used to provide an estimate of the FFB. Since the water content of FFB is constant in healthy individuals, oral administration of stable isotopes such as deuterium (^{2}H) or oxygen-18 (^{18}O) and calculation of their dilution within body fluids such as blood, urine or saliva can be used to estimate total body water.

Bioelectrical impedance

This is based on the assumption that a weak electric current will pass through the FFB rather than body fat. The impedance to electrical flow, therefore, will vary according to the amount of FFB. Although the impedance of FFB mass changes with age, making it potentially inaccurate in children, this technique has been validated in children against skinfolds and measurement of body water using isotope dilution (Gregory et al 1991).

Dual-energy X-ray absorptiometry (DEXA)

Although there are a number of different radiological techniques for measuring body composition, many are limited by radiation dose, inconvenience and cost. Dual-energy X-ray absorptiometry enables a low radiation non-invasive measurement of bone mineral density, in a number of body sites such as lumbar vertebra, forearm, or in the whole body. The latter are used to produce measures of bone mass, fat-free mass, fat mass and percentage body fat.

GROWTH CHARTS

Principles

Many organic variables such as height and weight are normally distributed, although others, such as skinfolds and BMI, have a skewed distribution. Prior to the age of 2 years this data is often plotted using a weekly or monthly grid, using chronological age corrected for gestational age. After this, true chronological age is used. Although some of the charts use a grid split into weeks or months, many use a decimal age. In calculating the decimal age for a child, the calendar year is divided into 10, and each date in the calendar is expressed in terms of thousandths of the year. Thus, a child born on June 1, 1988 would have a birthdate of 88.414, and would have an age of 10.263 years on September 5, 1998. This decimal age makes the calculation of velocities easier.

In order to interpret any biological variables it is important to make comparison with normal data for children of the same age and, where appropriate, sex. In producing this normal data it is important to remember that human variables often change with time (secular change), and vary within different groups and geographical areas (racial and geographical variation). It is therefore important to ensure that the data is representative of the population for which it is meant to be used. Once normal data has been produced for different ages and sexes, the spread of this data can be expressed as centiles or as standard deviations from the mean.

Centiles

These are lines delineating data into percentages. By definition, the 50th centile represents the average. Conventionally seven centile lines – the 3rd, 10th, 25th, 50th, 75th, 90th, 97th centiles – have been used for most data. In order to make the data comparable with the standard deviation Z-scores (see below), the newer charts have nine centile lines – 0.4th, 2nd, 9th, 25th, 50th, 75th, 91st, 98th, 99.6th centiles – with each line being two thirds of a standard deviation apart from the previous one.

Z-scores

As well as being given as a centile, the distance from the mean in normally distributed data can be expressed mathematically as a standard deviation score (SDS or Z-score). The Z-score is commonly used when statistical comparison is being made, as it enables children of different ages and sexes to be compared. By definition, a value on the 50th centile will have a Z-score of 0 SDS, whereas Z-score values of children on the 2nd and 98th centiles are -2 and +2 SDS respectively.

Height charts

The original growth charts in the United Kingdom were based on data from the 1950s and 1960s (Tanner & Whitehouse 1962), and although they were redesigned in 1976 the same data were used. By the early 1990s it was felt that these UK growth charts were out of date for two reasons:

◆ It was felt that there had been a secular trend over the decades towards increased height and earlier maturation.
◆ The data were not representative of the United Kingdom as a whole as they had been gathered from London and the south-east alone.

In 1991 a project was begun to compile new growth standards. Data from around 25 000 children measured as part of seven different growth studies between 1978 and 1990 were included (Freeman et al 1995). The data was cross-sectional (i.e. children were measured only once) unlike the Tanner–Whitehouse data which included not only cross-sectional but also longitudinal data (i.e. children were measured repeatedly over a period of time). Although when growth rates are relatively steady the cross-sectional data makes little difference, when the growth rate is changing rapidly (such as during adolescence) this has the effect of flattening out data. The 3rd, 50th and 97th centiles were found to be greater than the Tanner–Whitehouse standards at most ages for height, with an average increase of 1.5 cm during mid-childhood, and less for adults. Earlier maturation in both sexes was noted. A number of specialized disease-specific growth charts are also available, for example Turner's syndrome, Down's syndrome and achondroplasia.

Height velocity

These charts are based on the Tanner–Whitehouse data, and have not been subsequently updated. The data are based on a height velocity of at least a year, to take into account seasonal variation and accuracy of measurement. These charts also allow for early, normal and late developing children. Height velocity data taken over 6 months increase the distance between centile lines by approximately 1 cm. By definition a child growing along the 50th centile for height will have a height velocity over a year along the 50th centile. As tall children grow faster than average height children, who in turn grow faster than short children, children with heights on the 97th centile have a height velocity on the 75th centile, and children with heights along the 3rd centile have height velocities along the 25th centile. The Middlesex growth chart for height velocity screening uses the 25th to 75th centiles for height velocity for pre-pubertal children.

Infant growth charts

The 1988 Gairdner-Pearson record pooled data from a number of studies, with data on height, weight and head circumference from 24 weeks' gestation to 2 years of age. The chart is marked in weeks and months. Concerns have been expressed about the accuracy of measurements in infancy (especially length), and a study showed that 28.5% of recorded points were placed inaccurately, usually due to miscalculation of the age of the child (Cooney et al 1994). Despite a change in feeding practices over the last few decades, the updated data for the Cole charts shows little secular change for the period of infant growth.

Head circumference charts

These are from birth to 16 years of age and are based on data from Tanner and Whitehouse.

Weight charts

These are also based either on Tanner–Whitehouse or Cole data. The updated Tanner–Whitehouse data of 1975 showed children to be much fatter compared to the original data of 1962, especially in infancy. Compared to the Tanner–Whitehouse data of 1975, the Tanner–Buckler charts show that girls are lighter during childhood, heavier during puberty, and although the mean final weight is similar the spread in centiles is less. For boys the

pattern is similar although the 97th centile is lighter throughout, and the final weight for all centiles is less.

Weight velocity

Weight velocity charts are available, based on the Tanner–Whitehouse data (Tanner et al 1966). The velocity is calculated over a year, and for this reason these charts are not helpful in the assessment of short-term changes in weight.

Change in weight charts

In infants, although weight velocity charts are based on a shorter fixed time interval between measurements (such as 1 or 3 months), children are not usually measured at fixed time intervals, making these impractical. As a result, there has been a tendency to use centile crossing on the distance chart to ascertain changes in weight velocity. The Sheffield weight chart is a distance chart modified to interpret centile crossing, with extra channel lines spaced to ensure that just 5% of infants can be expected to shift up and down during a 2-week period, and by two channel widths in an 8-week period.

The Sheffield chart is, however, of no use for measurements taken more than 8 weeks apart. The phenomenon of regression to the mean, where there is a tendency for short children to show catch-up and large ones to show catch-down, also needs to be taken into account, as approximately 50% of babies cross at least one channel on the weight chart and 5% cross two channels between 6 weeks and 12 to 18 months of age. Charts which take this into account – so-called 'conditional references' – have now been produced for children aged 4 weeks to 2 years (Cole 1995). These three-in-one weight-monitoring charts contain the usual weight curves from 0 to 12 months, with superimposed thrive lines which cross the centiles downwards. A number of lines are required to cover the first year of life. These thrive lines are steepest from 4 weeks (once birthweight has been regained), then flatten at 6 months of age, and then become negative (indicating that weight loss at this stage is not abnormal). If the slope of weight gain over a 4-week period is less than the thrive line, then the weight gain is below the fifth percentile.

Body mass index (BMI) charts

Using height and weight data from the 1990 data set on almost 30 000 children aged from 33 weeks' gestation to 23 years of age, it has now been possible to produce BMI charts for the UK from birth to 20 years (Cole et al 1995). Like the other 1990 derived charts, there are nine centile lines, although unlike the growth chart there is significant skew, with the top centile channel being four times as wide as the bottom channel.

Skinfold charts

These are based on published data from Tanner and Whitehouse (1975). As these measurements do not have a normal distribution, they are often log-transformed before plotting. For both sexes there is a marked increase in skinfolds in the first year of life, a subsequent decrease to mid-childhood, and a gradual increase after this.

Assessment of growth

In order to assess the growth of a child, there are a number of steps which should be taken.

History

This should include enquiry regarding birthweight and early feeding practice, growth patterns (including familial history) and nutritional intake. Systematic review should include enquiry of feeding patterns and oromotor dysfunction, and gastrointestinal problems.

Examination

This should include measurement of height, weight and any other parameters of growth and nutrition. Examination should also look for signs of malnutrition, and endocrine and chronic disorders.

Plotting data

This should be done on appropriate charts to allow comparison with the population and with genetic targets (e.g., heights of parents).

Further investigation

This may include the estimation of skeletal maturity using bone age, confirmatory testing for other underlying disorders (including endocrine), and assessment of nutritional status and body composition.

Biochemical assessment of nutritional status

A number of biochemical measurements, usually of serum proteins, are used. None is ideal, as they have differing half-lives, and are all affected by other, non-nutritional physiological and pathological states. These are shown in Table 10.2.

There is little evidence that measurement of plasma amino acid concentrations has a role to play in the diagnosis and management of protein-energy malnutrition.

Importance of assessment of growth and nutrition

In conclusion, assessment of growth and nutrition is important, both in the diagnosis of primary nutritional and growth disorders and also in the diagnosis of chronic disorders.

This process may enable a diagnosis to be made, even at initial consultation. In the UK familial patterns of growth are the commonest cause of short stature, with endocrine problems being relatively uncommon. A diagnosis, however, may not be

Table 10.2 Half-lives of proteins	
Protein	**Half-life**
Albumin	18–20 days
Transferrin	8–9 days
Pre-albumin	2 days
Retinol binding protein	12 hours
Fibronectin	4 hours–24 hours
Amino acid profiles	Many

apparent on initial assessment, and further data are often required. Subsequent height measurements allow assessment of height velocity, but even if this is normal, significant pathology may be indicated by:

◆ extreme short stature
◆ inappropriately short stature for parents.

The role of the clinician is to try to distinguish those children who are normal, and consequently require no therapy, from those who have significant pathology requiring treatment. The present UK guidelines for growth monitoring in the community recognize the importance of early identification of all children with growth-related disorders (Hall 1996). The guidelines propose that all children are measured at least three times between the ages of 18 months and 5 years, and again between 7 and 9 years of age (either for all, or for selected children). A meeting was held in June 1998 to review growth-monitoring and a consensus statement is at present in preparation. It is possible, however, that in future there will be no formal pre-school growth-screening.

Growth guidelines

The current guidelines from the British Society for Paediatric Endocrinology and Diabetes (BSPED) for specialist referral are as follows (based on the Cole 9-centile charts):

◆ on single height measurement – to refer any child whose height falls either below the 0.4th or above the 99.6th centile
◆ on repeated height measurements – to refer any pre-school child whose height either moves upwards or downwards by the width of one centile band, or at school-age by two thirds of a centile band.

If the curve veers by two thirds in a pre-school, or one half in a school-age child then the child should be recalled in 6 months and remeasured.

FACTORS INVOLVED IN GROWTH

Whether an individual grows normally and achieves an appropriate final height and weight is

Table 10.3 Factors influencing growth

Influence	Examples
Familial	
Familial height	Familial short stature (FSS)
Familial growth patterns	Constitutional delay of growth and puberty
Genetic disorders/ syndromes	Turner's syndrome
Birth size	Intrauterine growth retardation (IUGR)
Chronic illness	
Respiratory	Asthma, cystic fibrosis
Cardiovascular	Chronic heart failure
Gastro-intestinal	Coeliac/inflammatory bowel disease
Renal	Chronic renal failure
Psychological factors	Psychosocial deprivation
Environmental	
Nutritional	Malnutrition
Socio-economic	Poverty
Endocrine disorders	
Growth hormone	GH-insufficiency
Thyroid hormone	Hypothyroidism
Corticosteroids	Cushing's syndrome
Sex steroids	Precocious puberty

dependent on a number of factors, both intrinsic and extrinsic, acting on the already genetically determined capacity for growth of that individual (Table 10.3).

Genetic influences on height

Once nutritional-dependent growth has run its course at 2 to 3 years of age, it is usual for the child's growth to continue along its own centile line. This correlates strongly not only with the final height centile, but also with the parental heights. In addition to genes determining growth potential and final height, there are also other genes which determine the rate of development. This pattern can be determined using both the bone age and pubertal ratings.

Mid-parental height

This is a way of assessing the adult genetic height potential of a child, and is calculated from the parental heights (preferably measured rather than reported). As men are on average 12.5 cm taller than women, when assessing a boy 12.5 cm should be added to the mother's height, and with a girl 12.5 cm should be subtracted from the father's height. The two heights are then added and averaged to produce the mid-parental height (MPH). The target centile range (TCR) with 95% confidence limits is a range plus or minus 10 cm either side of this.

Bone age

Although secretion of growth hormone continues throughout life, final height is achieved relatively early on when the growing ends of bones – the epiphyses – fuse. Assessment of the skeletal maturation (bone age) therefore quantifies the years of remaining growth, and enables an estimation of final height to be made. There are a number of different methods used to calculate this, such as Tanner and Whitehouse and Greulich & Pyle (1959). As the hand and wrist contain a number of epiphyses, it is common to use a radiograph of the non-dominant hand to estimate the bone age. As tall children mature faster than short ones, it is usual for the bone age to be advanced in tall children and delayed in short children. As the epiphyses are poorly formed in the hand prior to 18 months, the bone age is more difficult to assess in younger children. As the bone age reflects remaining growth, by combining it in an equation with height and growth it can be used to produce a final height prediction.

Tanner staging

Puberty is the phase of development of secondary sexual characteristics. Although the terms 'puberty' and 'adolescence' are often used interchangeably, puberty is usually used for the physical changes and adolescence for the psychological changes at this stage. Puberty itself is an ordered process with a specific consonance, deviation from which may suggest pathology. In females puberty starts at around 11 years of age with breast development, with subsequent pubic

Box 10.2 Tanner ratings for assessment of puberty

Both sexes: pubic hair

- ◆ Stage 1: Pre-pubertal.
- ◆ Stage 2: Sparse growth of long, downy hair, chiefly along the base of the penis or labia.
- ◆ Stage 3: Hair considerably darker, coarser and more curled, spreading sparsely over the junction of the pubes.
- ◆ Stage 4: Hair now adult in type, but area covered is still considerably smaller than the adult.
- ◆ Stage 5: Adult in quantity and quality, with spread to medial surface of the thighs.
- ◆ Stage 6: Spread of hair to linea alba.

Girls: breast development

- ◆ Stage 1: Pre-pubertal.
- ◆ Stage 2: Breast bud stage, with elevation of breast and papilla.
- ◆ Stage 3: Further enlargement of breast and areola, with no separation of their contours.
- ◆ Stage 4: Projection of areola and papilla to form a mound above the level of the breast.
- ◆ Stage 5: Mature stage, with projection of papilla only.

Boys: genital development

- ◆ Stage 1: Pre-pubertal.
- ◆ Stage 2: Enlargement of scrotum and testes.
- ◆ Stage 3: Enlargement of penis, initially in length. Further growth of testes and scrotum.
- ◆ Stage 4: Increased size of penis with growth in breadth.
- ◆ Stage 5: Genitalia adult in size and shape.

and axillary hair development. The peak height velocity is at mid-puberty, and by the time that menarche is achieved at an average age of 13 years, growth is slowing, with usually only a further 4 to 6 cm post-menarcheal growth.

In boys puberty does not start much later than in girls, with testicular enlargement. This is followed by growth of the penis and scrotum, followed by pubic and axillary hair development.

Puberty can be assessed using the Tanner ratings, which are shown in Box 10.2.

Racial/economic factors involved in height

In England and Scotland the factors most related to height are the father's social class and employment status, and the sibling size. The Cole data demonstrate that children are tallest in the south of England, becoming progressively shorter towards the north, although Welsh children are the shortest of all. Although studies from Birmingham have shown children of Pakistani origin to be comparable with the 1990 population standards (Kelly et al 1997), other groups have found that Sikhs are in fact taller than European children (Gatrad et al 1994). There are also differences in body proportions between ethnic groups; for instance, Caucasian and Afro-Caribbean children tend to have relatively longer legs than children of Japanese origin.

Despite these differences there are currently no growth charts for ethnic minority groups. These are not thought to be desirable for the following reasons:

◆ There are potential problems in recruiting sufficient numbers.
◆ Secular change in height in these children, with a tendency for their growth patterns to resemble the indigenous population, would mean that frequent revision would be required.
◆ The ethnic groups themselves show considerable variation (for example, there are a number of different racial groups from the Indian subcontinent).
◆ Noting genetic influences (for instance, by measuring parental heights) will often allow racial variations to be taken into account.

Nutrition

The next most important factor affecting growth is probably nutrition, and certainly worldwide malnutrition is the commonest cause of poor growth. The growth of children with severe nutritional deprivation such as kwashiorkor (malnutrition associated with loss of appetite and oedema) or marasmus (malnutrition associated with emaciation and preservation of appetite) is significantly disturbed, although less severe deficiencies may also cause growth problems. It can, however, be difficult to assess the influence of nutrition on poor growth since there are often other factors involved. In addition, deficiencies of vitamins and minerals (such as vitamin D and zinc) may also affect growth.

GROWTH PROBLEMS

The recommendations are that any child whose BMI falls above the top centile (99.6%) or below the bottom centile (0.4%) should be considered for referral even on the basis of a single measurement as these children are significantly over- or underweight; children in the next centile bands may also require referral. However, as there is little data that infant BMI correlates with later BMI it is suggested that infants on extreme centiles should be viewed conservatively, and action taken only if it continues well into the second year.

'Small for dates' and intrauterine growth retardation

'Small for dates'

This is a statistical term, and defines those babies who have birthweights below a specific level for sex and gestational age (some definitions also include maternal height). There is little consensus as to the level at which this should be taken, but a birthweight below the 10th centile for gestational age and sex is often used. In the UK birth length is rarely measured accurately.

Intrauterine growth retardation (IUGR)

This will usually include those children in the 'small for dates' group. However, whereas the 'small for dates' group will, by definition, include the smallest members of a population, IUGR implies that a pathological process is at work. Conversely, a child with a genetic potential at the top of the normal range may still have a weight within the normal range but be significantly growth-restricted. The recognition that children with low birthweights are more likely to develop diabetes mellitus, cardiovascular and respiratory disease, suggesting that factors acting in fetal life and infancy may be important in programming abnormal physiology, have stimulated interest in prevention and early treatment of IUGR.

Broadly, the differential diagnosis of IUGR involves a number of categories:

◆ environment
◆ maternal
◆ placental
◆ fetal.

Environmental factors include:
◆ ethnic
◆ racial
◆ socioeconomic status
◆ malnutrition.

Maternal factors include:
◆ short stature
◆ primiparity
◆ young maternal age
◆ chronic illness including heart, respiratory disease
◆ smoking
◆ alcohol
◆ drugs
◆ nutrition.

Placental factors include:
◆ placental insufficiency
◆ pregnancy-induced hypertension
◆ abrutio placenta.

Fetal factors include:
◆ congenital infection
◆ multiple pregnancies
◆ congenital malformations.

Environmental factors

Birthweight (as a reflection of intrauterine nutrition) is considered to be one of the indices of health within a country. In India, for example, the mean birthweight is 2771 g, with 29% of babies having birthweights below 2500 g. Birthweight tends to be

Table 10.4 The relative causes of IUGR (Dawes 1974)

Cause	Percentage
Vascular disease in mother	33%
Normal variations	10%
Chromosomal/congenital anomalies	10%
Maternal/fetal infections	5%
Drugs/smoking	5%
Placental/cord/uterine	<5%
Unknown	33%

greater in those of higher social class. Mothers of large babies tend to be taller and heavier than controls, and there is a positive correlation between a mother's pre-pregnancy weight and the weight of the fetus. It is also said that there are seasonal factors, with babies born in March to May being heavier than those born in June to August. Firstborn children tend to weigh around 110 g less than subsequent pregnancies, and girls tend to weigh approximately 150 g less than boys.

In a clinical study Dawes (1974) estimated the relative causes of IUGR. The results of the study are shown in Table 10.4.

Although hormonal abnormalities such as growth hormone and thyroid hormone deficiencies, and excess of cortisol and sex hormones are implicated in poor growth, these are relatively rare. As these hormones also have other metabolic functions such as in fat breakdown, as a rule these children are short and fat, whereas children with short stature secondary to chronic disorders are characteristically short and thin. Children with simple obesity are nearly always tall due to nutritionally derived growth factors.

This can be summarized as follows:

◆ endocrine abnormalities – short and fat
◆ chronic illness – short and thin
◆ simple obesity – tall and fat.

Chronic illness

Chronic disorders commonly cause impairment of growth to varying degrees. There are two major ways in which growth may be affected:

◆ growth delay
◆ absolute stunting of growth.

The former is common in normal children as well as in those with chronic disorders, and it also suggests a degree of reversibility in that the growth is put 'on hold'. The latter, on the other hand, suggests that the process is irreversible. In spinal irradiation for malignant disease, for instance, the loss of final height is 5.5 to 9 cm, depending on the age of irradiation (Shalet et al 1987). It is possible that the disease process initially produces growth delay, and that the absolute stunting only occurs when the disease process has been continuing for some time.

SUMMARY

◆ Growth is a critical indicator of child health.
◆ Growth is a complex process, involving a number of different factors, including environment, nutrition and illness.
◆ These factors affect an individual's ability to achieve his or her genetic potential.
◆ Growth failure may either be a primary problem or secondary to an underlying disorder.
◆ In assessing growth, it is important to realize that it is under different controls (both hormonal and nutritional) at different times of life.
◆ Measurements of growth and nutrition are usually simple to perform, inexpensive and reproducible.
◆ The term 'failure to thrive' is a term usually reserved for poor weight gain in the first years of life.

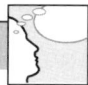

Questions

Answers are given in Appendix 2.

A 15-year-old boy has attended clinic for the last few years. His growth has been poor and his height is below the 3rd centile. There are no abnormalities except that he is pre-pubertal.

1. What further data would you require?
2. What initial investigations could be performed?
3. What is the likely diagnosis?

FURTHER READING

Cox L 1992 A guide to measurement and assessment of growth in children. Castlemead Publications, Ware

REFERENCES

Brook C 1971 Determination of body composition of children from skinfold measurements. Archives of Disease in Childhood 46:182–184

Cole T J 1995 Conditional reference charts to assess weight gain in British infants. Archives of Disease in Childhood 73:8–16

Cole T J, Freeman J V, Preece M A 1995 Body mass index reference curves for the UK, 1990. Archives of Disease in Childhood 73:25–29

Cooney K, Pathak U, Watson A 1994 Infant growth charts. Archives of Disease in Childhood 71:159–160

Dawes G S 1974 General discussion in size at birth. In: Elliot K, Knight J (eds) CBI Foundation Symposium 27. Associated Scientific, Amsterdam

Freeman J V, Cole T J, Chinn S, Jones P R M, White E M, Preece M A 1995 Cross-sectional stature and weight reference curves for the UK, 1990. Archives of Disease in Childhood 73:17–24

Gatrad A R, Birch N, Hughes M 1994 Pre-school weights and heights of Europeans and five sub-groups of Asians in Birmingham. Archives of Disease in Childhood 71:207–210

Gregory J W, Greene S A, Scrimgeour C M, Rennie M J 1991 Body water measurement in growth disorders: a comparison of bioelectrical impedance and skinfold thickness techniques with isotope dilution. Archives of Disease in Childhood 66:220–222

Greulich W W, Pyle S T 1959 Radiographic atlas of skeletal development of hand and wrist. Stanford University Press, California

Hall D M B 1996 Growth monitoring. In: Hall D M B (ed) Health for all children. Oxford University Press, Oxford

Kelly A M, Shaw N J, Thomas A M C, Pynsent P B, Baker D J 1997 Growth of Pakistani children in relation to the 1990 growth standards. Archives of Disease in Childhood 77:401–405

NHS Executive 1996 Child health in the community: a guide to good practice. NHS, London

Schilg S, Hulse T 1997 Growth monitoring and assessment in the community. Child Growth Foundation, London

Shalet S M, Gibson B, Swindell R, Pearson D 1987 Effect of spinal irradiation on growth. Archives of Disease in Childhood 62:461–464

Tanner J M, Whitehouse R H 1962 Standards for subcutaneous fat in British children. Percentiles for thickness of skinfolds over triceps and below scapula. British Medical Journal 1:446–450

Tanner J M, Whitehouse R H 1975 Revised standards for triceps and subscapular skinfolds for British children. Archives of Disease in Childhood 50:142–145

Tanner J M, Whitehouse R H, Takaishi M 1966 Standards from birth to maturity for height, weight height velocity and weight velocity for British children in 1965. Archives of Disease in Childhood 41:454–471

11 Nutritional support for children in the community

Chris Holden   Tracey Johnson   Debra Caney

Part I   Enteral Nutrition

KEY ISSUES

- Consequences of malnutrition
- Choice of feeds
- Continuous versus bolus feeding
- Equipment usage
- Home enteral feeding programme
- Monitoring and follow-up
- Family support

INTRODUCTION

Poor nutrition often complicates many childhood illnesses. Increasingly, home enteral feeding is being used to achieve growth and development and to ensure the child can be cared for in the home. Part 1 of this chapter focuses upon the indications for home enteral feeding and gives an overview of feeds in use, feeding equipment and procedures. Emphasis is placed upon training families and support initiatives required for home enteral nutrition. Case studies with questions and answers are used to develop the reader's skills and increase awareness of the issues facing the child and the family.

Enteral nutrition is the method of supplying nutrients to the gastrointestinal tract. It is the term often used to describe nasogastric, gastrostomy and jejunostomy feeding, although it can also include food and drink taken orally.

Enteral feeding is the preferred method of providing nutritional support to children who have a functioning gastrointestinal tract, with parenteral nutrition reserved for children with severely compromised gut function. It is safer and easier to administer than parenteral nutrition to children in hospital and at home, and can be adapted to meet the individual requirements of infants and children.

Some children require total nutrition via a nasogastric, gastrostomy or jejunostomy tube, whereas others require nutritional support to supplement their poor oral intake or to meet their increased nutritional requirements. Enteral feeding may be short term, but for many children it can be a long-term or even lifelong method of feeding. As a result of these diverse indications for enteral feeding, regimens need to be adaptable to ensure each child receives the vital nutrients he or she requires for normal growth and development.

CONSEQUENCES OF MALNUTRITION

Figures 11.1 and 11.2 show a child before and after enteral feeding. Undernutrition in children has a number of important consequences.

Impaired brain growth and development

The brain grows rapidly in the first year of life, and a poor nutrient intake at this crucial time can affect

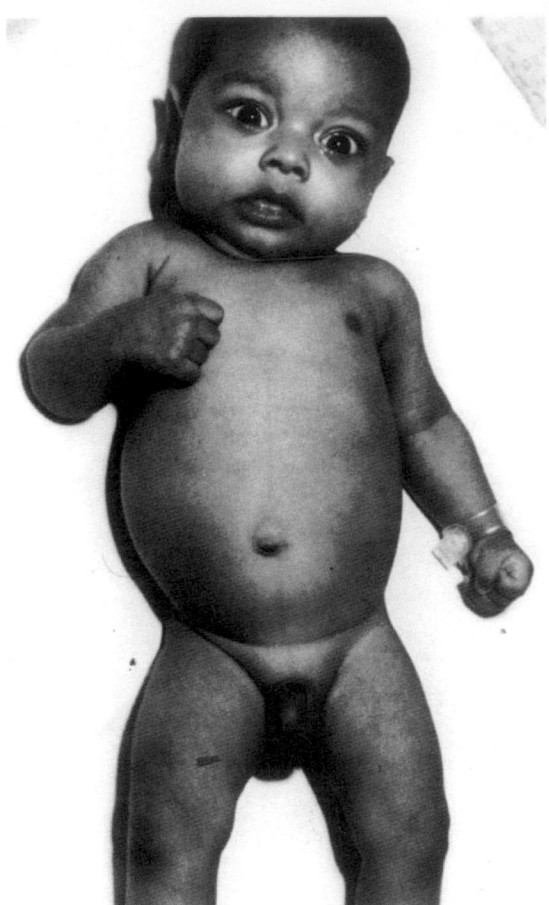

Figure 11.2 After enteral feeding. (Reproduced with permission of Birmingham Children's Hospital.)

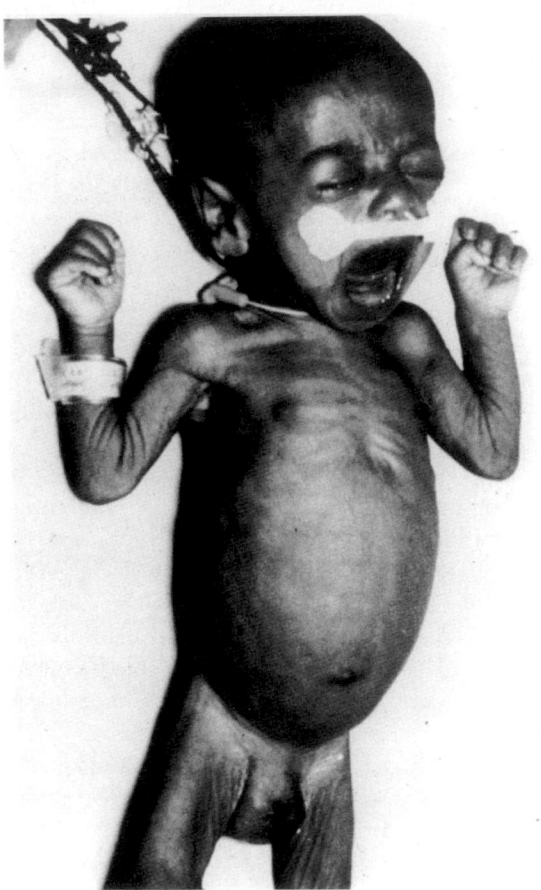

Figure 11.1 Before enteral feeding. (Reproduced with permission of Birmingham Children's Hospital.)

brain growth (Wigglesworth 1969, Winick 1987). In addition, gross motor development is significantly delayed in children who have been undernourished in the first year of life, although there are no long-term problems. Studies have also shown that poor nutrition, reflected in poor growth, affects cognitive development (Booth 1991). Improved nutritional status will reverse cognitive deficits with no long-term difficulties.

Impaired gastrointestinal function

Malnutrition can result in changes to gastrointestinal function. In severe cases there can be villous atrophy, reduced disaccharidase and pancreatic enzyme activity and altered intestinal bacteria, which can all lead to malabsorption and worsening failure to thrive.

Increased susceptibility to infection

Infections are more frequent in children with malnutrition, due to immunological abnormalities. These in turn can exacerbate the effects of poor nutrition with further loss of appetite, increase in metabolic rate and nutritional requirements, and diarrhoea. Catch-up growth becomes difficult to achieve, with each episode of infection leading to further deterioration in nutritional status.

Impaired growth and delayed puberty

The early effect of undernutrition is weight loss and wasting. More prolonged malnutrition can result in growth failure. This is seen commonly in children with chronic illnesses and severe developmental delay who have long-standing nutritional inadequacies. Undernutrition during adolescence delays puberty and the rapid growth spurt of the early teenage years.

Altered mood and depression

Children affected with malnutrition frequently become weak and apathetic. Good nutrition is essential to maintain the mental well-being of children whilst keeping them interested in their environment and able to benefit from the usual learning experiences of childhood.

Specific nutrient deficiencies

The majority of clinical micronutrient deficiencies in childhood are rare. Others, such as iron deficiency, are more commonly seen. Children with a globally inadequate nutritional intake will often show signs of iron deficiency anaemia resulting from a poor intake of iron-rich foods.

Table 11.1 shows indications for enteral feeding.

Table 11.1 Indications for enteral feeding

Indication	Examples
Inability to suck or swallow	Neurological handicap and degenerative disorders Severe developmental delay Trauma Ventilated child
Anorexia associated with chronic illness	Cystic fibrosis Inflammatory bowel disease Liver disease Chronic renal failure Congenital heart disease Inherited metabolic disease
Increased requirements	Cystic fibrosis Congenital heart disease Malabsorption syndromes (e.g. short gut syndrome, liver disease)
Congenital abnormalities	Tracheo-oesophageal fistula Oesophageal atresia Oro-facial malformations
Primary disease management	Crohn's disease Severe gastro-oesophageal reflux Short bowel syndrome Glycogen storage disease Very long chain fatty acid disorders

Table 11.2 Enteral feeding routes

Method	Advantages	Disadvantages
Nasogastric	Short-term feeding	Tube re-insertion may: • be distressing to child/family/carer and nurse • easily be removed by child/baby • entail risk of aspiration • cause discomfort to nasopharynx • have psychosocial implications
Nasojejunal	Less risk of aspiration Short-term feeding	Difficulty of insertion Radiographic check of position (Pobiel et al 1994) Risk of perforation Abdominal pain and diarrhoea if continuous feeding is not used Discomfort in nasopharynx Reflux of bile is facilitated
Gastrostomy	Cosmetically more acceptable to some children and families Easily hidden Long-term feeding	Increase reflux if present Local skin irritation Infection Granulation tissue Leakage Gastric distension Stoma closes within a few hours if accidentally removed
Gastrojejunal	Facilitates placement beyond ligament of Treitz Provides gastric decompression while feeding into jejunum	Precipitation of bile into stomach Regular gastric aspiration required
Jejunostomy	Reduced risk of aspiration Long-term feeding	Risk of perforation Constant infusion of feed required Bacterial overgrowth Dumping syndrome can occur

Routes of feeding

The main routes of feeding into the gastro-intestinal tract include nasogastric, nasojejunal, gastrostomy, gastrojejunal and jejunal feeding. Table 11.2 outlines the advantages and disadvantages of each route.

CHOICE OF FEEDS

There is a wide variety of nutritionally complete paediatric feeds available for enteral feeding. The feed needs to be selected to meet the specific requirements of each individual child. The choice of feed is dependent on a number of different factors:

◆ age
◆ gut function
◆ specific nutrient requirements
◆ dietary restrictions (e.g., milk-free, low protein)
◆ route of administration
◆ prescribability and cost.

Standard polymeric feeds are available as well as a wide range of highly specialized formulae for specific disease states (e.g., cow's milk allergy, lactose intolerance, liver disease, renal disease,

Table 11.3 Choice of feeds

	Normal gut function	Impaired gut function
Infants	Breast milk or normal infant formulae +/– calorie supplements or nutrient-dense infant formula (e.g., Infatrini, SMA High Energy)	Hydrolyzed protein formula +/– calorie supplements (e.g. Pregestimil, Peptijunior, Nutramigen) or modular feed
1–6 years (8–20 kg)	Standard paediatric enteral feed e.g. Nutrini, Paediasure (1 kcal/ml), Nutrini Extra (1.5 kcal/ml)	Hydrolyzed protein formulae +/– calorie supplements (e.g. Pepdite 2+, MCT Pepdite 2+) or modular feed
6 years + (>20 kg)	Standard adult enteral feed, e.g. Nutrison Standard, Osmolite, Ensure (1 kcal/ml), Nutrison Energy Plus, Fortisip, Ensure Plus (1.5 kcal/ml)	Hydrolyzed protein feeds +/– calorie supplements (e.g. Pepdite 2+, Nutrison-Pepti) or modular feed

inherited metabolic diseases and gastrointestinal disorders). Table 11.3 summarizes the choice of feeds.

Standard enteral feeds

Infants and children who require enteral feeding due to poor intakes alone will in most cases be fed with feeds based on a whole protein. The protein in commercially produced enteral feeds is usually cow's milk protein. Infants will have breast milk or a standard infant formulae (e.g., SMA Gold, Cow and Gate Premium). It may be necessary to increase the energy content of these formulae with the addition of calorie supplements, or to use a nutrient-dense infant formula such as SMA High Energy (SMA Nutrition) or Infatrini (Nutricia) (Clarke et al 1998).

Older children will have commercially produced standard enteral feeds. Special paediatric feeds are available for the 1 to 6 year age group who weigh between 8 and 20 kg. These feeds are also suitable for older children who are more than 6 years of age but fall within this weight range. For children over 6 years of age and weighing more than 20 kg, standard adult feeds are used to ensure a more appropriate intake of protein, vitamins and minerals. Both paediatric and adult feeds are available in concentrations between 1 kcal/ml and 1.5 kcal/ml.

Some adult feeds have a protein content of 6 g per 100 ml or more. Care must be taken when using these feeds, even in children who weigh more than 20 kg. Children troubled with constipation may benefit from an enteral feed supplemented with fibre, and commercial preparations are available for both 1 to 6 year-olds and older children, but only as 1.0 kcal/ml feeds. Given the large range of products available, it is important that children receiving enteral feeds receive supervision from a paediatric dietitian who will have the knowledge to decide on the most appropriate feed for individual children.

Hydrolyzed protein formulae

Infants and children with impaired gut function who do not tolerate whole protein formulae frequently benefit from the use of hydrolyzed protein feeds. Such feeds have lower allergenicity than standard formulae, and are free of cow's milk and lactose. Many of these formulae also have a proportion of the fat as medium chain triglycerides (MCT), which can be beneficial in children with fat malabsorption (e.g., liver disease, short gut syndrome, protracted diarrhoea). Examples of such formulae are Peptijunior (Cow and Gate) and Pregestimil (Mead Johnson).

A hydrolyzed protein feed is also preferred in children fed via a jejunostomy. In these children, feed enters the intestine distal to the site of release of pancreatic enzymes and bile, and malabsorption of standard feeds can occur as a result of inadequate digestion. In this situation, hydrolyzed feeds are tolerated well.

Modular feeds

If a commercial formula is unable to meet the specific requirements of an infant or child it is possible to formulate a feed from separate ingredients. This allows a choice of protein, fat and carbohydrate to meet the nutritional goals and to comply with the dietary restrictions of individual patients. These feeds are most commonly used in gastroenterology, hepatology, nephrology and inherited metabolic disease. Although modular feeds allow for flexibility, they are expensive and time-consuming to prepare and should be used only when dietary management with ready-made formulae is not possible. It can also take several days to establish a child on a full-strength modular feed.

There is a greater risk of bacterial contamination and mistakes during feed preparation. Ideally, feeds should be prepared in a dedicated special feed unit in hospital and parents should be carefully instructed on the preparation of feeds for home.

Feed thickeners

Gastro-oesophageal reflux is common in infancy and in children with neurological handicap. In combination with drug therapy and positioning, feed thickeners can be helpful in reducing vomiting. Feed thickeners can also be used as an addition to enteral feeds that would otherwise separate out when left to stand. For example, 0.5% Nestargel added to a comminuted chicken feed will keep the ingredients in suspension and allow it to be delivered as a continuous infusion without blocking the tube.

A number of feed thickeners that can be added to enteral feeds are available. Although many thickeners are stable, some continue to thicken over time and may be unsuitable if feed is delivered by continuous infusion. It may also be difficult to deliver a thickened feed via a gravity feeding system, and careful syringe feeding may be necessary. Table 11.4 lists some thickening agents.

CONTINUOUS VERSUS BOLUS FEEDING

Tube feeding can be given continuously via an enteral feeding pump, as boluses or a combination of both. A regimen should be chosen to meet the individual requirements of the child. In most cases it can be tailored to a practical method of feeding for home, to cause minimum disruption to the child's lifestyle and that of the family/carer.

Continuous feeding

Generally children will tolerate a slow, continuous infusion of feed better than bolus feeds, and this method is frequently chosen when enteral feeding is first started. Potentially there are fewer problems with intolerance when small feed

Table 11.4	Thickening agents					
	Instant Carobel (Cow and Gate)	**Nestargel (Nestlé)**	**Thixo-D (Sutherland Health)**	**Thick and Easy (Fresenius)**	**Nutilis (Nutricia)**	**Vitaquick (Vitaflo Ltd)**
Orally	Yes	Yes	Yes	Yes	Yes	Yes
Bolus	Yes	Yes	Yes	Yes	Yes	Yes
Continuous	Yes, but thickens slightly with time	Yes	Yes	Yes	Yes	Yes
Comments	Energy source 2.5 kcal/g	Needs to be boiled with water	Energy source 3.9 kcal/g	Energy source 3.6 kcal/g	Energy source 3.6 kcal/g	Energy source 4 kcal/g

volumes are infused continuously, and there is less time commitment for ward staff and for parents/carers at home. Mobility is also affected but is minimized by the use of portable feeding pumps, particularly for children who are on continuous feeding for longer than 12 hours.

There are situations where continuous feeding is essential. Feeds given through a feeding jejunostomy should always be delivered by continuous infusion. The stomach acts as a reservoir for food in the normally fed child, regulating the amount of food that is delivered to the small intestine. Feed given as a bolus into the jejunum can cause abdominal pain, diarrhoea and dumping syndrome, resulting from rebound hypoglycaemia. Other situations where continuous feeding is essential include the following:

◆ Severe gastro-oesophageal reflux can be managed with a slow continuous infusion of feed as an adjunct to anti-reflux medication and positioning.
◆ Infants and children with malabsorption will benefit from a continuous infusion of feed. This will slow transit time and may improve symptoms of diarrhoea, steatorrhoea and abdominal cramps and help to promote adequate weight gain.
◆ In children with protracted diarrhoea and short bowel syndrome, continuous enteral feeding with a specialized formula often forms the basis of medical management. Continuous tube feeding with an elemental formula is a well-established treatment option for children with Crohn's disease, to induce remission of disease.
◆ Infants and children with glycogen storage disease Type 1 require a constant supply of dietary glucose to maintain their blood glucose levels within normal limits. Continuous overnight nasogastric feeding is used to provide glucose overnight until children are established on cornstarch therapy at 2 to 3 years of age.

Intermittent bolus feeding

Bolus tube feeding is successfully used in many children requiring enteral feeding both in hospital and at home. Giving boluses three to four-hourly throughout the day via the nasogastric or gastrostomy tube mimics a physiologically normal feeding pattern and can be adapted to fit in with family mealtimes. It is more time-consuming than continuous feeding, but is the preferred method for many families with children on long-term feeding, as it gives them greater freedom and mobility.

Bolus feeding is recommended for children who have had a surgical anti-reflux procedure and are often unable to vomit. Large volumes of feed from a continuous infusion can accumulate in the stomach and remain undetected in children who have gastric stasis or poor gastrointestinal motility. This can lead to gastric rupture. Bolus feeding with a gravity feeding pack will prevent overfilling of the stomach. Tubes are routinely aspirated before each feed and feed will be prevented from entering the stomach from the feeding chamber if the stomach is already full.

Other situations where bolus feeding is recommended include the following:

◆ Children who frequently remove their nasogastric tube will also benefit from bolus feeding. Children can be constantly supervised during the feed, avoiding the risk of aspiration if the tube is inadvertently dislodged.
◆ Children with an oesophagostomy who are sham-fed should preferably receive bolus feeds to coincide with their oral feeds.
◆ Enteral feeds may interfere with the absorption of medication. Bolus feeding will provide a period of time before and after the medication to allow optimal absorption.

Therefore, certain situations dictate a preferred feeding regimen, but a flexible approach to feeding should be taken wherever possible. This enables the child to maintain his or her usual day-to-day activities and for the family/carer to experience minimal disruption to their lifestyle and routines. Flexibility is especially important in children with long-term feeding requirements who, as time passes, will need a feed that is appropriate to their age and changing nutritional requirements. A feeding regimen that is adaptable will help them grow and develop (Table 11.5).

EQUIPMENT USAGE

There is a huge amount of feeding equipment available on the paediatric market, so the discussion about products cannot be all-inclusive, but is intended as an overview for the reader. Enteral feeding tubes have evolved considerably over the last 10 years. It is important that the parent/carer and the child are aware of the options available to them and are given choices. It is also essential that the parent/carer is given written protocols and information regarding the specific care of tubes and button devices used and what to do if the devices accidentally fall out. (Appendices 11.1 and 11.2 detail the requirements for ideal tubes and buttons, and describe some products currently available for enteral feeding.)

Enteral feeding pumps

The availability of simple portable infusion pumps has enabled many families/carers to feed their child at home. Portable systems have revolutionized enteral feeding for children, enabling many children who require more than 12 hours of feeding to enjoy mobility, increased freedom and

Table 11.5 Choosing a suitable feeding regimen

Regimen	Example
Bolus top-up feeding	**Congenital heart disease** Bottle-feeds are not completed due to breathlessness and remaining feed is topped up via the nasogastric tube
Exclusive bolus feeding	**Long-term feeding for children with a neurological handicap** Daytime bolus feeding can allow flexibility and mobility and may provide a regimen that fits in with the family mealtimes **Post-fundoplication** Bolus feeding is the method of choice for children following a surgical anti-reflux procedure **Sham feeding** Children who are sham fed should receive a bolus feed to coincide with their oral feed
Combination of bolus and continuous feeding	**Chronic illness** Children with anorexia associated with chronic illness may receive a large proportion of their nutrition via a nasogastric or gastrostomy tube Daytime boluses allow for a normal meal pattern and overnight feeding with a feeding pump reduces the time commitment at night for parents/carer and ward staff
Overnight feeding only	**Supplementary nutrition** Children who require enteral feeding to supplement their poor oral intake or to meet their increased nutritional requirements are usually fed overnight only. This allows the children to maintain a normal daytime eating pattern, while still providing the nutritional support they require
Continuous feeding only	**Primary disease management** Gastro-oesophageal reflux Malabsorption syndromes (e.g. short gut) Crohn's disease Glycogen storage disease

independence. (Box 11.1 highlights features of an ideal pump for paediatric use.)

HOME ENTERAL FEEDING PROGRAMME

'Training of the family/carer is one of the key aspects of hospital pre-discharge care' (Holden & MacDonald 1997, p 218). Special needs of the child and family/carer should be identified, and arrangements should be made to fulfil these needs prior to hospital discharge. Compromise is usually necessary to adapt feeding regimens to suit the family's/carer's lifestyle, whilst ensuring the child receives sufficient nutrition. Townsley & Robinson

---

Box 11.1 Ideal enteral feeding pump

Features:

◆ Easy to operate
◆ Durable
◆ Small/lightweight
◆ Portable
◆ Accurate (5–10%) (constant infusion available)
◆ Option of bolus feeding available
◆ Easy to clean
◆ Suitability of controls
◆ Tamper proof
◆ Low noise level, particularly if nocturnal feeding
◆ Alarm: occlusion/empty and low battery
◆ Reliability essential

Teaching material available:

◆ Step-by-step guides to setting up the system
◆ Written instructions on side of pump and also in pamphlet form
◆ Pamphlet information
◆ Training video

Purchasing:

◆ Servicing – purchasers should identify servicing arrangements
◆ Information available from Medical Devices Agency
◆ Cost of pump and disposables to be considered

(1997) emphasize that families/carers should have one key person with whom they can liaise about all aspects of home enteral tube feeding. Prior to enteral feeding being established, all parents/carers should receive verbal and written information, not only regarding the practical aspects of tube feeding, but also the social and emotional impact it may have (Chaplen 1997).

Holden (1994) has identified that the social and emotional impact of tube feeding is often overlooked or grossly underestimated by health and social care professionals. It is helpful to focus on the effectiveness of communication skills in relation to the information provided for families (Bailey & Caldwell 1997).

Aims of a home enteral feeding programme

◆ Facilitate planned nutrition
◆ Facilitate patient and family autonomy and preference as to the route of feeding and plan of care
◆ Ensure safe, trouble-free maintenance of enteral feeding
◆ Maximize lifestyle as well as disease management (Sidney & Torbet 1995).

Teaching home enteral feeding

Programmes of care should be based upon detailed assessment, planning implementation and evaluation, with enteral feeding planned to fit in with the family's/carer's lifestyle. Holden et al (1997b) recommend that teaching sessions with the family/carer should be short to minimize stress. Increasingly, pictorial teaching aids have been used to help non-English speaking families/carers and those unable to read and follow written guidelines (Sexton et al 1996, Shah 1994).

Teaching programmes should include:

◆ detailed information about the necessity for home enteral feeding and likely duration
◆ safety aspects of care
◆ checking tube placement
◆ microbiological issues for consideration
◆ hand-washing techniques
◆ feed preparation
◆ familiarization with feeding equipment
◆ advice about social and practical implications of feeding for the child and family/carer

◆ problem-solving advice and what to do in an emergency

◆ advice regarding oral stimulation during feeding for families/carers with babies or small children

◆ telephone contacts of hospital and community staff

◆ detailed information about how to obtain equipment: for example, via home care companies or community staff.

Psychological preparation

Holden et al (1997a) reviewed the psychological preparation of 48 children undergoing home enteral nutrition by nasogastric tube. They emphasized that detailed preparation of families/carers takes time, and that passing of a nasogastric tube was seen as very distressing to both parents/carers and children. The authors concluded that children should be prepared for painful procedures and followed up sensitively according to their needs. Key areas likely to cause distress must be identified. A frank discussion and explanation should take place with regard to the length and degree of discomfort and pain of having a tube. Published literature incorporating the views and opinions of adolescents may be helpful (Paul et al 1993) (Figures 11.3–11.5). Information about problems with oral feeding, getting on with friends, sleeping at night with the pump and going to the toilet frequently should be discussed. Appendix 11.3 shows a checklist used as part of a home enteral teaching programme.

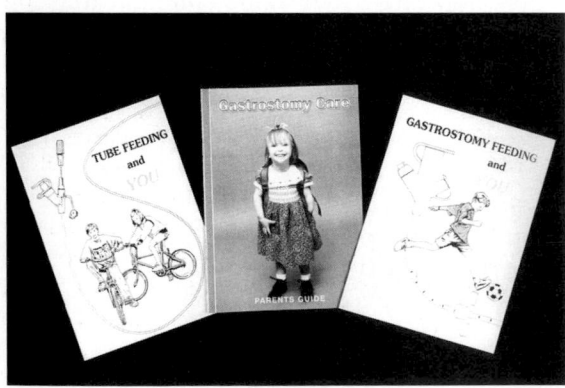

Figure 11.3 Psychological preparation (1).

For younger patients, it is important that, when children are prepared by play therapists, the procedure should be done immediately, as a delay may mean that the child becomes more upset (Holden et al 1997a). Parents/carers have commented that the play therapists helped their children through play, by providing them with an outlet for aggression and anger. Box 11.2 shows

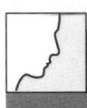

> **Box 11.2** Preparing a child for insertion of a nasogastric, gastrostomy or jejunostomy tube
>
> **Step One: Pre-preparation**
> Inform play therapist.
> Assemble materials: e.g. pens, paper and booklets.
> Greet child and introduce yourself (name, title and what you do).
> Explain the reason for meeting.
> Explore the child's hospital experience, past and present, by talking, drawing and playing.
>
> **Step Two: Preparation**
> Encourage the child to describe his or her own body (e.g. tummy, nose and mouth) by talking, drawing, pointing and using dolls.
> Direct the discussion towards nasogastric/ gastrostomy/jejunostomy tube feeding and the passing/insertion of the tube, saying when it will happen and who will be doing it.
> Check out and explore the child's knowledge of specific body parts and the functions of swallowing, breathing and digestion, by talking and drawing. Use the child's language, as well as the correct names for body parts, the equipment and the procedure.
> Look through the equipment with the child, encouraging questions, describing what it is for and how it might feel.
> Give the child clear information on how he or she can help to make the process easier. Encourage the child to think of ways of coping, e.g. deciding who to have with them. It is important for the child to decide what does or does not help. This step may require some suggestions from you.
>
> **Remember: Throughout the discussion always describe what is actually going to happen and how it may feel. Stick to the facts.**

some suggested guidelines for preparing a child for insertion of a feeding tube.

Implications for practice

Parents/carers often prefer gastrostomy feeding to nasogastric tube feeding as it avoids the psychosocial implications of re-passing nasogastric tubes, which both they and their child find distressing. Some children successfully pass their own nasogastric tubes at night and remove their tube in the daytime. This helps them retain control of the procedure.

Gastrostomy feeding is now widely used for long-term feeding. Whatever route is considered suitable, in-depth counselling for the child and family/carer is important, and advantages and disadvantages of treatment should be discussed (Holden et al 1997c).

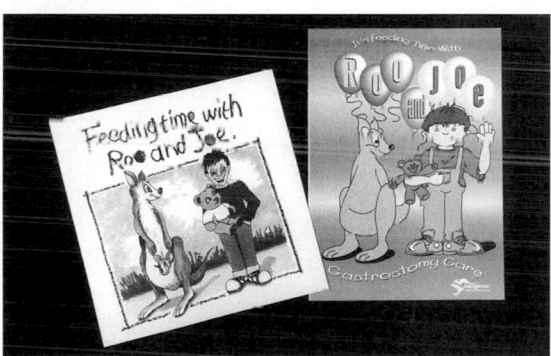

Figure 11.4 Psychological preparation (2).

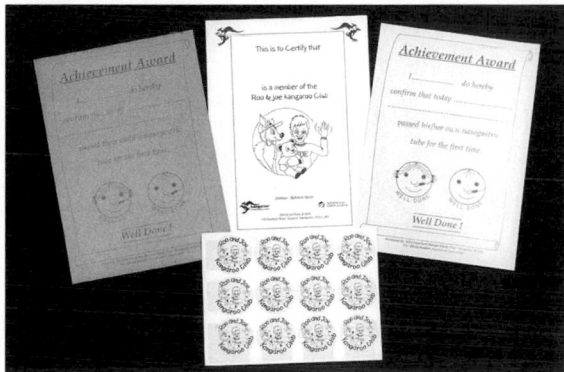

Figure 11.5 Psychological preparation (3).

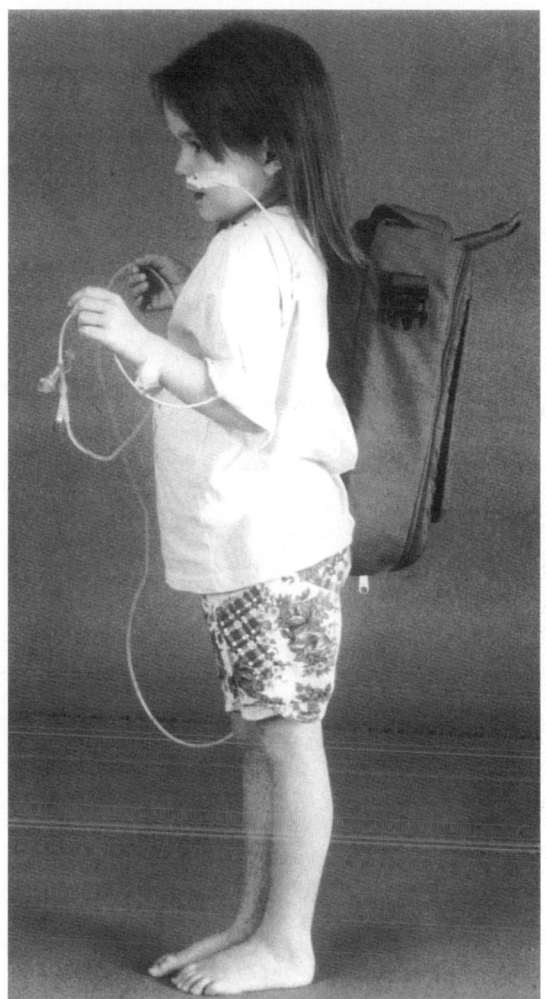

Figure 11.6 Home enterally fed patient with portable feeding system. (Reproduced with permission of Birmingham Children's Hospital.)

Pictorial assisted teaching tools for families

More and more children are successfully receiving enteral feeding in the home (Sidney & Torbet 1995), and teaching programmes are increasingly being devised to support this. It is clear that material used has a heavy bias towards written English, and is therefore not useful for families/carers who use other languages or who cannot understand written guidelines. The United Kingdom is a multicultural, multiracial, multireligion, multilingual society. The Action for

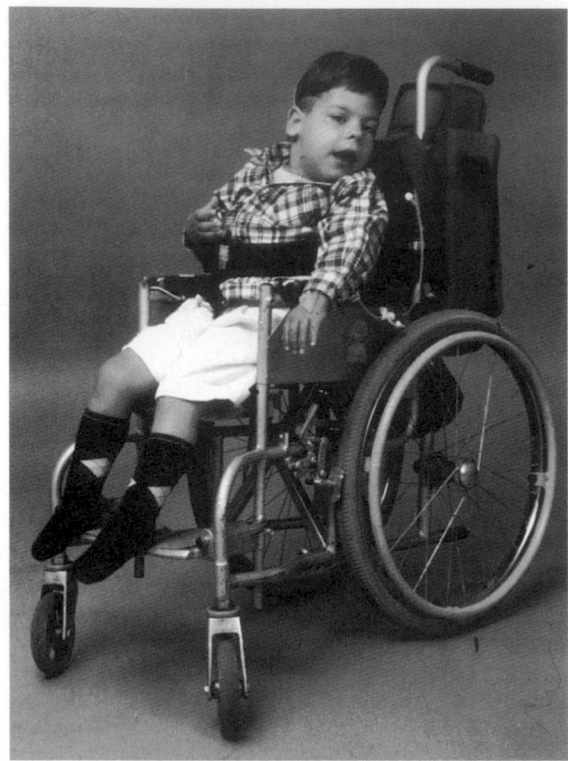

Figure 11.7 Home gastrostomy fed patient. (Reproduced with permission of Birmingham Children's Hospital.)

Sick Children Report 1993 has demonstrated that there are considerable communication difficulties for some families/carers. Effective training programmes must be developed with interpreters, to ensure equality of training for all. Sexton et al (1996) have developed numerous enteral pictorial teaching tools. And the management of all home nutritional programmes should be designed to ensure that the child and family are equal partners in care and that the family are active participants in all discussions.

Training models

Elaine Sexton and Chris Holden have developed a clear training model for parents/carers to show them how to insert nasogastric gastrostomy tubes. This was designed to enable parents/carers to visualize the correct positioning of nasogastric and gastrostomy tubes and buttons and also to practise insertion techniques in the training model.

Families have reported that this training model gave them invaluable practice and increased their confidence and understanding. Figures 11.8–11.10 show the model in use.

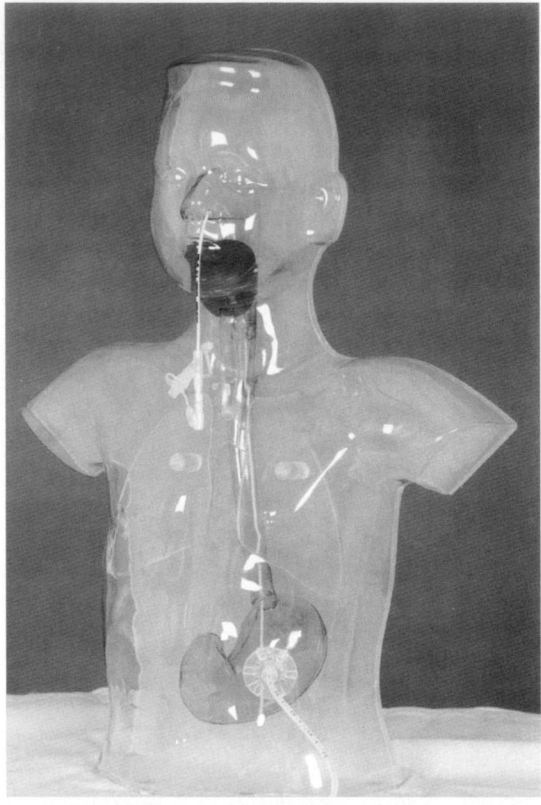

Figure 11.8 The training model. (Reproduced with permission of Birmingham Children's Hospital.)

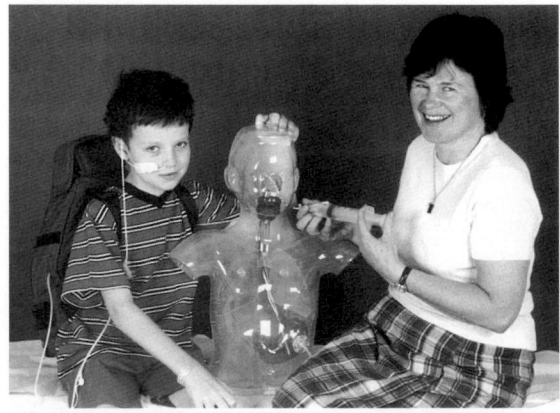

Figure 11.9 The use of a training model (1). (Reproduced with permission of Birmingham Children's Hospital.)

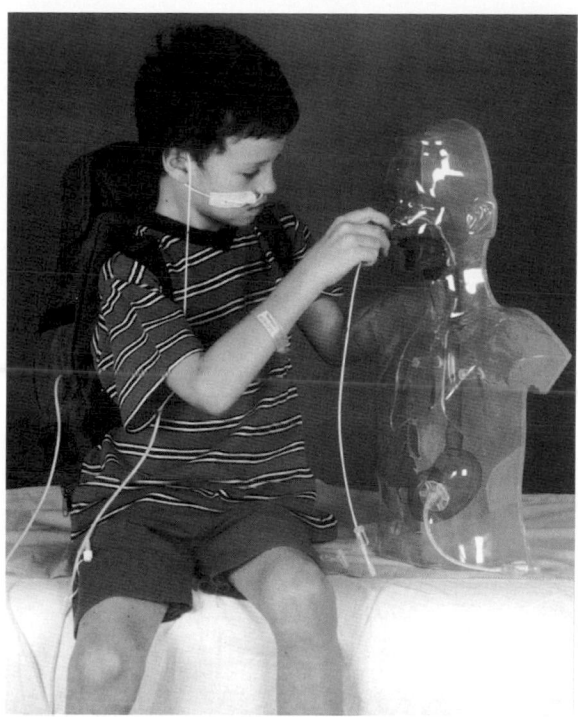

Figure 11.10 The use of a training model (2). (Reproduced with permission of Birmingham Children's Hospital.)

Discharge planning protocols should be developed to ensure effective home enteral feeding is achieved (see Appendix 11.4).

Microbiological issues regarding feeding

Studies have demonstrated that feed contamination is common in the home (Patchell et al 1994, Patchell et al 1998, Anderton & Nivgough 1991) and can lead to gastroenteritis and septicaemia. Training programmes must therefore include correct hand-washing procedures and clean handling of feeds. Manipulation and handling of feeding systems should ideally be kept to a minimum.

Feed intolerance

Gastrointestinal symptoms are the most common complications of enteral feeding and can lessen the effectiveness of enteral nutrition. With the wide choice of feeds, administration techniques

and enteral feeding devices, it should be possible to minimize gastrointestinal symptoms (Table 11.6).

Maintaining oral feeding skills

Even if children receive all their nutrition through a tube, it is still important to encourage normal feeding by mouth (Feeding Liaison Team 1998). With the exception of children who do not have a safe swallow, oral feeding gives children the chance to learn to like different tastes and textures and to use the lips and tongue. This is particularly important for young babies between 4 and 6 months of age, who are often more willing to taste different foods. If babies miss out on these early experiences of taste and texture they have difficulty accepting them later on. Even a small

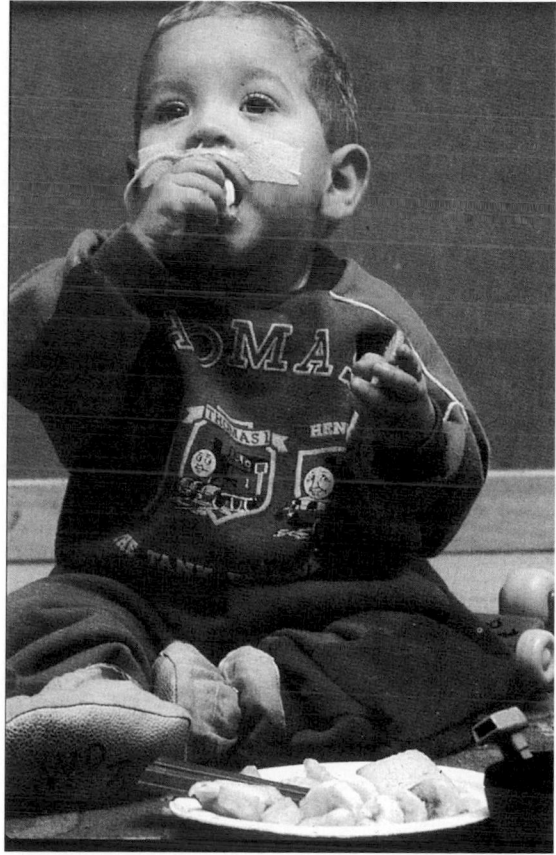

Figure 11.11 Maintaining oral skills. (Reproduced with permission of Birmingham Children's Hospital.)

amount of food will help to prevent the development of feeding problems.

MONITORING AND FOLLOW-UP

Children who are commenced on enteral feeding require monitoring. At the initiation of enteral feeding, goals will be set with respect to an improvement in nutritional status or control of symptoms. Regular follow-up is required to monitor both short-term and longer term progress. As children gain weight and get older their requirements change, and follow-up is essential to ensure they continue to receive adequate nutrition. Both hospital and community staff have a role to play in monitoring a child's progress and helping the family cope with tube feeding at home. The needs of a young infant are quite different to those of a toddler or teenager, and the individual needs of each child should be considered at different

Table 11.6 Feed intolerance

Symptom	Cause	Solution
Diarrhoea	Unsuitable feed in children with impaired gut function	Change to hydrolyzed formula or modular feed
	Excessive infusion rate	Slow infusion rate and increase as tolerated to provide required nutrition
	Intolerance of bolus feeds	Frequent, smaller feeds or change to continuous infusion
	High feed osmolarity	Build up strength of hyperosmolar feeds and deliver by continuous infusion
	Microbial contamination of feed	Use sterile commercially produced feeds wherever possible and prepare other feeds in clean environments
	Drugs (e.g. antibiotics, laxatives)	Consider drugs as a cause of diarrhoea before feed is stopped or reduced
Nausea and vomiting	Excessive infusion rate	Slowly increase rate of feed infusion
	Slow gastric emptying	Correct positioning and drugs
	Constipation	Maintain regular bowel motions with adequate fluid intakes and laxatives
	Medicines given at the same time as feeds	Allow time between giving medicines and giving feeds, or stop continuous feed for a short time when medicines are given
	Psychological factors	Review of feeding behaviour and possible psychology referral
Regurgitation and aspiration	Gastro-oesophageal reflux	Correct positioning, drugs, feed thickener, fundoplication
	Dislodged tubes	Secure tube adequately and test position of tube regularly
	Excessive infusion rate	Slow infusion rate
	Intolerance of bolus feeds	Smaller, more frequent feeds or continuous infusion

stages of the child's development: for instance, when the child attends school or enters adolescence.

Regular follow-up can also be important for the family. Home enteral feeding has a big impact on family life, resulting in both psychological and practical problems which should be addressed regularly (Holden et al 1991). Holden (1994) reviewed the reactions of families to home enteral feeding; the results of this review are summarized in Appendix 11.5. Fatigue, financial and communication problems were highlighted. Townsley and Robinson (1997) have highlighted similar support issues for disabled children requiring home enteral feeding.

Anthropometry

Weight is usually the best short-term indicator of an improvement in nutritional status. In infants this should be recorded daily while in hospital at the initiation of feeding, and on discharge should be monitored weekly and plotted on a centile chart. This allows inadequate or excessive weight gain to be recognized and addressed with appropriate feed changes. The health visitor is often the best person to monitor the weight in the community, using the same set of weighing scales at each visit. Close liaison with a dietitian is necessary to advise on feed changes. Older children should also have regular weight checks, initially weekly but less often in children who require long-term feeding. Disruption to schooling should be minimized and weight can be checked by school nurses. Length or height measurements should also be monitored to illustrate longer term improvements in nutrition and linear growth. Mid-arm circumference and skinfold measurements are also useful, particularly in severely disabled children in whom it is difficult to get accurate measurements of height.

Control of symptoms

Improvement in nutrition may not be the only goal. Enteral feeding may be an essential part of the disease management (see Table 11.1) and symptoms should be monitored (e.g., gastro-oesophageal reflux, diarrhoea).

Dietary assessment

It is useful to assess dietary intake with a 3-day food diary at regular intervals. In children who require very specific dietary requirements or restrictions (e.g., because of metabolic disease or renal disease) these assessments may need to be carried out several times a year, but an annual assessment is usually adequate for most children. This will allow the dietitian to assess the average intake of energy, protein, vitamins, minerals and trace elements and compare this with recommended intakes. It is also a useful tool to assess the proportions of nutrients from tube feeding and other food by mouth.

Blood monitoring

Enteral feeds are formulated to be nutritionally complete, but nutritional adequacy should be checked in children receiving long-term tube feeding with blood tests. Routine analysis of serum albumin, electrolytes and haemoglobin are useful as well as assessment of vitamin, mineral and trace element status. These are particularly important in children with high requirements or malabsorption (e.g., cystic fibrosis or short bowel syndrome). Blood tests can also be useful in assessing response to nutritional therapy in primary disease management. The success of feeding in children with active Crohn's disease can be assessed with monitoring of inflammatory markers (e.g., erythrocyte sedimentation rate (ESR), cero reactive protein (CRP)). In glycogen storage disease, the success of treatment can be measured by regular blood glucose monitoring.

FAMILY SUPPORT

Support groups

Patients receiving Intravenous and Nutritional Therapy (PINNT) is a support group for patients receiving parenteral or enteral nutrition therapy. HALF PINNT is the children's group. The group aims to promote public awareness and understanding of treatments. It also encourages contact between patients, with particular emphasis on the help and encouragement which patients' families/carer who have experience of treatment can give to new children and their families/carer. PINNT assists its members with anything they feel is important. This includes assistance with claiming benefits, an equipment bank which provides members with portable equipment for holidays, and a contact directory of its members for advice and support.

Funding

Health authorities and purchasers should take responsibility for funding and promoting training on home enteral tube feeding.

The funding of home feeding is very complex and remains a significant problem. Enteral feeds are prescribable by the General Practitioner; however, disposable equipment and support staff are generally funded either by specialist hospital departments or purchasing authorities. The funding of care for children with complex needs outside hospital has developed in a very ad hoc way. The British Association of Parenteral and Enteral Nutrition (BAPEN) continues to lobby government to ensure enteral feeding can be managed as a total package so that feeds and the equipment to give it are both prescribable items (Khair 1998). BAPEN encourages the use of homecare companies to provide feeds and equipment delivered to the family's/carer's home.

PART I SUMMARY

Enteral feeding continues to remain essential for some children. It is vital to ensure adequate growth and development. Multidisciplinary approaches to the care of these patients re-

main paramount to ensure children and their families/carers receive adequate support and care.

CASE STUDY: Gemma

Gemma is an 8-year-old child who suffers from severe gastro-oesophageal reflux. She lives with her mother and four younger siblings. Gemma's mum is a housewife. Gemma attends a normal school but misses school frequently as a result of chest infections. Her weight gain is extremely poor and her mother is only able to encourage her to have small amounts to eat. Gemma's Child Health Care growth record shows a gradual deterioration in height and weight. Her recent weight is 22 kg, and her height is 126 cm. Her growth chart is shown in Figure 11.12.

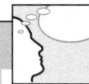

Questions

Answers are given in Appendix 2.

Think about Gemma in detail and answer the following questions.

1. Identify some reasons for giving Gemma enteral feeding.

2. What route would you consider?

3. Which feed would you use, taking into consideration the feeding route? How would feed be administered?

4. What issues do you need to think about when establishing home enteral feeding? For each issue, identify any specific points that need to be considered.

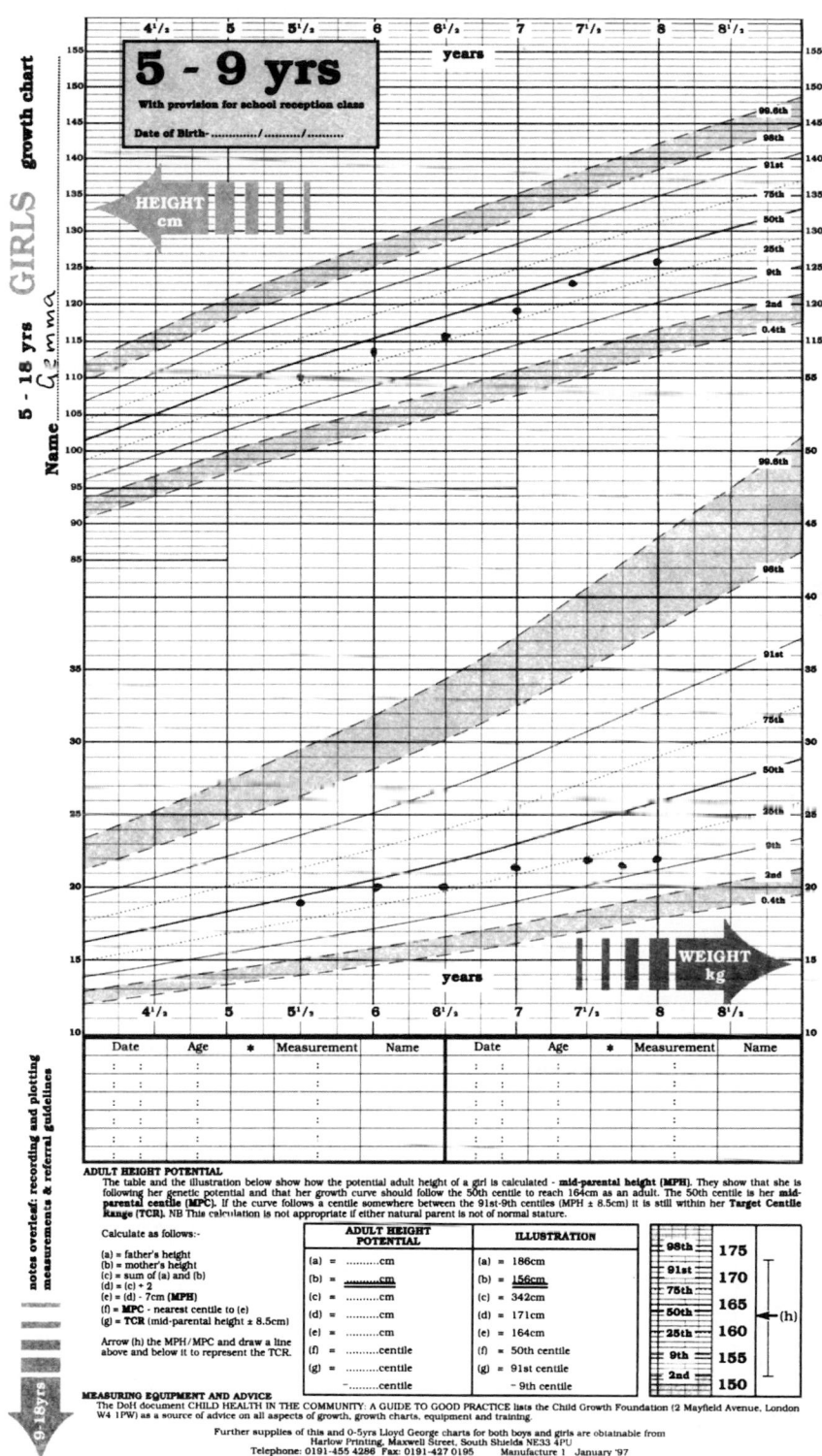

Figure 11.12 Growth chart – Gemma. (© Growth Foundation, reproduced with permission.)

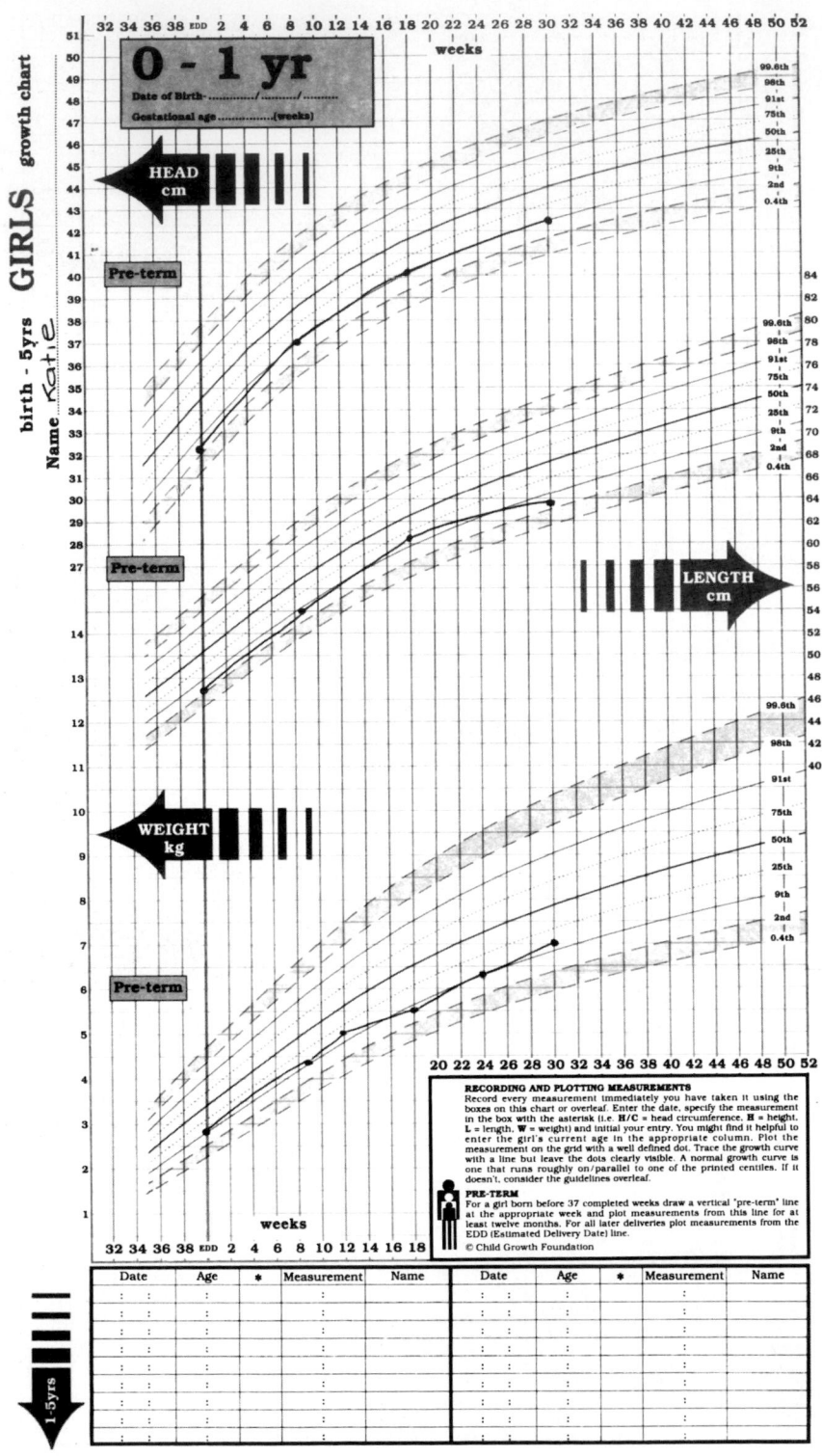

Figure 11.13   Growth chart – Katie (© Growth Foundation, reproduced with permission.)

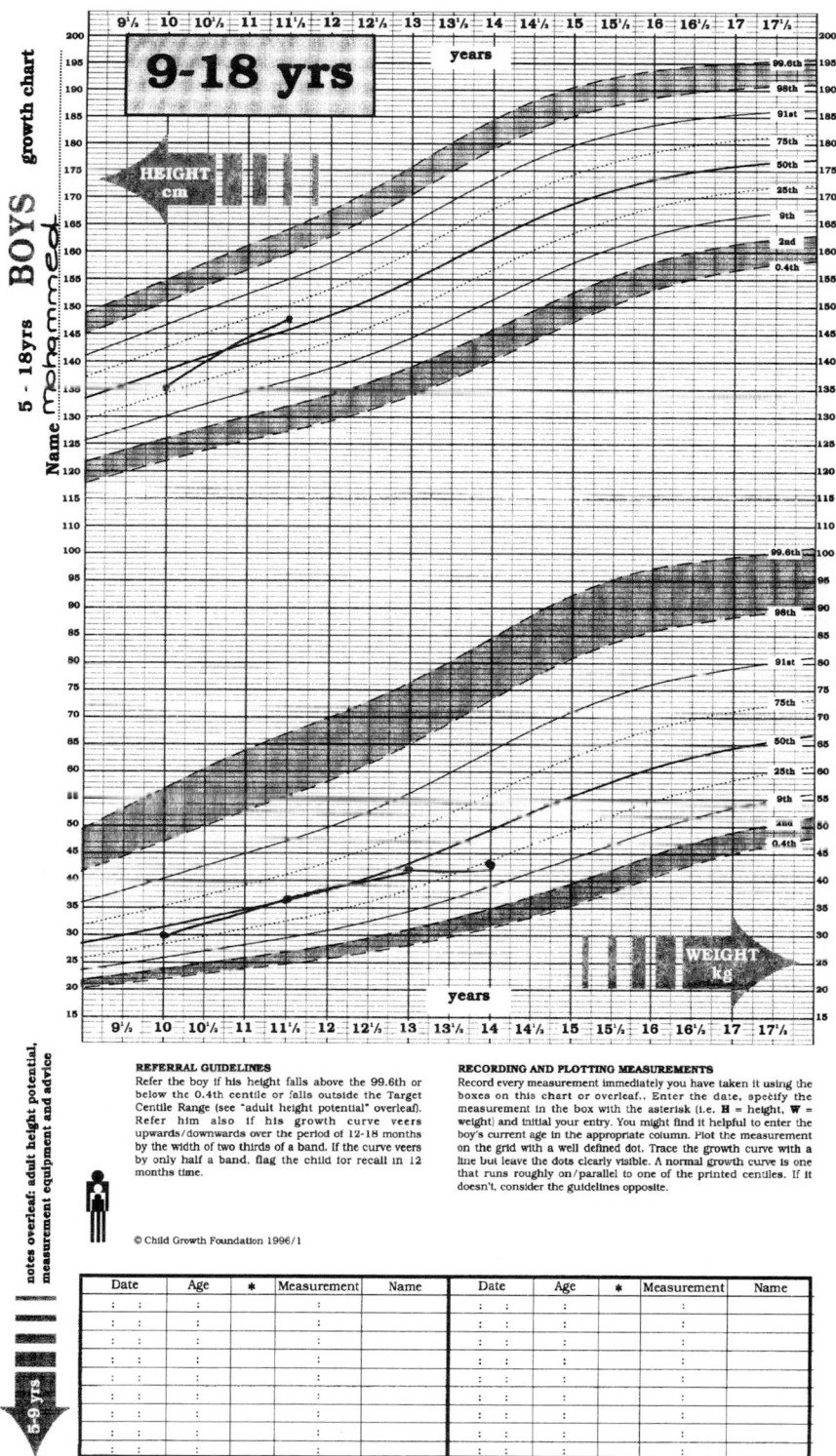

Figure 11.14 Growth chart – Mohammed (© Child Growth Foundation, reproduced with permission.)

CASE STUDY: Katie

Katie is a 6-month-old infant who has congenital heart disease and is awaiting surgery. She is getting increasingly breathless with feeds, but enjoys solids twice a day. Her parents are separated and there are no other siblings. Katie goes to a childminder during the day while her mother is at work. Katie weighs 7 kg (above the 9th centile), her length is 63.5 cm (below the 9th centile) and her head circumference is 42.5 cm (the 9th centile). Katie's growth chart is shown in Figure 11.13.

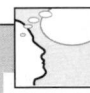

Questions

Answers are given in Appendix 2.

Think about Katie in detail and answer the following questions.

1. Which feed would you use?

2. How is the feed to be given?

3. What issues do you need to think about when establishing home enteral feeding?

CASE STUDY: Mohammed

Mohammed is a 14-year-old with a severe degenerative disorder and is confined to a wheelchair. He attends a special school. He has no swallowing or gag reflex and repeated attempts at oral feeding have resulted in aspiration. His mother is very concerned about recent problems she has had trying to feed him and about Mohammed's general deterioration. Mum speaks Urdu but is unable to understand English. Mohammed's father is in full-time employment. Mohammed's weight is 43 kg. It has not been possible to measure his height because of severe contractures. His growth chart is shown in Figure 11.14.

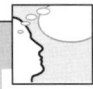

Questions

Answers are given in Appendix 2.

1. How would you assess Mohammed's nutritional status? (Refer to Chapter 10 on nutritional assessment for guidance.)

2. What route of feeding would you consider?

3. How would you monitor Mohammed's care in the community?

4. How would you facilitate safe training for this family?

Part 2 Parenteral Nutrition

INTRODUCTION

Home parenteral nutrition (HPN) is used for paediatric patients with intestinal failure, providing improvements in their quality of life. Patients receiving HPN require the expertise of a multidisciplinary nutritional care team at specialist centres (Beath et al 1995) and primary health care teams.

The objective of prolonged parenteral nutrition is to ensure the normal growth of the child and to offer to the child a quality of life as close as possible to that of other children of the same age, while waiting for an inflammatory syndrome to subside or for residual intestine to adapt, or pending an intestinal transplant (Ricour 1988).

HPN is complex and it carries risks which may be life-threatening. It is essential that detailed discussions with the family/carer occur to ensure that both the advantages and disadvantages of this treatment are highlighted. Avoidance of complications depends upon the child's care at home. Studies undertaken by Bisset et al (1992) and Carlsson et al (1997) emphasize that parents/carer are aware that the survival of their child is dependent upon their skill in delivering the HPN, and many find this a great burden. Despite these problems, all the parents/carer feel that caring for their child at home is very rewarding and infinitely preferable to the child remaining in hospital.

Whilst families/carers can manage the treatment at home, many psychosocial problems arise, and fatigue and financial problems are common. Information sources on a national level regarding this group of patients are run by the British Association for Nutritional Support (BANS), a subgroup of the British Association of Parenteral and Enteral Nutrition (BAPEN). The group's aim is to define the role of home parenteral nutrition in clinical practice (Wood et al 1995, Miller 1999). Data collected include audit of treatment and reviews of prognosis, treatment indications, cost and quality of life.

SUITABILITY OF CHILD AND FAMILY/CARER

Discussion with parents/carer, with the multi-disciplinary team and with a neutral ethical body should take place when permanent dependence on intravenous feeding is anticipated. The indications for home parenteral nutrition are detailed in Table 11.7.

The suitability of a child for home parenteral nutrition is dependent on both medical and social factors, and detailed discussion with the family is therefore essential. (These factors are shown in Box 11.3.)

Although home parenteral nutrition management is technical, the procedure can be successfully managed in the home. Parents/carers need to follow instructions precisely and diligently.

When home parenteral nutrition is considered, the multidisciplinary team must meet to discuss the special individual needs of both the children and family. Simple questions by families can often denote major fears and concerns which must be addressed (Liston 1987). Box 11.4 shows some of the advantages and disadvantages of home parenteral nutrition which should be discussed with the family/carer.

Additional issues when considering home parenteral nutrition include the following:

◆ rationale for home parenteral nutrition and discussion with family
◆ the aims and goals of treatment and expected duration of therapy
◆ financial, social and time commitments for families
◆ regular team meetings with the family are essential to exchange information and concerns
◆ discharge planning protocols for families are essential, detailing individual roles of the multidisciplinary team to facilitate a smooth transition for home (Holden et al 1996).

The main aims of any teaching programme should be to:

◆ teach the administration of home parenteral nutrition, so that it can be performed safely by the family/carer

---

Table 11.7 Indications for home parenteral nutrition. (Ball et al 1993, reproduced with permission of Fresenius Kabi.)

Neonates

Absolute indications	intestinal failure (short gut, functional immaturity, pseudo-obstruction)
	necrotizing enterocolitis
Relative indications	hyaline membrane disease
	promotion of growth in preterm infants
	possible prevention of necrotizing enterocolitis

Older infants and children

Intestinal failure	short gut
	protracted diarrhoea
	chronic intestinal pseudo-obstruction
	post-operative abdominal or cardio-thoracic surgery
	radiation/cytotoxic therapy
Exclusion of luminal nutrients	Crohn's disease
Organ failure	acute renal failure
	acute liver failure
Hyper-catabolism	extensive burns
	severe trauma

Box 11.3 Factors influencing the suitability of home parenteral nutrition

Medical issues

Completion of acute treatment:

◆ diagnostic and surgical procedures
◆ central venous catheter has been placed
◆ biochemistry values are within normal range
◆ the infant or child is free from infection.

Social issues

Parent/carer must be well and must be willing and able to undertake complex treatment.

A suitable home environment should be available:
◆ it should be clean
◆ ideally, the child should have his or her own bedroom
◆ adequate lighting in the bedroom
◆ safe electrical points for intravenous pumps
◆ lever arch or mixer taps available in bathroom for handwashing
◆ storage space for equipment (e.g., refrigerator for solutions)
◆ telephone in house
◆ family should have own transport – if not, an agreed emergency transport plan should be in place.

Box 11.4 Advantages and disadvantages of treatment at home rather than in hospital

Advantages

◆ Prevention of adverse effects of hospitalization for child
◆ Diminished risk of central venous catheter infections (Miller 1999).

Disadvantages

Life-threatening complications include (Puntis 1993, Holden et al 1996):

◆ line sepsis
◆ hepatic dysfunction
◆ loss of venous access
◆ pulmonary embolism.

(These complications can also occur in hospital.)

◆ educate the family/carer regarding potential complications of home parenteral nutrition (Puntis 1993)
◆ allow the baby/child and family/carer to return to as normal a lifestyle as possible.

TRAINING FOR FAMILIES

Individualized training programmes are essential. Ideally, families should be resident in hospital to enable them to get a true picture of all their child's needs in a 24-hour-period. Teaching sessions initially should be short, to help minimize stress and help assimilate information. Training booklets should be available with a section for parents/carers to write notes as training takes place. The training of families/carers should be undertaken by specialist nurses, ideally a nutritional care sister, to ensure highly skilled techniques of training are given. Specialist nurses must ensure up-to-date advice is available for the family/carer. Verbal and written programmes of education should be available (Holden et al 1993). Details of a training programme are shown in Box 11.5.

Teaching videos of parents setting up parenteral nutrition at home can prove invaluable in helping improve parent/carer confidence.

Parents/carer should keep accurate detailed records, recording all treatments. Increasingly, hand-held records, detailing the child's care, are used. This information should include:

◆ medical summary (updated summaries should be sent to parents/carer following each clinic visit)
◆ central venous line (CVL) history
◆ CVL care protocols
◆ feed prescription information
◆ techniques for heparinizing CVL
◆ unblocking CVL
◆ protocol for line sepsis
◆ how to respond to emergency situations
◆ list of hospital and community contacts
◆ growth charts
◆ biochemical monitoring.

Realistically, few treatment options are available for families/carers whose child requires

Box 11.5 Training programme for parents and carers

Anatomy and physiology

◆ Child's underlying diagnosis/disease
◆ Placement and function of central venous catheter
◆ Possible complications of treatment, which may include:
  – catheter-related infections
  – embolism
  – liver dysfunction, cholestasis.

Feeding solutions

◆ General overview of nutrients used to provide parenteral nutrition
◆ How to set up the solutions of parenteral nutrition
◆ How to adjust flow rates.

The use of intravenous pumps

◆ Maintenance and problem-solving advice re alarms

Care of central venous catheter

◆ Aseptic techniques for central venous line and skincare

Emergences procedures

◆ How to deal with, and be aware of, possible emergency situations:
  – air in the line
  – line infection
  – blocked central venous catheter (Cottee 1995)
  – hypoglycaemia
  – torn central venous catheter.

Monitoring

◆ Urine testing
◆ Blood glucose monitoring techniques.

Issues for the family

◆ Social implications of the therapy
◆ Emergency contact numbers detailed
◆ Addresses of support groups locally/nationally.

long-term parenteral nutrition. Home parenteral nutrition allows children to grow and develop normally at home. Unfortunately, support services, respite centres and alternatives to hospitalization remain a limited resource for these children and require improvement in the UK. Ethical dilemmas continue to occur when permanent dependence is anticipated, as complications of this therapy can be life-threatening.

MONITORING

Ideally, the nutritional care sister observes the family setting up the intravenous feeding on the first night at home. Graded discharges promote confidence and families/carers should be given the opportunity to return to the hospital if major problems occur. It is essential that the follow-up of home parenteral nutrition patients is initiated by the same person who has done the training (Wilcox et al 1991). Availability of a hospital bed is essential if problems occur.

Specialist nurses should monitor medical and social issues and provide the consultant with up-to-date information, prior to clinic visits. Holden et al (1995) have developed an outpatient record form to highlight preliminary information provided from home visits to the consultant. Families/carers have commented that this information is useful because it means that the consultant is aware of issues of concern for families/carers prior to clinic (Holden 1994). Home parenteral nutrition families have also commented that it is helpful if all patients are seen in a specialized clinic so that they can exchange views with other families/carers and so that all team members are available for questions and advice.

Clinic members include a consultant, a specialist registrar, a dietitian, a pharmacist and a nutritional care nurse. Consultation with a psychologist and a speech therapist can be arranged as necessary. Monitoring patients receiving home parenteral nutrition requires specialist knowledge (Table 11.8). Routine blood tests for biochemical monitoring and growth

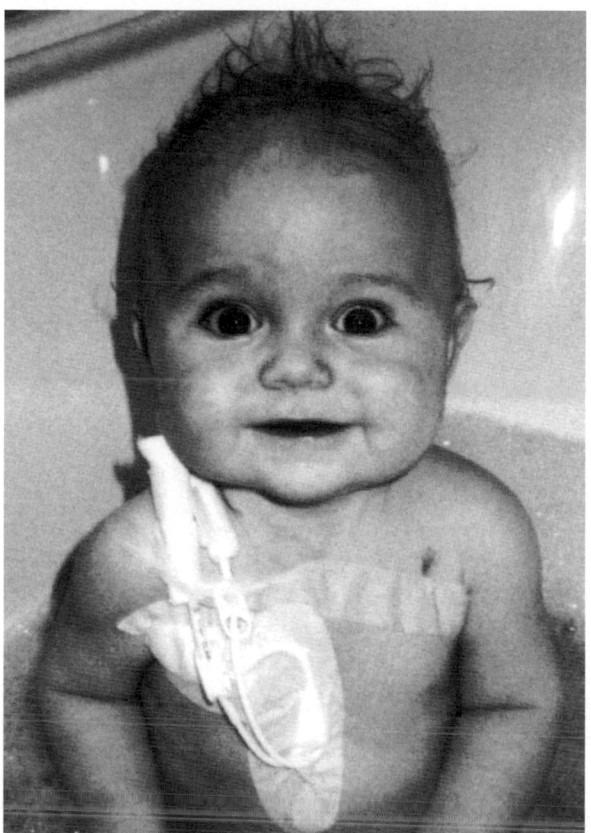

Figure 11.15 Home parenterally fed patient. (Reproduced with permission of Birmingham Children's Hospital.)

monitoring are routinely undertaken by a specialist nurse for the child (Table 11.9).

INTRAVENOUS DEVICES FOR THERAPY

Home parenteral nutrition must be given via a central venous catheter as the parenteral nutrition solutions are irritant to peripheral veins. The catheter tip should be in superior vena cava or right atrium. Current access devices are shown in Appendix 11.6.

Metabolic complications of parenteral nutrition include:

◆ infection
◆ hypo- and hyperglycaemia
◆ electrolyte disturbances

Table 11.8 Monitoring of home parenteral nutrition patients

Anthropometry	Height, weight, head circumference, mid-arm circumference, triceps skinfold, subscapular skinfold measurements
Haematology } Biochemistry }	See Table 11.9
Radiology	VQ scan
Cardiology	Echocardiography
Psychology	Developmental assessment 6-monthly

Table 11.9 Home parenteral nutrition bloods

	Analyses
Clinical chemistry	
	Electrolytes
	Urea
	Phosphate
	Magnesium
	Calcium
	ALT, AST, ALP, albumin
	Bilirubin
	Cholesterol
	Triglycerides
	Selenium
	Vitamins A and E
	Vitamin D
	Zinc
	Manganese
	Copper
	Red cell transketolase activity (for thiamine status)
	Aluminium
Haematology	
	Full blood cell count
	White cell count
	Platelets
	Differential
	B_{12}
	Folate
	Ferritin
	PT
	PTT

◆ hypophosphataemia
◆ anaemia
◆ thrombocyte and neutrophil dysfunction
◆ trace element deficiencies
◆ hyperammonaemia
◆ essential fatty acid deficiency
◆ hepatic dysfunction
◆ metabolic acidosis.

Table 11.10 shows complications which may be associated with home parenteral nutrition.

Feeding regimens

Parenteral nutrition solutions are complex and it is essential that all the following trace elements are added to parenteral nutrition. (Nutrients required are shown in Table 11.11, while the clinical consequences of deficiency are shown in Table 11.12.)

Detailed information regarding prescribing can be obtained from a booklet written by Ball et al (1993). The booklet details the daily intravenous requirements of children requiring nutrition

Table 11.10 Complications of home parenteral nutrition	
Sepsis	Low sepsis rates are achieved by families/carers at home (Holden 1991, Bisset et al 1992, Carlsson et al 1997). Most infections are due to gram positive organisms, especially staphepidermis (Puntis et al 1990). Systemic antibiotics and/or antibiotic locks instilled into the catheter are used to treat infections. Tunnel infections and yeast infections will require removal of catheter or implantable device.
Line occlusions	Results from a build-up of blood, fibrin, fat or mineral deposits or combination of all four (Cottee 1995). Strategies/protocols should be developed by the team. Drugs commonly used to prevent occlusions include urokinase-blood fibrin (Baranowski 1993), lipid-ethanol flushes (Pennington & Pithie 1987).
Cholestasis	Inability to utilize the gut with enteral feeding leads to: ◆ mucosal atrophy ◆ decrease in intestinal hormones ◆ abnormal enterohepatic circulation of bile salts ◆ abnormal biliary motility contributes to liver damage ◆ sepsis also contributes to liver damage. **Prevention of parenteral nutrition-related cholestasis is essential.** The following information may be helpful in its reduction: ◆ avoid line sepsis ◆ treat bowel overgrowth ◆ try to stimulate intestinal growth and biliary function by giving: – small amounts of enteral feeding – glutamine – growth hormone (Beath et al 1995).
Trace element deficiencies	Routine blood tests are taken to monitor vitamins and minerals. Adequate provision of trace elements is essential for the optimal utilization of amino acids and energy substrates. The most important are probably zinc, copper, selenium and iron (Puntis 1995).
Psychosocial development	Lack of oral stimulation will lead to severe feeding difficulties and food rejection. Essential to provide some oral feeding programmes, to be developed with help of dietitian and speech therapist. Schooling: whenever possible, child should attend normal school.

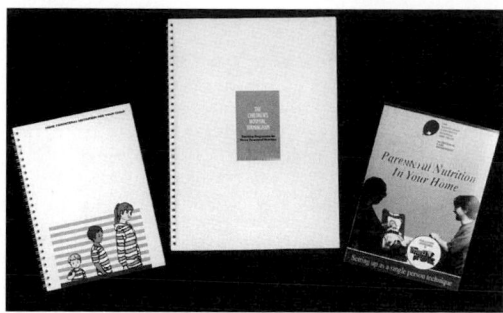

Figure 11.16 Information booklets for families – home parenteral nutrition.

and describes some commercially available products for use.

Intravenous pumps

Equipment designed for use in hospital may be inappropriate for home use. Specially designed portable infusion pumps do much to increase freedom and improve quality of life (Wardley et al 1997). The Medical Devices Agency reviews the selection and use of intravenous pumps for ambulatory application.

Table 11.11 Parenteral nutrition solutions. (From Holden & Kelcey 1997, with permission of Nursing Times.)

Carbohydrate
Glucose is the carbohydrate of choice. It is readily utilized by red cells, brain and cardiac muscles.

Lipid
Lipid solutions are calorie-dense and rich in essential fatty acids.
They are a rich source of essential fatty acids: linoleic and α-linolenic acids.

Nitrogen source
A clear colourless to straw-coloured solution of amino acids in the physiological L-form. They are used in conjunction with glucose and electrolytes for intravenous nutrition.

Micronutrients
In addition to amino acids, fat and carbohydrate, children receiving parenteral nutrition require a supply of vitamins, electrolytes and trace elements in order to maintain or restore body composition.

Trace elements
Peditrace or (Additrace if child is over 40 kg) is added to amino acid or glucose solution. It is a clear, colourless solution containing the following:
◆ zinc
◆ copper
◆ manganese
◆ selenium
◆ iron
◆ potassium iodinate.

Vitamins
Vitlipid N Infant is a white oil in water emulsion, containing fat-soluble vitamins A, D_2, E and K in the oil phase of emulsion. It is added to the lipid bag.
Solivito N contains the following water-soluble vitamins:
Vitamin B_1
Vitamin B_2
Nicotinamide
Vitamin B_6
Pantothenic acid
Biotin
Folic acid
Vitamin B_{12}
Vitamin C

Table 11.12 Clinical consequences of trace element deficiency (Ball et al 1993)

Trace element	Main symptoms of deficiency state
Zinc	Peri-orificial crusting dermatitis with bullae on hands and feet Alopecia Diarrhoea Growth failure
Copper	Refractory hypochromic anaemia Neutropenia Osteoporosis, sub-periosteal haematoma, soft tissue calcification
Selenium	Cardiomyopathy Skeletal muscle myopathy with pain and tenderness
Chromium	Hyperglycaemia and glycosuria Peripheral neuropathy Encephalopathy
Manganese	Reddening of hair Weight loss Hypocholesterolaemia
Molybdenum	Tachycardia Central scotomata Irritability Coma

In particular, ambulatory systems are essential when feeding is undertaken over a 10-hour period. However, the price of intravenous sets for ambulatory use is high and this may preclude their use in some areas.

Delivery of equipment and solutions

Funding of home parenteral nutrition is arranged with the local authority as a total package of care. The responsibility for prescribing parenteral nutrition now rests with the hospital-based team, and specialist hospital teams should provide training for community teams and respite centres. There are many specialist home care companies which can deliver disposable equipment and parenteral nutrition to the family's/carer's home. Some companies also have specialist paediatric trained nurses to help facilitate the transition from hospital to home.

ISSUES FOR FAMILIES

High technology home care is a reality in today's health care system. Nutritional care teams should be available for both families/carers and community teams (Beath et al 1995). Liaison with paediatric community nurses (if available) is essential, as they are in a prime position to respond sensitively to family needs, whilst mobilizing local resources available to them. Arrangement of clinical waste disposal, and contact with services such as electric, gas and water companies are essential to ensure services are maintained.

Holden (1994) identified major issues of concern for families/carers whose children receive this complex therapy. These include:

◆ uncertainty about child's future
◆ the unpredictability of hazardous events which may occur
◆ trying to balance domestic and work responsibilities

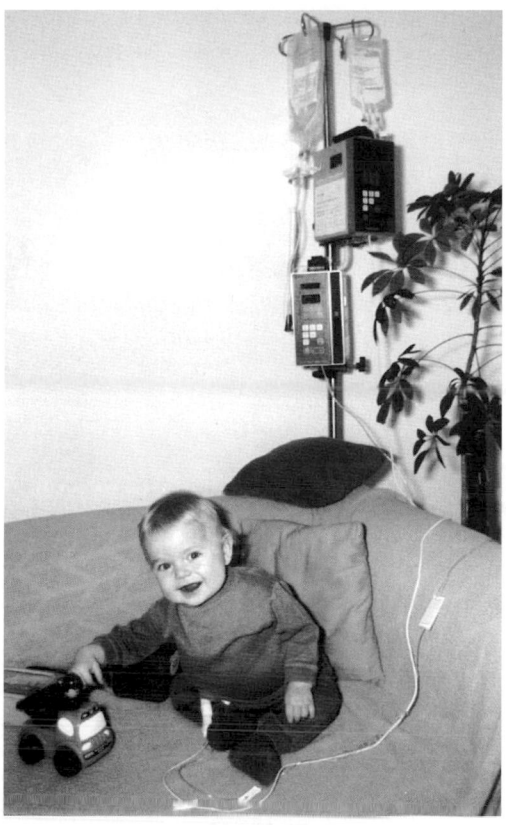

Figure 11.17 Home parenterally fed patient. (Reproduced with permission of Birmingham Children's Hospital.)

◆ exhaustion associated with sleepless nights
◆ lack of trained respite services
◆ financial problems
◆ education.

For those children whose intestinal failure is irreversible, small bowel transplantation is now an option (Kelly & Buckels 1995). It is essential that parents and children are given choices and that appropriate counselling is offered. Some children may require a combined transplantation for irreversible liver disease, secondary to parenteral nutrition and loss of vascular access with significant liver disease. Timing of assessment and listing for transplantation is crucial and early referral is essential. Specialist team members should be available at all times for families (Brooks 1998).

Holden (1994) identified different coping strategies of families/carers whose child received home parenteral nutrition. Some of these are shown in Table 11.13.

As medical technology advances, more children with complex illness can be supported at home. However, it is becoming increasingly important for health care professionals, both inside and out

Table 11.13 Parental coping strategies

Social support	Sharing the burden of their child's chronic illness with friends, relatives, professionals and self-help groups
Normalization	Attempts made by parents to try and minimize differences between children in the family Integration of child into normal family life to provide a sense of hope
Feeling in control	Parents mastered specific demands imposed by their child's illness Feeling of decreased anxiety as parents achieved a sense of being in control Availability of up-to-date and accurate information
Acceptance and understanding	Trying to attribute meaning to the experience of their child's illness
Communication	Families who were able to communicate freely and openly between themselves and other siblings appeared to cope better
Problem-solving and positive thinking	Families who balance positive and negative views of the situation and tended to choose the positive views, enabling them to draw on their own resources and to feel less overwhelmed

of hospital, to develop strategies for addressing parental concerns:

> The psychological care of the sick child in the community involves not only the needs of the child, but also the whole family. It is, therefore, important to view the management of the child's illness as part of a family process. Members of the family are affected by the child's condition and in turn, the way in which the family copes will affect the course of some illnesses. (Douglas 1993, p.51)

Negotiation

Chronic illness, such as intestinal failure with its characteristics of irreversibility and incurability, presents a situation of long-term negotiation between parent/carer and multidisciplinary team. Liston (1987) describes the issues for families nursing a child with home parenteral nutrition.

The National Health Service targeted families/carers, emphasizing the need for them to cope with home care. Financial resources and respite services should be made readily available to families/carers. Ideally, patients should have open access to the hospital and a 24-hour on-call service. Health care purchasers have a responsibility to recognize the standards of care required by children receiving home parenteral nutrition (Elia 1994, Wood et al 1995).

High technology home care is a reality (Smith et al 1993). Nurses should therefore be asked to recognize the ability of the patient and family/carer to physically or emotionally manage the therapy at home. For the patient or carer, learning to give care and treatment for their child is part of the process of adjustment and acceptance.

Bisset et al (1992) emphasized that reduced line sepsis rates and prolonged line survival of home patients almost certainly relates to the consistent care the child receives at home. Some parents/carers feel trapped by the needs of the child, but find that when they seek help from support agencies there is no understanding of the medical problems of the child or the social or emotional needs of the parents/carer.

Ricour et al (1990) reviewed 112 children in France who received home parenteral nutrition and emphasized:

> HPN provides a remarkable improvement in the quality of life of children on prolonged parenteral nutrition. It is none-the-less a complicated technique which is not without risk. Both medical and psychological follow-ups are necessary to prevent complications and interruptions of treatment.

PART 2 SUMMARY

Parenteral nutrition has given life to patients with chronic intestinal failure. Children requiring this intense nutritional support require the support of a multidisciplinary paediatric nutritional care team. The treatment is a huge commitment by the family/carer.

 FURTHER READING

Baker S B, Baker R D, Davis A (eds) 1994 Paediatric enteral nutrition. Chapman and Hall, London

This book identifies the rationale for feeding paediatric patients by tube and describes what can be accomplished with a practical approach to the delivery, monitoring and management of enteral nutrition.

Ball P A, Booth I W, Holden C E, Puntis J W L 1993 Paediatric parenteral nutrition. Pharmacia & UpJohn, Milton Keynes

This is a concise reference book, detailing general principles of initiating paediatric parenteral nutrition and establishing a nutritional support service.

Bard Access Systems 1994 Nursing procedure manual detailing the use of Hickman Leonard and Broviac Catheters. Bard Access Systems, Salt Lake City

Bravery K, Hanna J 1997 The use of long-term central venous access devices in children. Paediatric Nursing 9(10):29–35

This is a continuing education article, run in conjunction with the Royal College of Nursing Institute. The article focuses mainly on the technical issues of central venous access devices.

Clayden G, Lissauer T (eds) 1997 Illustrated textbook of paediatrics. Mosby, London

Highlights and gives an overview of paediatric conditions. The book follows a lecture-note style, using short sentences and lists of important features. Case histories have been chosen to describe paediatric conditions.

Elia M (ed) 1994 Enteral and parenteral nutrition in the community. British Association for Parenteral and Enteral Nutrition (BAPEN), Maidenhead

An overview of current issues related to home enteral and parenteral feeding.

Holden C E, Ball P A, Paul L et al 1993 Home parenteral nutrition for your child. Blackwell Masters, North Yorkshire

This is a guide for families written by The Birmingham Children's Hospital NHS Trust, the Institute of Child Health, the University of Birmingham and the University of Leeds.

McLaren D S, Burman D, Belton N R 1991 Textbook of paediatric nutrition. Churchill Livingstone, Edinburgh

A comprehensive book reviewing the role of nutrition in paediatric patients.

Queen P M, Long C E 1993 Handbook of paediatric nutrition. Aspen Publishers, ML

Informative book reviewing paediatric nutrition.

Wardley B J, Puntis J W L, Taitz L S 1997 Handbook of child nutrition. Oxford University Press, Oxford

This book is a guide in respect of child nutrition for nurses, health visitors, community nurses, midwives and general practitioners. Key sections include growth in children, feeding the premature infant, enteral tube feeding and parenteral nutrition. Particular reference to feeding methods in the community are included in this informative text book.

REFERENCES

Anderton A, Nivgough C E 1991 Problems with the re-use of enteral feeding systems. A study of design of enteral feeding sets. Journal of Human Nutrition and Dietetics 4:25–32

Bailey R, Caldwell C 1997 Preparing parents for going home. Paediatric Nursing 9(4):15–17

Ball P, Puntis J W L, Booth I W, Holden C E 1993 Paediatric parenteral nutrition. Pharmacia & UpJohn, Milton Keynes

Baranowski L 1993 Central venous access devices. Journal of Intravenous Nursing 16(3):167–194

Beath S V, Booth I W, Murphy M S et al 1995 Nutritional care and candidates for small bowel transplantation. Archives of Disease in Childhood 73:348–350

Bisset W M, Stapleford P, Long S, Chamberlain A, Sobel B, Miller P J 1992 Home parenteral nutrition in chronic intestinal failure. Archives of Disease in Childhood 6:109–114

Booth I W 1991 Continuous enteral feeding in childhood. British Journal of Hospital Medicine 46:111–113

Brooks G 1998 Quality of life issues: parenteral nutrition to small bowel transplantation. A review. Nutrition 14(10):813–816

Carlsson G, Hakansson A, Rubensson A, Finkey Y 1997 Home parenteral nutrition (HPN) in children in Sweden. Paediatric Nursing 23(3):272–274

Chaplen C 1997 Parent's views of caring for children with gastrostomies. British Journal of Nursing 6(1):34–38

Clarke S E, MacDonald A, Booth I W 1998 Impaired growth and nitrogen deficiency in infants receiving an energy supplement standard infant formula. Proceedings of Royal College of Physicians Child Health Annual Spring Meeting. Abstract G132:2–75

Coalfield M P 1994 Percutaneous endoscopic gastrostomy placement in children. Gastrointestinal Endoscopy Clinics of North America 4(1):179–193

Cottee S 1995 Heparin lock practice in total parenteral nutrition. Professional Nurse 11(1):25–29

Douglas J 1993 Psychology and nursing children. Macmillan, Basingstoke

Elia M (ed) 1994 Enteral and parenteral nutrition in the community. British Association for Parenteral and Enteral Nutrition (BAPEN), Maidenhead

Feeding Liaison Team 1998 Parents' positive action for feeding. The Birmingham Children's Hospital NHS Trust, Birmingham

Holden C E 1991 Home parenteral nutrition. Paediatric Nursing 3(2):13–17

Holden C E 1994 Enteral and parenteral nutrition:feeding at home – impact on family life and the implications for home care. MSc thesis, Wolverhampton University

Holden C E, Kelcey H 1997 Fluid systems. Nursing Times 93(8):61–64

Holden C E, MacDonald A 1997 Nutritional support at home: emotional support and composition of feeds. Current Paediatrics 7:218–222

Holden C E, Puntis J W L, Charlton C P J, Booth I W 1991 Nasogastric feeding at home: acceptability and safety. Archives of Disease in Childhood 66:148–151

Holden C E, Ball P A, Paul L et al 1993 Home parenteral nutrition for your child. Blackwell Masters, Yorkshire

Holden C E, Murphy S, Booth I W 1995 Parenteral nutrition outpatient record. The Birmingham Children's NHS Trust, Birmingham

Holden C E, Brook G, Wills J, Paul L, Sexton E 1996 Home parenteral nutrition: present management, future options. British

Journal of Community Health Nursing 1(6):347–353

Holden C E, MacDonald A, Ward M et al 1997a Psychological preparation and support of children undergoing enteral nutrition: an evaluation. British Journal of Nursing 6:376–385

Holden C E, Sexton E, Paul L 1997b Enteral nutrition for children. Nursing Standard 11 (32):49–56

Holden C E, Fitzpatrick G, Paul L et al 1997c Gastrostomy care: parents' guide. Nutritional Care Team, The Birmingham Children's Hospital NHS Trust, Birmingham

Kelly D, Buckels J 1995 The future of small bowel transplantation. Archives of Disease in Childhood 72:447–451

Khair J 1998 Wishful thinking. Nursing Times 94(33):75

Liston L 1987 Paediatric HTPN: a father's view. Intensive Therapy and Clinical Monitoring 8:186–196

Metheny N, Reed L, Wiersema L, McSweeney M, Wehrle M A, Clark J 1993a Effectiveness of pH measurements in predicting feeding tube placement: an update. Nursing Research 42(6):324–331

Metheny N, Reed L, Worsek M, Clark J 1993b Equipment guide. How to aspirate fluid from small-bore feeding tubes. American Journal of Nursing May:86–88

Miller P 1999 Current perspectives on paediatric parenteral nutrition. British Association for Parenteral and Enteral Nutrition (BAPEN), Maidenhead

Patchell C J, Anderton A, MacDonald A, George R H, Booth I W 1994 Bacterial contamination of enteral feeds. Archives of Diseases in Childhood 170:327–330

Patchell C J, Anderton A, Holden C, MacDonald A, George R H, Booth I W 1998 Reducing bacterial contamination of enteral feeds. Archives of Disease in Childhood 78:166–168

Paul L, Holden CE, Smith A et al 1993 Tube feeding and you. Nutritional Care Team, The Birmingham Children's Hospital NHS Trust, Birmingham

Pennington C R 1996 Current perspectives on parenteral nutrition in adults. A report by a working party of the British Association for Parenteral and Enteral Nutrition (BAPEN). British Association for Parenteral and Enteral Nutrition, Maidenhead

Pennington C R, Pithie A D 1987 Ethanol lock in the management of catheter occlusion. Journal of Parenteral and Enteral Nutrition 11:507–508

Pobiel R S, Bisset G S, Pobiel M S 1994 Nasojejunal feeding tube placement in children: four years cumulative experience. Radiology 1901:127–129

Ponsky J L, Gaunder M W, Stellab T A, Aszedi A 1985 Percutaneous approaches to enteral alimentation. American Journal of Surgery 149:102–105

Puntis J W L 1993 Update on intravenous feeding in children. British Journal of Intensive Care 3(8):299–305

Puntis J W L 1995 Paediatric parenteral nutrition. In: Payne-James J (ed.) Artificial nutrition support in clinical practice. Edward Arnold, London

Puntis J W L, Holden C, Smallman S, Finkel Y, George R H, Booth I W 1990 Staff training: a key factor in reducing catheter sepsis. Archives of Diseases in Childhood 66:335–337

Ricour C 1988 Total parenteral nutrition in children. Annales Nestlé 46:61–72

Ricour C, Gorski A M, Goulet O 1990 Home parenteral nutrition in children: 8 years of experience with 112 patients. Clinical Nutrition 9:65–71

Rollins I I 1998 Managing enteral feeding tubes at home. Clinical Nutrition Update 2(3):3–4

Sexton E, Paul L, Holden C E 1996 A pictorial assisted teaching tool for families. Paediatric Nursing 8(5):24–26

Shah R 1994 Practice with attitude: questions in cultural awareness training. Child Health 1(6):245–249

Sidney A, Torbet S 1995 Enteral feeding in community setting. Paediatric Nursing 7(6):21–24

Singer L, Farkas L K 1989 The impact of infant disability on maternal perception of stress. Family Relations 38:444–449

Smith C E, Moushey L, Ross H J A, Gieffer C 1993 Responsibilities and reactions of family care givers of patients dependent on total parenteral nutrition at home. Public Health Nursing 10(2):122–128

Stein R, Riessman L 1980 The development of an impact on family scale: preliminary findings. Medical Care 18:465–472

Townsley R, Robinson C 1997 Online support: effective support services to disabled children who are tube fed. The Norah Fry Research Centre, Bristol

Wardley B L, Puntis J W L, Taitz L S 1997 Nutritional management in chronic disease. In: Wardley B L, Puntis J W L, Taitz L S (eds) Handbook of child nutrition. Oxford University Press, New York

Wigglesworth J S 1969 Malnutrition and brain development. Developmental Medicine and Child Neurology 11:791–803

Wilcox H, Armstrong J, Cottee S, Neale G, Elia M 1991 Artificial nutrition support for patients in the Cambridge Health District. Health Trends 23:93–100

Winick M 1987 Long-term effects of kwashiorkor. Journal of Paediatric Gastroenterology and Nutrition 6:833–835

Wood S, Shaffer J, Wheatley C 1995 Home parenteral nutrition. Quality criteria for clinical services and the supply of nutrient fluids and equipment. British Association for Parenteral and Enteral Nutrition (BAPEN), Maidenhead

Appendix 11.1 Ideal feeding tubes and devices

Nasogastric tube

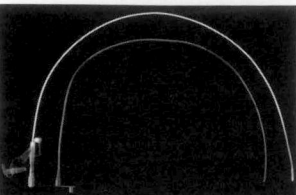

Conforms to British Standards BS 6314 (should have a male luer and anti-intravenous female connection)
Small FG with a large internal diameter
Comfort: cosmetically acceptable
Tip: soft with no dead space; scooped end to avoid suction of the tip onto the stomach wall; aids aspiration and reduces blockage
Guidewires should be stiff to ensure easy insertion; flexible to avoid damage to the tube and should not coil
Connectors should be durable and fit any giving set or syringe with or without a suitable adapter
Radio-paque

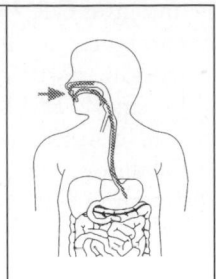

Nasojejunal feeding tube

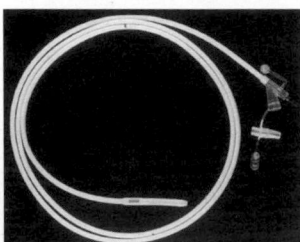

Tube and guidewire should be radio-opaque to help confirm position
Biocompatible polyurethane tube tungsten weighted may be helpful
Open distal end promotes good fluid flow
Comfort: cosmetically acceptable

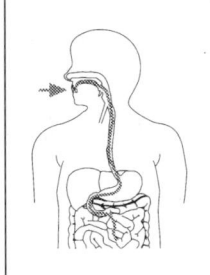

Percutaneous endoscopic gastrostomy tube – (PEG tube)

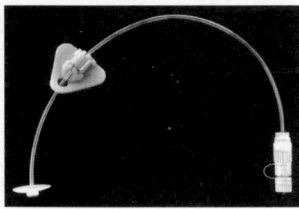

Bumper bar and tube should be made of pliable, biocompatible silicone; this material easily passes down the oesophagus and helps maintain a healthy stoma
Bumper bar helps to resist inadvertent removal and migration into stoma tract
Connections compatible with external feeding systems to minimize separation and leakage

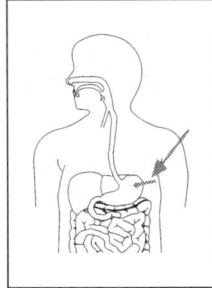

Gastrostomy tube

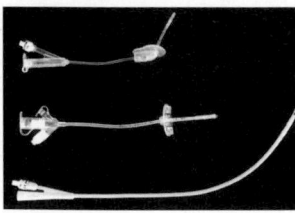

Medical grade silicone material, biocompatible and flexible for patient comfort
Y-port connector to allow easy flushing and giving of liquid medication without disconnecting feeding sets
Centimetre graduations to allow assessment of potential tube migration
Securing disc lifts easily for cleaning of stoma site/prevents tube migration
Translucent to facilitate assessment of stoma
Holes to promote airflow for a healthy stoma site
Gastric balloon expands evenly to maintain a secure, comfortable fit and to minimize leakage
Balloon inflation port is safely marked with the maximum balloon volume and the words 'inflation' to prevent accidental over-inflation and administration of medicines
Open distal end promotes good fluid flow

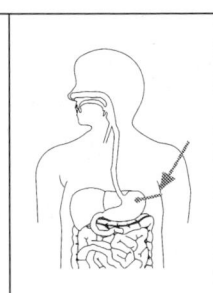

Gastrostomy button

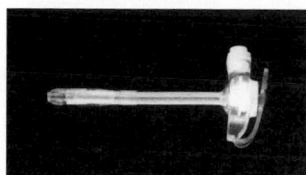

Low-profile device makes it suitable for children, who may be self-conscious of standard gastrostomy tube
Anti-reflux valve prevents leakage of feed when tube is not in use
Balloon inflation to facilitate removal/replacement

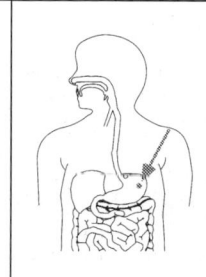

Stoma measuring devices for buttons

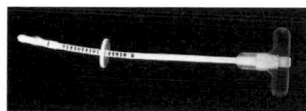

Depth of tract required is measured by a stoma measuring device
Measuring device packed separately to the button

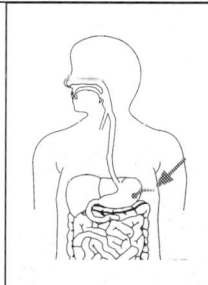

Transgastric jejunal feeding tube

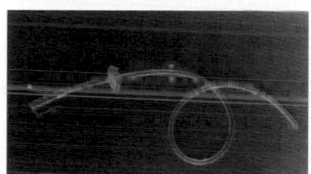

Facilitates placement of tube beyond the ligament of Trietz for endoscopic and radiologic procedures
Provides gastric decompression while simultaneously feeding into the jejunum
Multiple feeding ports improve flow of feed and minimize clogging
Sliding ring balloon system prevents the tube migrating and controls gastric leakage
Built-in universal connectors help minimize feeding set disconnections

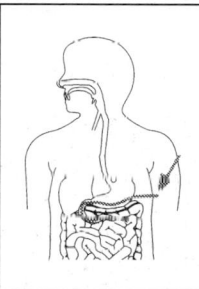

Jejunal feeding tube

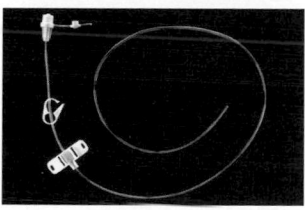

Flexible medical grade clear silicone to minimize site irritation
Radio-opaque allows verification of tube position

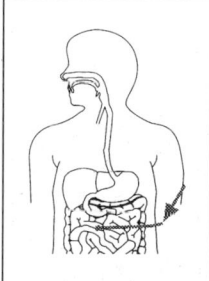

Appendix 11.2 Equipment for tube feeding

Device	Usage	Complications	Specific care
Nasogastric tubes Polyvinyl chloride, e.g. (Vygon), (Portex) (Simms)	Short-term Bolus or continuous	Tube stiffness over time Tissue damage may occur if used > 10 days Sinusitis can be a problem Psychosocial implications	Easy to aspirate Test tube aspirate for acid reaction – (Metheny et al 1993a, Rollins 1998) Requires regular flushing to prevent bacterial contamination
Polyurethane (fine bore tube) made of soft polyurethane or silicone elastomer. Fine bore tubes may have wire stylets to give the tube rigidity, when passed (Merk) (Flocare) (Medicina)	Long-term Continuous (bolus feeds can take a long time to give) Older children can be taught to insert tube	High risk of continuous tracheal intubation in children with impaired swallowing or children requiring ventilation Tube may be displaced in child prone to vomiting Tissue damage rare Nasal polyps may obstruct passage of tube Psychosocial implications	Collapses down when aspirating Test aspirate for acid reactions – (Metheny et al 1993b) Blocks easily – use of carbonated liquids to flush tube helps clear/prevent build-up of feeds Pancreatic enzyme can be used to unblock tube Guidewire is removed following insertion
Gastrostomy tubes Without retaining disc Examples include: • Foley • Bard • Malecot	Open procedure (Stamm) Short-term use	No retention disc Easily migrates into duodenum Risk of perforation and misplacement of tube Skin problems, infection, granulation tissue leakage around site	Requires strapping securely in place to prevent tube migration Clean site daily with warm normasol and dry thoroughly Air to be removed from the stomach by opening port prior to feeding
Gastrostomy tubes MIC, MEDICINA, Flocare (Nutricia), Ballard (Vygon), Kangaroo (Kendall), MIC (Vygon), Medicina	Use following: Open procedure (Stamm) Short/long-term use	Risk of necrosis if retention disc is tight Skin problems, infection, granulation tissue leakage around site Misplacement of tube Stoma closes down within a few hours if accidental removal	Clean site daily with warm normasol Clean/check retention disc Dry thoroughly Allow air to be removed from the stomach prior to feeding
Percutaneous inserted gastrostomy tubes (PEG) BARD (Ballard), MIC (Vygon), Bower (E Merck Ltd.), Medicina	Endoscopic placement using flexible telescope (Coalfield 1994, Ponsky et al 1985) Long-term tube Cross bar/bumper bar holds tube in position	Previous abdominal surgery can prevent use of this technique Risk of bowel perforation Misplacement of tube Risk of necrosis around stoma site if bumper bar is too tight Removal of PEG is dependent on individual design. Usually removed endoscopically in children	
Skin level devices low profile e.g., MIC Key (Vygon UK) BARD button	Long-term feeding	Leakage can occur if tract is not established Heavy sedation/anaesthetic required to remove button Taping of connector needed in small children	A stoma measuring device is used to determine length of stoma prior to the insertion of the button Feeding connectors used to access device Rotate device daily to avoid tube adhering to tissue Clean site with warm normasol Dry stoma site thoroughly Allow air to be removed from the stomach de-gassing prior to feeding Stoma closes down within a few hours if removed accidentally Replace button immediately

Device	Usage	Complications	Specific care
Gastrojejunal tubes e.g., MIC tubes (Vygon UK)	Long-term feeding	Reflux of bile into the stomach Dumping syndrome Risk of bacterial overgrowth	Continuous feeding required pH paper to check placement
Jejunostomy e.g., MIC (Vygon UK), Frekajejunal PEG (Fresenius)			Aseptic technique when handling catheter Use of sterile water when flushing tube Repair kit available for some tubes

Home Enteral Feeding Teaching Programme
Birmingham Children's Hospital NHS Trust

Patient's name:　　　　　**Reg:**　　　**DoB:**　　　**Ward:**

Consultant:　　　　**Nutritional Care Sister:**

The following sections have been designed to ensure that all aspects of tube feeding are discussed and demonstrated to parents/carers. Parents should set up feeding systems daily until competent, so it can be performed safely at home. Please sign programme training as objectives achieved.

	Date discussed	Parents aware	Further discussion required
Psychological preparation of parent and child			
Reasons for enteral feeding discussed with parent/carer/child	☐	☐	☐
Discussion of emotional and psychosocial aspects of feeding	☐	☐	☐
Visual aids to support training can include: 　child's/parent's/carer's booklet 　videos	☐	☐	☐
Play therapist to support preparation of children	☐	☐	☐
Safety aspects			
Explanation of anatomy related to gastrointestinal/respiratory tract	☐	☐	☐
Complications related to tube misplacement	☐	☐	☐
Microbiological contamination of feed discussed	☐	☐	☐
Explanation of importance of oral stimulation			
Written information to be provided	☐	☐	☐
Community			
Community staff contacts	☐	☐	☐
Support groups available to families	☐	☐	☐

	Date shown	Date practised	Date practised	Date practised	Date completed	Evaluation of care given/required Comments
Hygiene issues						
Reasons for handwashing discussed	☐	☐	☐	☐	☐	_____
Handwashing demonstration	☐	☐	☐	☐	☐	_____
Cleaning work surfaces with household cleaner (e.g. Milton) discussed	☐	☐	☐	☐	☐	_____
Feed preparation						
Parents are confident in preparation of feed	☐	☐	☐	☐	☐	_____
Parents visit Special Feed Unit, if necessary	☐	☐	☐	☐	☐	_____
Parents understand different feed components	☐	☐	☐	☐	☐	_____
Decanting of feeds	☐	☐	☐	☐	☐	_____
Storage of feed	☐	☐	☐	☐	☐	_____
Equipment						
Familiarization with pump and equipment	☐	☐	☐	☐	☐	_____
Alarm systems identified	☐	☐	☐	☐	☐	_____
Running feed set through	☐	☐	☐	☐	☐	_____
Storing equipment	☐	☐	☐	☐	☐	_____
Tube care						
Care of feeding tube	☐	☐	☐	☐	☐	_____
Tube replacement	☐	☐	☐	☐	☐	_____
Aspiration technique	☐	☐	☐	☐	☐	_____
Flushing of tube	☐	☐	☐	☐	☐	_____
Care of skin	☐	☐	☐	☐	☐	_____
Tube change, if applicable	☐	☐	☐	☐	☐	_____

Parent information:

Telephone numbers:

Evaluation of Training at
Birmingham Children's Hospital NHS Trust

Patient's name: **Reg:**   **DoB:**   **Ward:**

Consultant: **Nutritional Care Sister:**

At the end of a teaching programme parents should answer verbally the following questions. Please complete for every patient prior to discharge. Return the form to the Nutritional Care Sister.

	Dates discussed	Date achieved	Evaluation of care given/ requested Comments
Safety aspects of feeding			
The foodpipe and windpipe are very close together. How do you know if the tube is being passed down into the windpipe?	☐	☐	_____
What would you do if your child's colour deteriorated and child was coughing when passing a feeding tube?	☐	☐	_____
How do you check that the feeding tube is in the correct position?	☐	☐	_____
How would you position your child at night during feeds?	☐	☐	_____
What is the correct temperature for the feed to be given?	☐	☐	_____
Why is it important to check the rate of the feed?	☐	☐	_____
What would you do if too much feed went through too quickly?	☐	☐	_____
If your child vomited what would you do?	☐	☐	_____
Hygiene			
How can bacteria/germs enter your child's feed?	☐	☐	_____
How can you prevent bacteria entering the feed?	☐	☐	_____
If your child developed diarrhoea, what would you do?	☐	☐	_____
General tube care			
Why is it important to flush the feeding tube?	☐	☐	_____
How often should a feeding tube be flushed?	☐	☐	_____
Why should the feeding tube be changed?	☐	☐	_____

	Dates discussed	Date achieved	Evaluation of care given/ requested Comments
What attention should be paid to the skin and taping of the feeding tube?	☐	☐	_____
Problem solving advice Who would you contact if there were any problems with tube feeding?	☐	☐	_____
What problems do you perceive with feeding? Discussion to take place	☐	☐	_____

Parent's signature ....

Nurse's signature ....   **Date** ....

Discharge Planning Protocol for Home Enteral Feeding from Hospital to Home

24 hours before discharge, the parent/carer will have the knowledge, skills and support necessary to provide safe, effective nutrition at home for their child/baby

Plan of care	Implementation	Evaluation of care
A written referral plan by medical/dietetic colleagues regarding initiating enteral training for families is required to facilitate discharge planning	The medical staff will fill in referral detailing: child's nutritional status reasons for enteral feeding expected aims of nutritional support likely duration	Psychosocial support is given and home circumstances reviewed. Training is given to families which require home enteral feeding Discharge planning is facilitated
There is a written protocol for doctors and nurses who are likely to be involved in the management of home enteral nutrition	Nursing staff and Nutritional Care Sister (NCS) have the necessary experience and have undergone specific training in order to educate the patient	The parent/carer/child feels confident that the feeding system will be appropriate for the child's individual needs
Written learning goals are available in the format of a training programme	The ward nurses teach the patient according to his or her individual capacity for learning	The parent/carer/child is able to demonstrate required skills and achieve all learning and nursing goals. Evaluation of training is done by: questionnaire discussion observations of setting up feeds
Detailed psychological preparation	The child receives psychological preparation for insertion of nasogastric/gastrostomy/jejunostomy tube	The child is prepared according to cognitive development
A suitable nasogastric/gastrostomy/jejunostomy tube is inserted for use	The parent/carer is made aware of the choices available for their child	The parent/carer is competent in looking after the tube/button and feeding equipment
A suitable feed is given to baby/child	Dietetic staff will prescribe feed and feed volumes for baby/child. Parent/carer will visit Special Feed Unit and be given instruction regarding making up feed, if appropriate	The parent/carer is competent in making required feed
There is an instruction manual	The NCS will ensure that literature is available within the parent's/carer's homes for use by health care/community staff	The parent/carer will have written instruction regarding their child's care
The discharge planning documentation will include sections on domestic and family issues and way of life	The NCS will evaluate the patient's domestic and social circumstances and adapt the feeding programme accordingly with dietetic colleagues	The parent/carer feels secure that the feeding system will be appropriate to their child's individual needs
Nursing staff will assess competency of parent/carer	Written/verbal assessment is undertaken to ensure safe practice	The parent/carer will be confident and safe

Plan of care	Implementation	Evaluation of care
Information required for community agencies, for example: paediatric community nurses community nurses General Practitioners health visitors school nurses community dietitians community physiotherapist/speech therapy/occupational therapist	Telephone contact made Written information and training given, as required	Community agencies have up-to-date information regarding child's care
A list of all equipment required for parent/carer will be given to ward nursing staff. Parent/carer will be provided with 7 days' worth of equipment from ward stock	NCS will provide a list of equipment for community staff. Liaise with Home Care Company to deliver feed and equipment to the parents'/carer's home. Liaise with the community re funding	The parent/carer will know how supplies will be delivered and safely stored at home
Child's nutritional status will be monitored by dietetic colleagues and NCS	NCS will initially assess child's growth in detail. This should include skinfolds, height, weight (head circumference of children under 2 years), mid-arm circumference	Evaluation of child's growth to ensure baby/child is thriving
Monitor enteral feeding in community	Dietetic colleagues/NCS will telephone parent/carer weekly. Home visits arranged as necessary. Liaison with community nursing staff/community dietitian	Review home enteral feeding. Audit/monitor complications. Continued assessment of care and nutritional status of child.

(Adapted from British Association of Parenteral and Enteral Nutrition (BAPEN) recommendations)

Percentages of agreement for responses to modified impact on family scale (H.E.N.) = 40
(Stein & Riessman 1980, Singer & Farkas 1989)

	Strongly agree %
My partner and I discuss my child's problem together	85
Additional income is needed to care for my child	82.5
Learning to manage my child's disability/illness has made me feel better about myself	80
Because of what we share, we are a closer family	77.5
It is hard to find a reliable person to take care of my child	77.5
Sometimes I feel in turmoil when my child is acutely ill; OK when things are stable	77.5
Fatigue is a problem for me because of my child's illness	75
My relatives have been helpful and understanding with my child	75
Sometimes we have to change plans about going out at the last minute because of my child's condition/state	75
I do not have much time left over for other family members after caring for my child	72.5
The disability/illness is causing financial problems for the family	72.5
Our family gives up things because of my child's disability	70
Travelling to the hospital is a strain on me	67.5
I worry about what will happen to my child in the future	65
I thought about not having more children because of my child's illness/disability	64.8
We see family and friends less because of my child's illness	50
We have little desire to go out because of my child's disability/illness	40
Sometimes I wonder whether my child should be treated specially or the same as a normal child	40
Nobody understands the burden I carry	48
Time is lost from work because of medical appointments	42.5
I am cutting down the hours I work to care for my child	42.5
Because of the disability/illness, we are not able to travel	37.5
People in our town treat us specially because of my child's disability/illness	35
I live from day to day and do not plan for the future	35

Ambulatory infusion devices for parenteral nutrition

◆ A maintainable accurate delivery of fluids
◆ A visual indication of the total volume infused
◆ Appropriate protection against air embolism
◆ Suitable provisions against tampering or misuse
◆ An occlusion alarm
◆ An end-of-infusion alarm
◆ A low and depleted battery alert
◆ Small and low-weight
◆ Availability to taper parenteral nutrition rates to suit individual requirements.

Equipment used in home parenteral nutrition

In-line filters

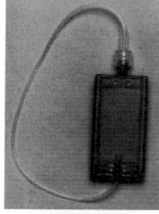 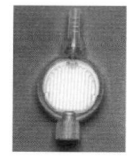

Filters remove endotoxins and particulate matter from parenteral fluids

Closed intravenous connection systems – for example Interlink (Becton and Dickinson), Bionnector (Vygon UK Ltd.)

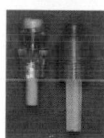

Hub manipulation is reduced and this is thought to be helpful in reducing catheter-related sepsis

Central venous access devices for home intravenous

Device	Description	Advantages	Disadvantages
Partially implantable devices **For example: Broviac Line** 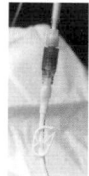	◆ Silicon, radio-opaque, flexible catheter with open or closed ends ◆ Dacron cuff on catheter enhances tissue ingrowth to secure catheter	◆ Dacron cuff ◆ Easy to use ◆ Easily removed ◆ Able to be repaired ◆ Groshong catheters are available. They have an anti-reflux valve which prevents blood flow up the catheter	◆ Requires regular heparin flushes (weekly). A Groshong catheter requires only normal saline to flush ◆ Must be clamped at all times (with exception of Groshong catheter)
Totally implanted devices **For example: Port-a-cath Vascuport** 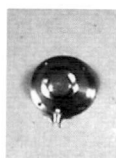	◆ Totally implantable metal or plastic device ◆ Consists of self-sealing injection port with pre-connected or attachable silicon catheter that is placed in a large blood vessel	◆ Reduced risk of infection ◆ Placed completely under the skin ◆ No limitations on most physical activity ◆ No dressing required ◆ Increased patient acceptance	◆ More difficult to access ◆ Must pierce skin for access ◆ Removal more complex ◆ Catheter may become dislodged from port

12

Feeding children on special diets

Carolyn Patchell   Tracey Johnson

INTRODUCTION

For all children the provision of good nutrition is of utmost importance. For most children, diet should be a varied and balanced mixture of foods that will provide sufficient energy and nutrients to maintain growth and good health. For children who require a special diet, food may have an even bigger role to play.

Special diets can be necessary for a number of reasons and they can take many forms. Certain foods may need to be increased or decreased, avoided or included, and requirements may change, necessitating regular monitoring and alteration of regimens. Avoidance of certain foods is commonly required, such as in coeliac disease where management of the disease is with a gluten-free diet. This is also seen in food allergy, renal disease and inherited metabolic diseases where diet forms the mainstay of treatment.

Chronic illness in childhood is frequently associated with anorexia. For this reason, special diets are often not only associated with dietary restrictions, but may also include nutritional supplementation to ensure adequate calorie intakes and optimum growth and development.

Many children have to follow special diets for many years and sometimes for life. Although the principles of the diet are often the same for all age groups, regular follow-up of children on special diets is essential. This not only helps to maintain compliance and ensure nutritional adequacy, but also allows the diet to be be modified to meet the changing needs of children as they grow. Children who only need a special diet temporarily also require regular follow-up. They, too, need regular assessment of compliance and nutritional adequacy, but in addition these children will need food challenges to avoid unnessary adherence to a restricted diet.

Although many individuals will have a role to play in caring for children on a special diet, it is essential that the treatment is coordinated by a specialist paediatric dietitian. A paediatric dietitian will be able to offer comprehensive advice on a child's special diet, and will also be experienced in meeting the changing nutritional requirements from infancy through childhood and into adolescence.

SPECIAL DIETS IN HOSPITAL

Special diets are generally managed at home but children may require special diets in hospital. This may be an admission related to their condition, or may be an admission for routine surgery or an unrelated childhood illness.

When a child is admitted to hospital the dietitian should be notified so that arrangements can be made for the provision of a special diet. Ideally, special diets should be prepared in a diet kitchen or diet bay by catering staff who have received formal training from a dietitian.

In hospital, diets need to be monitored accurately by nursing staff, and regular weight and height measurements are also vital for a full assessment. Children may be admitted during the evening and require food before being seen by a dietitian. It is therefore essential that nursing staff have regular training on the fundamentals of the special diets they may encounter, so they can make appropriate choices from the foods available. It is also necessary to have some simple written guidelines which can be followed before the patient can be assessed by the dietitian.

DIABETES MELLITUS

Incidence

One in 500 children in the United Kingdom will develop diabetes. It is the third most common condition in childhood.

KEY POINTS

- ◆ Peak presentation is at 11 to 12 years of age.
- ◆ Diagnosis is by urinalysis, followed by blood glucose levels.
- ◆ The aims of the diabetic diet are to maintain normoglycaemia, achieve normal growth and development, and minimize the risk of diabetic complications.
- ◆ The dietary emphasis is on an increase in complex carbohydrate and fibre and a reduction in fat and sugar intake.
- ◆ Dietary extremes should be avoided and regular meals and snacks are encouraged.

Presentation

Children commonly present with polydipsia, polyuria, lethargy, weight loss and anorexia. The onset of diabetes is frequently triggered by an intercurrent illness or a stress such as starting a new school, or changes within the family. Onset may be insidious with the child presenting with mild symptoms, diagnosis being made on urine analysis and venous blood glucose levels, or more rarely may be acute with the child presenting in ketoacidosis. Peak presentation is at the time of starting or changing school, around 4 to 5 years of age and 11 to 12 years of age.

Aims of the diabetic diet

Box 12.1 shows the aims of a diabetic diet.

Dietary energy intake should be sufficient for growth and for exercise, but should not be excessive to avoid obesity. Growth should be plotted on growth charts at regular intervals. Poor growth

Box 12.1 Aims of the diabetic diet

- ◆ To meet normal nutritional requirements.
- ◆ To maintain normoglycaemia (4–7 μmol/1).
- ◆ To minimize the risk of diabetic complications.
- ◆ To achieve normal growth and development.

and development can be a result of poor diabetic control. Obesity can develop, with adolescent girls being most at risk. Early detection and dietetic advice is vital.

Recommendations for the diet of diabetics have been made in two reports published by the British Diabetic Association, 'Dietary recommendations for people with diabetes' (1992) and 'Dietary recommendations for children and adolescents with diabetes' (1989). These are summarized below.

Carbohydrate

In excess of 40% of energy should come from carbohydrate. The formula 120 g carbohydrate plus 10 g for every year of life can be used as a guide, but consideration must be given to a child's body weight and activity. A child who has a weight and height over the 50th centile will require more energy and carbohydrate than a child on the 3rd centile.

Fibre

A general guideline is that children should have 1 g per 100 kcal per day. This may require considerable modification of the child's diet and may need to be done gradually. It can be achieved by the use of wholemeal bread, high fibre breakfast cereals such as Weetabix, Shreddies and Shredded Wheat, and fruits and vegetables, particularly pulse vegetables such as baked beans, peas, sweetcorn and red kidney beans.

Fat

Approximately 35% of energy should come from fat. This can be achieved by the use of:

◆ grilled rather than fried foods
◆ lean meats, fish and poultry
◆ lower fat crisps
◆ reduced-fat cheeses, for example Edam
◆ semi-skimmed milk for children over 2 years of age and skimmed milk for children of 5 years and over.

Fat is an important source of fat-soluble vitamins and essential fatty acids, and over restriction should therefore be avoided.

Protein

Children with diabetes have normal protein requirements. Most children take around 15% of dietary energy from protein (Department of Health 1991).

Sugar

Sugar may be used as part of a mixed meal and will not have a detrimental effect on blood glucose control. Sugar is absorbed more rapidly than complex carbohydrate and may result in a rapid rise in glucose levels if eaten by itself. However, it can be given at the end of a main meal when the response will be less. The inclusion of sugar in controlled amounts, given with meals, is helpful as it improves compliance and palatability.

Exercise

Extra carbohydrate will be required for prolonged strenuous exercise. The child should take rapidly absorbed carbohydrate, such as glucose drinks, as a top-up during exercise.

In general, complex carbohydrate can be given prior to exercise, although children will often prefer a simple sugar snack. The amount of carbohydrate needed depends on the duration and intensity of exercise. Initially, children should take a blood sugar reading before, during and after exercise so that the amount of carbohydrate required can be decided.

Special foods

The use of diabetic products should be discouraged as they are expensive and contain sorbitol which may cause osmotic diarrhoea. Low sugar and low calorie drinks are extremely useful in the diet of diabetic children, as are low sugar jams and diet yoghurts. However, special foods in general should be discouraged and the emphasis should be on healthy eating. Artificial sweeteners such as aspartame may be used on cereals, in drinks and desserts. Saccharin is generally not popular due to its bitter aftertaste. Sorbitol and fructose are not recommended as sweeteners.

Table 12.1	10 g carbohydrate exchanges
Bread $\frac{1}{2}$ large/1 small slice	
Breakfast cereal	
Weetabix	1 biscuit
Porridge	7 tablespoons
Cornflakes	5 tablespoons
Potatoes	
Boiled	1 small
Mashed	1 scoop
Chips	5
Baked	1 medium
Rice	3 tablespoons – cooked
Pasta	3 tablespoons – cooked
Digestive	1
Crisps	1 packet
Fruit	
Apple, orange, banana	1
Grapes	10
Beans in tomato sauce	5 tablespoons
Milk	$\frac{1}{3}$ pint
Yoghurt diet/natural	1 carton
Fruit yoghurt	$\frac{1}{2}$ carton

The diet

Initially, a detailed diet history should be taken to show the child's normal intake and the pattern of eating in the home. Carbohydrate should provide 40 to 50% of energy and should be taken at regular intervals with a pattern of three meals and three snacks a day. Meals should be eaten within 30 minutes of taking an insulin injection. The dietary fat should be kept as low as possible, and the fibre should be increased gradually to achieve as high an intake as practical.

Carbohydrate exchanges

In the past, a 10 g carbohydrate exchange system was often used (Table 12.1). A child was given a daily allowance and a suggestion was made of the distribution of carbohydrate throughout the day.

The British Diabetic Association recommends that foods are not measured, but that a meal or snack of approximately equal carbohydrates is given at regular intervals. The meal is assessed by eye and no measures are made. This method is useful for adults, and is being introduced increasingly for children, with the emphasis on healthy eating with a regular high complex carbohydrate intake over the day.

Hypoglycaemia

Hypoglycaemia may occur if insufficient carbohydrate is eaten, if there is a delay between injection and eating or after exercise. Symptoms include irritability, pallor and fatigue. 10 to 20 g of refined carbohydrate should be given, followed by another dose 10 to 15 minutes later if necessary. Glucose drinks, glucose tablets, jam or syrup can be used.

If hypoglycaemia occurs just before a meal, the meal should be given after the rapidly absorbed carbohydrate. If the next meal is not due for a while, a food containing complex carbohydrate such as a piece of fruit or a slice of bread should be given. If hypoglycaemia occurs regularly, the insulin regimen and diet should be reassessed.

Illness

Insulin injections should be given throughout illness. Blood glucose levels will generally be high throughout illness. The usual diet may be refused and it may not be necessary to replace it all. Small, frequent doses of rapidly absorbed carbohydrate should be given. Glucose drinks are often useful.

Infants

The normal feeding pattern of small frequent feeds is ideal. The infant with diabetes may be breast or bottle-fed and should be fed on demand at a normal intake of 150 to 200 ml/kg/day. Breast or formula milk should be continued until 12 months of age.

Solids can be introduced at the normal age of 4 to 6 months. Initially, puréed vegetables should be given, and once the child has established a good solid intake, carbohydrate-containing solids can be introduced. Breast or formula milk will continue to be the major source of carbohydrate, but the emphasis will shift throughout the first year as more solids are introduced. Vitamin supplements, as recommended for all infants, should be given.

Hypoglycaemia may be difficult to detect in infants. Extra milk with additional sugar or Ribena can be given. If hypoglycaemia occurs at night when the infant stops night-time feeds, a supper should be given or a milk feed and cereal at bedtime to maintain normoglycaemia overnight.

Toddlers

The erratic eating pattern and food fads of toddlers may cause anxiety for parents due to the risk of hypoglycaemia. Children should not be force-fed, as hypoglycaemic symptoms, if they develop, will make the child hungry and so more likely to eat. The normal recommendations for feeding toddlers should be followed. Semi-skimmed milk can be introduced at 2 years of age, provided the child is growing normally and has a varied diet. Skimmed milk can be introduced at 5 years of age.

School children

The British Diabetic Association's School Pack and Coping with Diabetes at School provide useful advice for teachers.

Children are advised to carry glucose tablets at school, and teachers should have a glucose drink to hand should it be needed. Advice should be given to teachers on the symptoms of hypoglycaemia and its treatment. Children should take extra carbohydrate prior to exercise, and physical education teachers should understand the signs of hypoglycaemia and its treatment. Children may need to carry extra carbohydrate for use during prolonged exercise.

Special school meals are not necessary and the usual school meal main course will be suitable. The dessert should be replaced by diet yoghurt or fresh fruit. Older children should be taught to select suitable foods if the meal is of a cafeteria style. Snacks such as crisps, peanuts, fresh fruit and raisins should be used in preference to sweets or chocolates.

 CASE STUDY

A 3-year-old girl is diagnosed with diabetes. She is started on once daily long acting insulin.

Her dietary pattern before and after diagnosis are shown in the table below:

	Pre-diagnosis	Post-diagnosis
Breakfast: 7.30 am	5 tablespoons Rice Krispies Sugar $\frac{1}{3}$ pint milk $\frac{1}{2}$ slice white toast + butter	7 tablespoons porridge $\frac{1}{3}$ pint milk $\frac{1}{2}$ slice wholemeal toast + poly unsaturated margarine
Mid-morning: 10.30 am	Chocolate covered biscuit Orange squash	10 grapes + 1 digestive biscuit Sugar-free squash
Lunch: 12.30 pm	5 tablespoons baked beans on 1 slice white toast with butter 1 banana	5 tablespoons baked beans on 1 slice wholemeal toast with polyunsaturated margarine 1 banana
Mid afternoon: 3.00 pm	Packet chocolate buttons Orange squash	1 biscuit Sugar-free squash
Dinner: 5.30 pm	5 tablespoons spaghetti bolognaise Chocolate bar	5 tablespoons spaghetti bolognaise 3 tablespoons stewed apple + sugar-free custard
Bedtime:	$\frac{1}{3}$ pint milk	$\frac{1}{3}$ pint milk $\frac{1}{2}$ slice wholemeal toast + polyunsaturated margarine

Adolescents

There is a tendency for adolescent girls, particularly, to become overweight. Weight control can be achieved by cutting out crisps and fried foods. The amount of carbohydrate should not be reduced. Advice should be given about the hypoglycaemic effect of alcohol.

CYSTIC FIBROSIS

Cystic fibrosis occurs in 1 in 2500 live births in Caucasian populations and is the most common recessively inherited disease (British Paediatric Association 1988). The disease is characterized by dysfunction of the exocrine glands, resulting in pancreatic insufficiency, pulmonary disease, intestinal obstruction, liver disease, diabetes and infertility. Survival rates in the UK up to 1985 were 50% surviving to the age of 20 years and 25% surviving to the age of 30 years.

KEY POINTS

◆ Incidence of 1 in 2500 live births in Caucasian populations.
◆ Main characteristics are pancreatic insufficiency, pulmonary disease, intestinal obstruction, liver disease, diabetes and infertility.
◆ Improved nutritional status is thought to improve survival.
◆ Dietary energy and protein intakes are increased by around 20 to 30% by increasing dietary fat and sugar intakes.
◆ Dietary supplements are frequently required and overnight enteral feeding is increasingly used.
◆ 90% of cystic fibrosis patients are pancreatic insufficient, requiring pancreatic enzyme replacement therapy.
◆ Diabetes is common. Two percent of cystic fibrosis patients develop diabetes between 10 and 15 years of age, 12% by 25 years, and 17% over 25 years.

Dietary management

Improving nutritional status of cystic fibrosis patients is thought to improve survival by improving a depressed immunological system, enhancing growth, and increasing respiratory muscle strength (Knowles 1988). Malnutrition is common in cystic fibrosis. The causes are outlined below.

Malabsorption

90% of patients with cystic fibrosis are pancreatic insufficient. There is also reduced duodenal bicarbonate and pH, gastric hypersecretion, disorders of bile salt metabolism and abnormal gastric motility. Pancreatic enzyme supplements are used. Even with correct use of enzymes, however, there may be significant loss of energy in the stools (Murphy et al 1991).

Increased energy expenditure

Resting energy expenditure is higher in cystic fibrosis than in healthy age-matched controls due to the increased effort of breathing and increased metabolic rate as a result of chronic infection.

Poor dietary intake

Children with cystic fibrosis have reduced dietary intake, resulting in poor energy intake. This is due to chronic respiratory infection, recurrent vomiting and abdominal pain. Parental anxiety and excessive focus on food and weight gain can result in behavioural food refusal, force-feeding and undue pressure at mealtimes. Media pressure and peer pressure to follow a low-fat, low-sugar diet, inappropriate weight-reducing diets, vegetarian diets and dislike of fatty foods all contribute to a poor dietary intake, as can the inappropriate use of dietary supplements.

Nutritional support

There are three levels of support:

◆ high protein/high energy diet
◆ dietary supplements
◆ enteral feeding.

High protein/high energy diet

Energy requirements are thought to be increased in cystic fibrosis, but individual requirements vary depending on age, activity and clinical status. Adequate intake should be monitored by weight gain and growth. Energy-rich foods, particularly foods which are high in fat and sugar, are encouraged. The diet should be based on a good routine with the inclusion of foods from all food groups, but the emphasis is on foods with a higher fat and sugar content. Full-cream milk, butter or margarine, cheese, meat, full-cream yoghurt, milk puddings, cakes and biscuits are encouraged. Foods should be fried or basted with oil. Butter can be added to potatoes and vegetables. Cream or full-cream milk can be used in soups and sauces. Snacks are encouraged between meals, but children should not replace meals with sweets or snacks.

Many parents, school teachers and some health professionals may find it difficult to accept the dietary recommendations as they directly oppose current recommendations for the general population.

Protein. It is recommended that protein provides 15% of the total energy to compensate for loss of protein in stools and sputum. A high protein intake can be achieved without extra supplementation.

Fat. Between 35 and 40% of energy should be provided by fat. Fat is the most concentrated source of energy and by increasing fat intake in the face of anorexia, an adequate energy intake can be achieved.

Carbohydrate. From 45 to 50% of total energy should be derived from carbohydrate as a combination of starchy foods and sugary foods. High-fibre foods may be helpful in reducing abdominal symptoms, particularly abdominal pain, but they can be filling and may reduce energy intake if used excessively.

Table 12.2 Vitamin supplementation in cystic fibrosis	
Vitamin	**Daily supplement**
Vitamin A	8000–10 000 iu (2400 µg–3000 µg)
Vitamin D	20 µg or 800 iu
Vitamin E	50 mg – infants 100 mg – children aged 1–10 years 200 mg – 10 yrs +
Vitamin K	In cystic fibrosis liver disease
Water-soluble vitamins	Not necessary

Table 12.3 Vitamin preparations used in cystic fibrosis	
Preparation	**Daily dose**
Abidec	1.2 ml/day
BPC multivitamins	3 tablets
A & D capsules	2 capsules
Separate vitamin E supplements	

Table 12.4 Salt supplementation in cystic fibrosis	
Age	**Salt supplementation**
0–1 year	2 mmol/kg
1–5 years	2 × 300 mg sodium chloride tablets (10 mmol Na+)
6–10 years	2 × 600 mg sodium chloride tablets (20 mmol Na+)
11 years +	3–4 × 600 mg sodium chloride tablets (30–40 mmol Na+)

Vitamin and mineral supplements. Fat-soluble vitamin deficiencies have been reported due to the loss of fat-soluble vitamin in the stools. Supplementation is required in all pancreatic insufficient patients, and should be considered in the 10% of patients who are pancreatic sufficient (Tables 12.2 and 12.3).

Sodium. Salt depletion may occur in hot weather or during strenuous exercise. A salt supplement is generally recommended in all infants under 1 year of age and for older children during summer months (Table 12.4).

Dietary supplements

Dietary supplements are frequently used as an additional source of energy and protein if adequate growth and weight gain are not achieved by diet alone and food intake is poor during a respiratory infection.

A wide range of supplements may be prescribed. Useful supplements fall into three main categories: fortified milk shakes, fortified fruit drinks and glucose polymers. The cartoned fortified milk shakes, such as Ensure Plus, Fortisip and Fresubin, and juice drinks such as Provide Xtra, Fortijuce and Enlive are popular with children and are particularly useful in packed lunches. They provide an additional source of energy and protein, and are fortified with vitamins and minerals. They are particularly useful in children with a poor quality diet where the additional minerals, particularly iron and zinc, may be useful.

Glucose polymer powders (e.g., Maxijul, Polycal and Caloreen) provide additional energy only and are easily incorporated into drinks at a concentration of 15 to 20% glucose. They are tasteless and so are useful in children who get bored of one flavour or type of drink and may reject cartoned milk shake or juice drinks for this reason. Concentrated glucose drinks, such as Polycal and Hycal, may also be diluted with water or lemonade and provide additional energy only.

Some children prefer the taste of milk shakes prepared with fresh milk. Scandishake (SHS International) is a useful supplement for this group of children. It provides 600 kcal when one sachet is added to 240 ml of fresh milk. It does not provide additional vitamins or minerals. Home-made and commercially available milk shakes are useful, but they are not fortified and can be expensive.

Inappropriate use of dietary supplements may reduce the appetite for normal foods and care should be taken in the quantity and timing of supplements. They should be given two or three times daily, after meals or at bedtime. The quantity recommended is dependent on age, older children being capable of taking larger volumes without affecting appetite.

Dietary supplements available in the UK

Fortified milkshakes

◆ Ensure Plus (Ross) (not suitable for children under 5 years)
◆ Fortisip (Nutricia)
◆ Fresubin (Fresenius)
◆ Entera (Fresenius).

Fortified juice drinks

◆ Enlive (Ross)
◆ Fortijuce (Nutricia)
◆ Paediasure (Ross)
◆ Provide Xtra (Fresenius).

Table 12.5 Recommendations for the use of dietary supplements

Age	Daily energy from supplements
1–2 years	200 kcal
3–5 years	400 kcal
6–11 years	600 kcal
12 years +	800 kcal

Glucose polymer drinks

◆ Polycal (Nutricia)
◆ Maxijul liquid (SHS International).

Glucose polymer powders

◆ Maxijul (SHS International)
◆ Caloreen (Clintec)
◆ Polycal (Nutricia).

Milkshake powders for use with fresh milk

◆ Scandishake (SHS International).

Table 12.5 shows recommendations for the use of dietary supplements.

Enteral feeding

Enteral feeding is being used increasingly as a means of achieving adequate nutritional status in patients with cystic fibrosis, the incidence being highest in adolescents and young adults. Feeding is usually given overnight by continuous infusion through a nasogastric or gastrostomy tube.

Enteral feeding is known to increase body fat and lean body mass, to improve strength and to trigger the development of secondary sexual characteristics. It is associated with reduced weight loss during respiratory infection and improved body image (Ramsey et al 1992). Guidelines on when to start feeding include failure to gain weight over 6 months or a weight for height of 80% or less (MacDonald et al 1991), failure to gain weight over 3 months or a weight for height of 85% or less (Ramsey et al 1992).

Enteral feeding is usually long-term, although some children benefit from a 2- or 3-week course of enteral feeding during inpatient episodes for the administration of intravenous antibiotics. This may be sufficient to maintain nutritional status, and should be considered if enteral feeding at home is not possible (Pierce et al 1990). Choice of feed preparation varies across different cystic fibrosis centres from elemental and semi-elemental to polymeric feeds. Elemental feeds are said to be better absorbed in cystic fibrosis, and some centres do not give pancreatic enzymes with elemental feeds. There is little published data to compare the effects of elemental versus polymeric feeds, and elemental feeds are expensive and have a lower energy density than polymeric feeds.

Most children will tolerate the less expensive option of polymeric feeds, provided that an appropriate dose of pancreatic enzymes is given. The method of administering pancreatic enzymes varies across cystic fibrosis centres, with some centres preferring to give enzymes at the start of the feed, others splitting the dose into two and giving some at the start and some midway or at the end of the feed. The dosage of enzyme required is estimated by using the amount needed for a meal and comparing its composition with that of the feed.

Nasogastric, gastrostomy and jejunostomy tubes have been used, gastrostomy and nasogastric tubes being used more commonly. The choice of tube is influenced by the likely duration of feeding and the preferences of the child and family. There are advantages and disadvantages to each route and these should be fully discussed with the family.

Pancreatic enzyme supplementation

A range of pancreatic enzymes are available as enteric coated microspheres:

- The enzyme is released in the duodenum and can achieve 90% fat absorption. The exact dose of pancreatic enzyme depends upon the amount of food eaten and the fat content. High-fat foods require more enzymes.
- Pancreatic enzymes are required with all fat-containing meals, snacks and drinks.
- A useful starting dose is half a capsule per feed for an infant and 2 to 3 capsules per meal for a 2 to 3-year-old child.
- The enzyme should be opened and the granules given mixed in fruit purée for infants and in fruit purée or jam for toddlers.

- Children should be encouraged not to crush or chew the granules and to take the enzymes whole as soon as possible.
- The dose should be adjusted to achieve minimal steatorrhoea following concerns regarding overuse of enzymes.

The Committee on Safety of Medicines recommended that a dose of 10 000 iu lipase per kg of body weight should not be exceeded unless there is evidence by faecal fat measurements of continued steatorrhoea. The majority of children will achieve good fat absorption on doses of less than 10 000 iu lipase per kg per day.

Adjunctive therapy to pancreatic enzymes

H_2 receptor antagonists have been used to enhance the effect of pancreatic enzymes. They reduce the volume and acid concentration of gastric secretions and reduce acid deactivation of enzymes. They may help increase the effect of enzymes and should be considered in children requiring large doses or with uncontrolled steatorrhoea.

Box 12.2 shows some guidelines on the use of pancreatic enzymes.

Box 12.2 Guidelines for the use of pancreatic enzymes

- Give with a meal rather than before or after.
- Give extra enzymes with fatty or large meals and snacks.
- Give enteric coated microspheres whole where possible. In infants the capsule may be opened and mixed with fruit purée.
- Do not crush or chew granules.
- Do not mix enzymes directly with food.
- Do not give enzymes with squash, fizzy drinks, fruit, boiled or jelly sweets.
- Increase the dose if stools are loose, fatty or more than twice a day.

Infant feeding

Many infants with cystic fibrosis have failure to thrive and hypoproteinaemia; this is true even of those identified early by neonatal screening. There may be reduced body fat, body mass and length, and low fat-soluble vitamin, serum protein and potassium levels. Appropriate dietary supplementation and pancreatic enzymes should enable most infants to achieve their optimum growth potential.

Feeds suitable for the infant with cystic fibrosis include breast milk, normal infant formula and protein hydrolysates.

Breast milk

There are several advantages to breastfeeding an infant with cystic fibrosis. Breast milk lipase may help to compensate for pancreatic insufficiency, it provides some immunological protection and enhances the mother–child bonding process. Infants with cystic fibrosis have been shown, with adequate use of pancreatic enzymes, to grow satisfactorily when breastfed.

The low sodium content of breast milk may lead to sodium depletion, and additional sodium supplements may therefore be required. Urinary and serum electrolyte tests will identify infants in need of additional sodium.

Weight gain should be monitored weekly and breast milk may be fortified with extra energy if necessary.

Normal infant formula

Normal infant formulae, both whey and casein dominant, are used successfully in infants with cystic fibrosis. The low sodium content may mean that infants require additional sodium, and energy supplements should be added if weight gain is poor.

Protein hydrolysates

Protein hydrolysates are used routinely in the USA, where it has been demonstrated that infants with cystic fibrosis show better growth on a casein hydrolysate feed than breast-feeds or normal infant formula (Farrell et al 1985). Protein hydrolysates are, however, more expensive and unpalatable and are used in the UK, only where there has been surgery for meconium ileus and a secondary disaccharide intolerance has developed. Pancreatic enzymes are still required with protein hydrolysates.

Weaning

Infants with cystic fibrosis should be weaned at the usual time of 4 to 6 months, and weaning should follow the normal practice. Parents may select home-prepared or commercial baby foods. Dried commercial baby foods may be prepared with infant formula or expressed breast milk instead of water and home-prepared foods may be supplemented with additional milk or butter. By 6 months of age the infant should be eating three meals a day, and milk puddings and custard made with cow's milk may be introduced. Adult yoghurts may also be used. Parents should be encouraged to go through the usual progression to lumpy and mashed foods, and introduce finger foods and drinks from a beaker from around 6 to 8 months of age.

Enzyme administration in infants

Enteric coated microspheres are the most effective preparation to use in infancy. They may be given off a spoon in a small amount of expressed or formula milk, or may be more effective mixed in a little fruit purée. These methods are effective even in infants of a few weeks of age. Dosage will vary, but one scoop of Creon for children or 0.5 of capsule preparations per breast-feed or formula feed of 90 ml is a good starting dose.

Toddlers

The emphasis on adequate weight gain and a good nutritional intake may lead the parents to focus excessively on a child's food intake. Mealtimes may become tense and behavioural food refusal is common. Parents may, in an attempt to get the child to eat, resort to force-feeding, which will in turn result in more severe food refusal. In severe cases, referral to a psychologist may help. There are a number of strategies, however, which may be helpful, and referral to a psychologist may be done if these are unsuccessful:

◆ Do not force-feed.
◆ Offer small regular meals.
◆ Provide a reward for good feeding by positive verbal reinforcement and smiling.
◆ Take uneaten food away without comment and do not give alternative foods instead.
◆ Do not discuss the child's feeding behaviour in front of him or her.
◆ Be consistent.
◆ Try to make mealtimes pleasant and relaxed.
◆ Time the meal to last for 20 to 30 minutes.
◆ Encourage the child to eat with others.
◆ Reassure the parents that the child will not be harmed in the short term by food refusal.

COELIAC DISEASE

Coeliac disease is defined as a disease of the small intestine characterized by an abnormal small intestinal mucosa associated with a permanent intolerance to gluten. Removal of gluten from the diet results in a full clinical and histological remission.

The prevalence of coeliac disease varies in different countries, but is about 1 in 1500 in the United Kingdom and Europe, although in Ireland it can be as high as 1 in 300. Approximately 3000 people are diagnosed with coeliac disease each year in the UK but the incidence in children has fallen (Stevens 1987).

KEY POINTS

◆ Commonly presents with gastrointestinal symptoms and failure to thrive.
◆ Diagnosis made by small intestinal biopsy and demonstration of clinical remission on a gluten-free diet.
◆ Treatment is with a lifelong gluten-free diet.
◆ Gluten challenge is recommended in children diagnosed under the age of 2 years.

CASE STUDY

A 6-month-old infant is diagnosed with cystic fibrosis. He is found to be pancreatic insufficient and at the time of presentation has six bulky offensive stools daily. He is failing to thrive: his weight is below the 3rd centile and his height is on the 25th centile.

Diet before diagnosis

6.00 am	200 ml infant formula feed
9.00 am	Cereal and milk + $\frac{1}{4}$ slice buttered toast
1.00 pm	Puréed chicken Potatoes and vegetables Stewed apple Baby juice
4.00 pm	Jar of commercial baby food 200 ml infant formula feed
8.00 pm	200 ml infant formula feed
11.00 pm	200 ml infant formula feed

Diet after diagnosis

6.00 am	200 ml high-energy infant formula feed $\frac{1}{2}$ capsule pancreatic enzyme
9.00 am	Cereal made with high-energy infant formula + sugar Buttered toast + jam 200 ml high-energy infant formula $1\frac{1}{2}$ capsules pancreatic enzyme
1.00 pm	Puréed chicken Potato + vegetables extra butter added Stewed apple + custard Baby juice 1 capsule pancreatic enzyme
4.00 pm	Jar of commercial baby food, yoghurt or other dessert 200 ml high-energy infant formula $1\frac{1}{2}$ capsules pancreatic enzyme
8.00 pm	200 ml high-energy infant formula $\frac{1}{2}$ capsule pancreatic enzyme
11.00 pm	200 ml high-energy infant formula $\frac{1}{2}$ capsule pancreatic enzyme

Symptoms

Infants and young children commonly present with gastrointestinal symptoms and failure to

Table 12.6 Symptoms of coeliac disease

Common symptoms	Less common symptoms
Failure to thrive	Vomiting
Growth failure	Constipation
Diarrhoea or steatorrhoea	Hypoalbuminaemia
Abdominal pain	Other micronutrient
Abdominal distension	deficiencies
Buttock wasting	Mouth ulcers
Pallor	Delayed puberty
Mood change	Increased appetite
Reduced appetite	
Anaemia	

thrive. This can occur any time after the first introduction of gluten-containing foods. Older children, like many adults, may have non-specific symptoms and have entirely normal growth and no obvious abnormalities in gastrointestinal function. Table 12.6 summarizes the symptoms of coeliac disease.

Diagnosis

Classical symptoms and anti-gliadin and anti-endomesial antibody studies may point towards a diagnosis, but guidelines state that a small intestinal biopsy demonstrating mucosal atrophy is necessary to confirm coeliac disease (ESPGAN 1992). For this reason it is essential that a gluten-containing diet be continued prior to the biopsy, even if a diagnosis of coeliac disease is suspected.

The next step in the diagnosis is the demonstration of remission of clinical signs on a gluten-free diet. If the clinical response is equivocal then a second biopsy to verify the response to dietary intervention is necessary, but usually relief of all symptoms is enough evidence to make a diagnosis. Recovery is often very rapid, with good weight gain, better mood and improvement in stools within as little as 2 weeks from commencement of treatment.

In children who are diagnosed under 2 years of age it is recommended that a gluten challenge takes place to demonstrate relapse on a gluten-containing diet. This is important to rule out other enteropathies such as cow's milk sensitivity and post-gastroenteritis syndrome with transient gluten intolerance. This challenge usually takes place about 2 years after the initial diagnosis and it is often helpful to complete the challenge by 5 years of age so a definitive diagnosis is established before the child attends school.

Gluten-free diet

The treatment for coeliac disease is a strict, lifelong, gluten-free diet. Gluten is a type of protein found in wheat, oats, rye and barley and foods made from any of these cereals. Some studies have shown that there is no clinical relapse in adult patients who include oats in their diet (Srinivasan et al 1996) but current UK guidelines recommend that oats continue to be excluded. The diet can be divide into three main groups of food: fresh foods, manufactured foods and special gluten-free products.

Fresh foods

Many foods are naturally gluten-free and can be included freely in the diet. Maize, rice, tapioca and buckwheat are cereals that do not contain gluten and are suitable to include in the diet. Fresh meat, fresh fish, milk, cheese, eggs, fruit and vegetables are also free from gluten.

Manufactured foods

Many everyday foods such as bread, flour, biscuits, cakes and pasta contain wheat flour and need to be avoided. Other less obvious foods such as sausages, sauces and ready-prepared meals may also contain hidden sources of gluten and these too must be excluded. Parents and children are advised to look carefully at food labels to recognize any possible sources of gluten. Many commercially produced baby foods contain gluten and parents should be careful to avoid such products. The Coeliac Society publishes a list of gluten-free manufactured foods to help families identify suitable products. A new list is produced every year, with twice-yearly updates in the society newsletter and weekly updates on Ceefax. It is essential that families use current information as manufacturers frequently change food ingredients.

Special gluten-free products

To make the diet more varied and easier to follow there are a number of specially prepared gluten-free foods available on prescription. These include flour, bread, plain biscuits, crackers, pasta and pizza bases. Other luxury items such as cakes, chocolate-coated biscuits, pastry and ready-prepared meals cannot be prescribed but can be bought from health food shops, from chemists and by mail order.

Table 12.7 shows some guidelines for a gluten-free diet.

Children who are diagnosed with coeliac disease should be advised on a gluten-free diet by a state registered dietitian who has an important role to play in helping the child and his or her family to establish a strict gluten-free diet. Although the principles of the diet are the same for all age groups, children often need to achieve catch-up growth and to continue to maintain normal growth throughout childhood and adolescence, and the advice of a paediatric dietitian is preferable.

Comprehensive advice should be given on basic dietary principles as well as information on prescribable products, manufactured foods and recipes with specific advice tailored to individual families. Help with holidays and eating out can also be useful.

The diet may require more food to be home-cooked from fresh ingredients, which can have financial and time implications for families. In addition, families who may have done very little baking will need to learn to cook with gluten-free flour, which may require help with recipes and cooking techniques. Many commercial companies provide special gluten-free recipes and videos to help with gluten-free cookery. Very young children will also require close supervision at mealtimes to ensure they do not share food with siblings or friends. It is

Table 12.7 Basic guidelines for a gluten-free diet

Type of food	Examples of food allowed	Examples of food to avoid unless known to be gluten-free
Meat, poultry and fish	Fresh meat, chicken, turkey and fish	Processed foods e.g. sausages, burgers, chicken nuggets, fish fingers
Bread, biscuits and cakes	Gluten-free bread, biscuits and cakes	Bread, biscuits and cakes made with wheat flour, oats, rye or barley
Breakfast cereals	Rice Krispies, Cornflakes, Frosties	Weetabix, Muesli, Ready Brek, Shredded Wheat
Flours, grains and pasta	Gluten-free flour, potato and soya flour, rice, sago, cornflour, buckwheat, gluten-free pasta	Wheat flour, oats, rye, barley, semolina, pasta
Milk and dairy foods	Milk, cream, butter, cheese, yoghurt	Cheese spread, processed cheese, muesli, yoghurt
Eggs	Boiled, fried, scrambled, poached	Scotch egg
Fats and oils	Butter, margarine, lard, oil, dripping	Packet suet
Vegetables	Fresh, frozen, tinned and dried	Croquette potato, potato waffle, vegetables in a sauce
Fruit	Fresh, frozen, tinned and dried	Fruit pie fillings
Puddings and desserts	Jelly, fruit, pies and crumbles made with gluten-free flour	Mousses, instant desserts, ice cream, pies, sponges, crumbles
Drinks	Milk, tea, coffee, squash, fruit juice, fizzy drinks	Horlicks, Ovaltine, barley water
Miscellaneous	Salt, herbs, freshly ground pepper, bicarbonate of soda, vinegar	Mixed spices, ground pepper, baking powder, curry powder

CASE STUDY

Adam has recently been diagnosed with coeliac disease. Changes have been made to his current intake to fit into a gluten-free diet. Changes are shown in italics.

	Normal diet	Gluten-free diet
Breakfast	Weetabix with milk and sugar	*Cornflakes* with milk and sugar
	Toast and butter	*Gluten-free toast* and butter
	Orange juice	Orange juice
Mid-morning	Digestive biscuit	*Gluten-free biscuit*
	Milk	Milk
Lunch	Cheese sandwich	*Gluten-free cheese sandwich*
	Kit Kat	*Bar of milk chocolate*
	Apple	Apple
	Orange squash	Orange squash
Mid-afternoon	Swiss roll	*Cake made with gluten-free flour*
	Tea	Tea
Tea	Roast chicken	Roast chicken
	Gravy	*Gluten-free gravy*
	Mashed potato	Mashed potato
	Peas and carrots	Peas and carrots
	Apple pie and cream	*Apple pie (made with gluten-free pastry)* and cream
Bedtime	Toast and butter	*Gluten-free toast* and butter
	Milk	Milk

advisable to teach children as young as possible about their diet. At diagnosis they may have been too young to understand the diet, so as soon as they are old enough it is important that children are taught which foods they can and cannot eat.

Long-term dietary compliance is essential for children with coeliac disease, and helping the family fit the diet around normal family meals and routines increases the likelihood of compliance. Teaching should involve as many family members as possible. Parents, siblings and grandparents all need to know the principles of a gluten-free diet to avoid dietary indiscretions. Childminders and nurseries also need to be advised on the importance of a strict gluten-free diet.

School meals

It is usually possible to arrange suitable gluten-free meals at school. This may be through the local school meal service or by direct liaison with schoolteachers and school cooks. The dietitian will be able to provide help with diet sheets, menus and recipes, and supplies of gluten-free flour, bread and pizza bases for the school will also help with providing a more varied menu. Canteen-style school meals present additional problems, but it may still be possible to provide special foods or give advice on choosing gluten-free items from daily menus.

Coeliac Society

The Coeliac Society was formed in 1968 to promote the welfare of children and adults with coeliac disease. All families are advised to join the Coeliac Society, which offers excellent information and help to members. There are local branches nationwide that can offer support and enable children and their families to meet others with coeliac disease.

Monitoring

Regular dietetic and medical follow-up is essential for all children with coeliac disease. This is particularly important during the first few weeks and months after diagnosis, when families require further support and dietetic advice in establishing the diet. It is important to document a clinical response to a gluten-free diet and complete resolution of symptoms. Children who present with weight loss or growth failure should have regular weight and height measurements to demonstrate catch-up, and blood tests may also be necessary to look at coeliac antibodies and to demonstrate resolution of hypoalbuminaemia, anaemia and other nutritional deficiencies. Failure to respond to the diet could indicate a wrong diagnosis or poor dietary compliance and should be investigated further.

Once the diet has become established the level of dietetic follow-up can be reduced as the child and family become more familiar with the regimen. Medical follow-up also becomes less frequent with children often returning to clinic for an annual review. It could be argued that the diet becomes a way of life and children may not require long-term follow-up, but studies suggest that dietary compliance is poor in the long term (Bardella et al 1994). Follow-up is recommended at a minimum of 6- to 12-monthly intervals to assess symptoms and dietary compliance and should be maintained throughout the patient's life (British Society for Gastroenterology 1996). Regular dietary assessments by a dietitian will help to monitor nutritional adequacy and dietary compliance. Continuing support may be particularly important when children start school or enter adolescence. Additional support can be provided by health visitors and school nurses who have a role to play in monitoring growth and maintaining dietary compliance when hospital follow-up is less frequent.

A strict, lifelong gluten-free diet is necessary to avoid the risk of developing complications and it is important to maintain dietary compliance even in the absence of symptoms. Studies suggest an increase in malignant lymphoma (Walters 1994) and osteoporosis (Holmes 1997) in patients with undiagnosed coeliac disease and those who do not keep to a strict gluten-free diet. Infertility can also be a problem in untreated patients (Collin 1996). Early diagnosis and good dietary compliance is therefore essential to safeguard against these complications.

Related conditions

The association of coeliac disease with other disorders is well documented. These include Down's syndrome, cystic fibrosis and insulin-dependent diabetes. Prevalence rates of coeliac disease in insulin-dependent diabetes mellitus have been reported between 4–6% (Sigurs 1993) and it has become routine to screen patients with insulin-dependent diabetes mellitus for coeliac disease.

FOOD ALLERGY AND INTOLERANCE

Intolerance to food is frequently described in children. Although it is seen more often in infants and young children than in adults, adverse reactions to food are medically proven in only a small percentage of cases, and perceived food intolerance and over-diagnosis of food allergy is common.

Food allergy is described as an abnormal immunological reaction to a food and is mediated through IgE mechanisms. There are many foods that can cause an allergic reaction, the commonest in children being cow's milk, egg, wheat and nuts. Symptoms may be trivial (e.g., urticaria or eczema), but in severe cases the allergic reaction may be life-threatening. An adverse reaction to food that is not immune-mediated is known as a food intolerance. Although symptoms are usually less severe, they can still be troublesome.

It is important that children are not placed unnecessarily on a restricted diet, so a clear diagnosis should be made before foods are permanently excluded. The first stage is to demonstrate an improvement in symptoms by excluding suspected foods from the diet. The second stage is to demonstrate a reproducible reaction to the food when it is reintroduced into the diet.

KEY POINTS

- Food allergy is an abnormal immune response to a food.
- Food intolerance is an adverse reaction to a food that is not immune-mediated.
- Symptoms range from trivial to life-threatening.
- Dietary treatment excludes foods that cause a reaction. Advice should be comprehensive and tailored to each individual child.
- Diets should be nutritionally adequate.
- Children should be monitored regularly.
- Most cases of food allergy and intolerance are temporary so it is important to challenge children regularly so they do not remain unnecessarily on a restricted diet.

Once a diagnosis has been reached the child should be started on a diet that excludes the foods that have caused adverse reactions. Following an exclusion diet is a big undertaking for the family and it is important to establish that the diet is not worse than the symptoms. Whilst there is no doubt that children at risk of anaphylaxis need to adhere rigidly to a diet, a child with mild eczema may tolerate his or her symptoms better than a highly restricted diet. Parents and children must be highly motivated and given comprehensive information so they are able to follow the diet. It is also of vital importance that the diet remains nutritionally adequate. In some cases, avoiding a food has no nutritional consequences, such as the case of children with nut intolerance. In other cases, such as cow's milk intolerance, there are significant nutritional implications and care needs to be taken to maintain a nutritionally adequate diet. It is essential that children who are to follow a restricted diet are referred to a pediatric dietitian who can provide appropriate dietary advice for the child and the family, ensuring that the diet remains nutritionally complete and allows for normal growth.

Many cases of food allergy and intolerance are temporary. Children often grow out of their intolerances, and for this reason it is important to challenge children regularly so that they do not remain unnecessarily on a restricted diet. Food challenges are advisable for nearly all adverse reactions to foods, but should be carried out with care in children who have had severe life-threatening reactions.

Each child's diet will vary according to his or her particular dietary restrictions, but there are common features to all elimination diets:

◆ Parents and children need to know how to recognize obvious and hidden sources of forbidden foods.
◆ Food alternatives need to be provided if the restriction has nutritional implications for the child's diet.
◆ Parents need advice on how to alter the child's existing diet to cause minimal disruption to family mealtimes and routines.
◆ Particular help is also needed with provision of school meals, children's parties and eating out.

The problems of a restricted diet for food intolerance will be illustrated in detail using milk intolerance as an example, with details specific to other special diets being described briefly.

Milk intolerance and milk-free diets

Milk is one of the commonest foods to cause intolerance in children. It may occur in young infants and also in older children, but in most cases it is not a lifelong problem. Intolerance may be to the protein in milk, and this is often referred to as cow's milk protein intolerance. Intolerance to the milk sugar is called lactose intolerance and is most commonly seen as a complication of gut surgery or gastroenteritis. Symptoms of milk intolerance are varied but include diarrhoea, bloody stools, abdominal pain, iron deficiency anaemia, failure to thrive, urticarial skin rash, asthma and eczema. Both cow's milk protein intolerance and lactose intolerance require total exclusion of milk from the diet.

Milk substitutes

Infants rely solely on a milk source to provide all their nutrition in the first 4 months of life, and even at 2 years of age milk remains a major source of energy, protein, calcium and vitamins (Francis 1987). All normal infant formulae are based on cow's milk, and even babies who are breastfed can exhibit signs of cow's milk protein intolerance due to transference of allergens through the mother's milk. It is essential that all infants and young children are provided with a nutritionally complete

Table 12.8 Nutritionally complete soya formulae

Milk substitute	Manufacturer
Infasoy	Cow and Gate, Nutricia
Wysoy	SMA Nutrition
Farleys Soya	Farleys Health Products
Prosobee	Mead Johnson Nutritionals
Isomil	Ross Laboratories

Table 12.9 Nutritionally complete protein hydrolysate formulae

Milk substitute	Manufacturer
Pregestimil	Mead Johnson
Nutramigen	Mead Johnson
Peptijunior	Cow and Gate, Nutricia
Alfaré	Nestlé
Prejomin	Milupa
Pepdite 0–2	SHS International

milk substitute. There are many suitable milk sub-stitutes available, including soya formulae (Table 12.8) and protein hydrolysate formulae (Table 12.9). There is a high cross-reactivity between soya and cow's milk formulae in children who have gastrointestinal symptoms of cow's milk pro-tein intolerance (ESPGAN 1992), and in children less than a year old a nutritionally complete pro-tein hydrolysate formula is the feed of choice. Soya formulae are, however, perfectly adequate for older children and for those with simple lactose intolerance. All these feeds are ACBS listed and available on prescription.

There are many soya milks that can be bought from supermarkets and health food shops. These are not nutritionally complete, and are therefore unsuitable for infants and young children. They may, however, be a suitable milk substitute for older children, providing such children eat a varied and balanced diet. Some of these soya milks are fortified with calcium. Goat's milk and ewe's milk are also widely available but they, too, are not a suitable substitute for infants and young children.

Milk-free diets

Infants should be weaned on to a milk-free diet and parents should be given advice on suitable commercially produced weaning foods and milk-free foods that they can prepare themselves. For older children all manufactured foods need to be carefully checked for sources of milk, and parents are advised to check all labels very carefully.

Milk products are found in a wide variety of manufactured foods and may be listed on labels in many ways. All of the following are milk-contain-ing components:

- ◆ milk
- ◆ skimmed milk powder
- ◆ casein and caseinates
- ◆ whey
- ◆ lactose
- ◆ butter
- ◆ milk sugar
- ◆ cheese and cheese powder
- ◆ cream
- ◆ yoghurt.

The use of milk-free baby food lists and milk-free manufactured food lists can be very helpful. These are available from a dietitian, who will be able to supervise the milk-free diet and make sure that the diet meets the child's nutritional needs. Comprehensive advice should be given on basic dietary principles as well as information on pre-scribable products, manufactured foods, and recipes with specific advice tailored to individual families.

The diet may require more food to be home-cooked from fresh ingredients, which can have financial and time implications for families. Very young children will also require close supervision at mealtimes to ensure they do not share food with siblings or friends. If they are old enough, it is

 CASE STUDY

Emma has cow's milk protein intolerance and has been prescribed a soya formula as a milk substitute. Her diet has been changed to fit in with a milk-free diet. Changes are shown in italics.

	Normal diet	Milk-free diet
Breakfast	Ready Brek with milk	Ready Brek with *soya formula*
	Toast and butter	Toast and *milk-free margarine*
	Orange juice	Orange juice
	Chocolate biscuit	*Biscuit known to be milk-free*
Mid-morning	Milk	*Soya formula*
	Cheese sandwich	*Ham sandwich*
Lunch		*(milk-free margarine)*
	Fruit yoghurt	*Jelly and tinned fruit*
	Orange squash	Orange squash
Mid-afternoon	Swiss roll	*Cake known to be milk-free*
	Tea	*Tea made with soya formula*
Tea	Fish in batter	*Grilled fish*
	Chips	Chips
	Baked beans	*Baked beans known to be milk-free*
	Banana custard	*Banana custard made with soya formula*
Bedtime	Toast and butter	Toast and *milk-free margarine*
	Milk	*Soya formula*

important that children are taught about their diet so they can learn which foods they can safely eat. Parents, siblings, grandparents and childminders all need to know the principles of a milk-free diet to avoid dietary indiscretions, and teaching should involve as many family members as possible.

Compliance with the diet is essential and can become difficult for children who are deprived of many popular children's foods. The dietitian can also offer advice on milk-free alternatives for favourite foods, and ideas to keep the diet varied and interesting. Trying to fit the diet around normal mealtimes and routines will also help compliance, and liaison with health visitors can offer additional support to families. Regular follow-up is important to check the nutritional adequacy of the diet and to ensure children grow and gain weight normally.

Eating outside the home

Children who are required to follow a milk-free diet must adhere to their diet at all times. It is possible to arrange milk-free meals at school and at nursery, and teachers and school cooks should be advised about the diet and given help with menus. Children's parties pose a difficult problem. Warning parents ahead of time can help but it is still usually necessary to be careful, as popular party foods such as sandwiches, cakes, biscuits, crisps and ice cream are all potential sources of milk and milk derivatives. It is usually necessary for children to take their own food with them and supplement with safe party foods such as plain crisps and jelly.

Eating out in restaurants can be difficult. There may be suitable milk-free choices but it is not always possible to identify them from the menu. Some larger chains of restaurants may produce information about which foods are milk-free; alternatively, the chef may be able to advise on milk-free choices.

Milk challenges

Milk intolerance is usually a temporary condition and it is important that children do not remain on a restricted diet longer than necessary. Lactose intolerance, with the exception of rare congenital alactasia, resolves after a maximum of 3 to 4 months and reintroduction of cow's milk can be tried at home. Cow's milk protein intolerance persists for much longer and children are usually advised to stay on a milk-free diet for a minimum of 2 years. Children with cow's milk protein intolerance can have a severe reaction to cow's milk and reintroduction of milk is usually done under medical supervision.

Calcium supplements

Children who do not take adequate amounts of milk substitute, either as a drink or incorporated into their diet, may require a calcium supplement to ensure they meet the recommended dietary intake for their age. This is quite common in older children who refuse a nutritionally complete milk substitute. Breastfeeding mothers who are required to follow a milk-free diet may also require a calcium supplement. Calcium supplements are available in many forms and are available on prescription (Table 12.10).

Table 12.10 Commonly used calcium supplements in paediatrics

Preparation	Calcium dose
Calcium Sandoz Syrup (Sandoz)	108 mg/5 ml
Sandocal 400 (Sandoz)	400 mg/tablet
Calcichew (Shire Pharmaceuticals)	500 mg/tablet
Sandocal 1000 (Sandoz)	1000 mg/tablet

RENAL DISEASE

Special diets have an essential role to play in the management of children with impaired renal function. The kidneys have three main functions:

1. Excretion of waste products (e.g., urea, creatinine, phosphate).
2. Regulation of water and electrolyte content of the body.
3. Metabolic control (e.g., production of erythropoetin and 1,25-dihydroxycholecalciferol).

Disorders that affect the kidney's ability to maintain these functions are managed with dietary modifications in addition to medical management.

Children with renal failure often have very poor appetites resulting in a poor dietary intake. Anorexia increases as blood urea rises and is the main contributing factor in failure to thrive. Vomiting is also a common problem in children with renal failure and can have a significant effect on nutrition. Dietetic management must therefore aim to implement the necessary dietary restrictions, but must also maintain an adequate nutritional intake for growth. Dietary supplements are commonplace to meet nutritional requirements, but enteral feeding is also frequently required either via the nasogastric or gastrostomy route (Coleman & Watson 1992). This is usually provided by continuous infusion overnight, allowing the maintenance of oral feeding during the day. Children with renal disease are likely to continue with poor appetites until they have had a successful kidney transplant, which may not happen for several years. It is therefore important that children learn oral feeding skills even if oral feeds contribute very little to the overall nutritional intake. Weaning should be at the normal time, and a wide range of tastes and textures should be offered so children learn to feed normally.

Poor linear growth is also frequently seen, particularly in children who have developed renal failure in the first few years of life. Maximizing nutritional intake is an important part of management but children may still fail to grow normally despite correction of dietary and metabolic problems. Catch-up growth after kidney transplantation can occur but will depend on the age of the child, the extent of growth retardation and the effects of immunosuppressive drugs (steroids).

Kidney disorders in childhood that require special diets can be divided into three main categories:

1. Acute renal failure.
2. Chronic renal failure.
3. Nephrotic syndrome.

Acute renal failure

This is a sudden deterioration in renal function. The most common cause is haemolytic uraemic syndrome. Children may sometimes be managed conservatively, but short-term dialysis is commonly required. Full recovery of renal function usually occurs but acute renal failure may lead to chronic renal failure.

Chronic renal failure

Chronic renal failure is the final pathway in a number of different diseases of the kidney in children. The most common causes are glomerulonephritis and reflux nephropathy. Chronic renal failure will proceed to end-stage renal failure, and dietary management of chronic renal failure involves delaying this progression, minimizing uraemia and ensuring adequate nutrition to maintain growth. End-stage renal failure is inevitably reached, after which time the introduction of dialysis becomes necessary and transplantation is required.

Nephrotic syndrome

This condition is characterized by heavy proteinuria, hypoalbuminaemia, hyperlipidaemia and gross oedema. Minimal change nephrotic syndrome accounts for the majority of cases of the disease. The primary treatment is with steroids, and if children are responsive to treatment there

---

KEY POINTS

- ◆ Nutritional management in children with abnormal renal function should implement the necessary dietary restrictions but also maintain growth.
- ◆ Anorexia is common and consequently calorie supplementation and enteral feeding is often necessary.
- ◆ The main nutrients that require modification are protein, potassium, calcium and phosphate.
- ◆ Fluid restriction is usually necessary for patients on dialysis.
- ◆ Treatment should be tailored to the needs of each individual child.

are few dietary problems and the prognosis is good. If response is poor and children relapse frequently, they may become steroid-dependant, and dietary intervention then has a greater part to play both in maintaining nutritional status and in preventing steroid-induced obesity. If children are unresponsive to steroids and proteinuria continues they may go on to develop chronic renal failure, and this is also the inevitable end progression of congenital nephrotic syndrome. Growth can be affected in children on prolonged steroid therapy, and obesity commonly becomes a problem (Rees et al 1988). If children are not responsive to steroids they exhibit growth failure due to inadequacy of protein and energy intake as anorexia is a common problem. A high-energy diet will minimize catabolism, but to control oedema many children are also advised to follow a low-salt regime which makes the diet unpalatable.

Dietary manipulation requires attention to the following nutrient intakes:

◆ energy
◆ protein
◆ calcium and phosphate
◆ fluid
◆ potassium
◆ sodium
◆ vitamins.

Table 12.11 summarizes the dietary restrictions associated with renal disease.

Energy

The provision of adequate energy is essential to promote growth in all children. In children with renal disease it is particularly important, when protein intake is restricted, in order to 'spare' the protein for anabolism. Anorexia is common in children with renal disease, and consequently calorie supplements are widely used to improve energy intake with the aim of providing the appropriate energy intake for age (Department of Health 1991). In nephrotic syndrome that is sensitive to treatment with steroids, there may be rapid weight gain and it may be necessary to advise children on sensible healthy eating to prevent obesity.

Protein

The kidneys have a major role to play in the excretion of end products of protein metabolism. Poor kidney function leads to a raised urea and creatinine and can be controlled with dietary protein restriction. This is usually necessary when the glomerular filtration rate falls below 50 ml/min/m^2. The degree of restriction depends on a number of factors and will vary according to the nature of the kidney disease, biochemical assessment, and the age and weight of the child. Dialysis treatment will also affect the protein allowance, with more generous amounts of protein allowed on dialysis than pre-end stage renal disease. The aim would be to keep plasma urea levels below approximately 20 mmol/l. Many children self-restrict their protein intake due to their poor appetite, and minimal restrictions to food intake may be necessary. If their appetite remains good, children are given daily protein allowances. Infants may require specially modified formulae, and older children on enteral feed may also require specially modified feeds. A range of special low-protein products can be used to add variety and provide extra energy.

A high-protein diet has been used in the past to treat nephrotic syndrome, but there is no evidence to suggest that high dietary protein increases plasma albumin levels (Al-Bander & Kaysen 1991) and it may in fact accelerate the progression of chronic renal failure.

Calcium and phosphate

The maintenance of a normal serum calcium and phosphate is important to achieve normal bone growth and prevent rickets and hyperparathyroidism. Impaired phosphate excretion leads to an alteration in the balance of calcium and phosphate which can seriously affect the bones, so dietary phosphate restriction is frequently necessary in chronic renal failure. Whey-based infant formulae are lower in phosphate than casein-based formulae and are therefore encouraged in infancy. If phosphate levels remain high it may be necessary to commence infants on Kindergen Prod (SHS), a commercially prepared low phosphate infant

Table 12.11 Summary of dietary restrictions

	Age	Energy	Protein g/kg/day	Phosphate restriction	Potassium restriction	No added salt diet	Fluid restriction
Acute renal failure (conservative management)	0–2 years			<400 mg/day			
	2–9 years	>EAR	1.0–1.8	<600 mg/day	Low	Yes	Yes
	> 9 years			<RNI			
Acute renal failure (peritoneal dialysis)	0–2 years		2.0–2.5				
	2–9 years	>EAR	1.0–2.5	<RNI	Low	Yes	Yes
	> 9 years		1.0–2.5				
Acute renal failure (haemodialysis)	0–2 years		1.5–2.1				
	2–9 years	>EAR	1.0–1.8	<RNI	Low	Yes	Yes
	> 9 years		1.0–1.8				
Chronic renal failure (conservative management)	0–2 years		1.5–3.0				
	2–9 years	100–120% EAR	1.5–2.0	<RNI	Possible	Possible	No
	> 9 years		1.0–1.5				
End-stage renal failure (peritoneal dialysis)	0–2 years		2.0–3.0				
	2–9 years	EAR	2.5	<RNI	Moderate	Yes	Yes
	> 9 years		1.5–2.0				
End-stage renal failure (haemodialysis)	0–2 years		1.5–2.0				
	2–9 years	EAR	1.0–1.5	<RNI	Very low	Yes	Yes
	> 9 years		1.0–1.5				
Nephrotic syndrome (unresponsive)	All ages	100–120% EAR	2.0–4.0	None	None	Yes	Yes
Nephrotic syndrome (steroid responsive)	0–2 years		2.0				
	2–9 years	<EAR	1.5	RNI	None	Yes	Yes
	> 9 years		1.0–1.5				

EAR = estimated average requirement, RNI = recommended nutrient intake for age formula. For older children it is necessary to restrict milk and dairy products as well as other protein-containing foods that are also rich in phosphate. Commercially available low-protein milk substitutes are also low in phosphate and may be a suitable alternative to cow's milk.

If dietary restriction fails to control serum phosphate levels children may require phosphate binder tablets. The binders contain calcium carbonate and are prescribed to be taken with meals and snacks to minimize absorption of phosphate. Many preparations are available, including a solution that can be added to infant formulae and enteral feeds.

Fluid

Fluid restriction is rarely needed pre-dialysis. Many children with kidney disease may in fact be polyuric in the early stages when they lose the capacity to concentrate urine. It is important to maintain an adequate fluid intake in these children. If the disease progresses urine output will decrease as the glomerular filtration rate falls, ultimately resulting in end-stage renal failure and the need for fluid restriction. Fluid restriction is also necessary in the oedematous phase of nephrotic syndrome. Fluid restrictions will vary and are based on urine volume plus insensible losses. Children with nephrotic syndrome require only temporary fluid restriction, but children with end-

stage renal disease will require a longer term restriction. Compliance can be difficult for children who are anuric or oliguric and may be the most difficult part of their dietary management. This is particularly difficult in children who are receiving part of their daily allowance as nasogastric or gastrostomy feeds. Despite concentrating the feed up to as high as 2 kcal/ml, oral fluid allowances may be very small. Daily peritoneal dialysis allows for a more generous fluid allowance than haemodialysis.

Potassium

Potassium restriction becomes necessary when children are approaching end-stage renal failure and is associated with a reduced urine output. Reduced potassium excretion in the urine results in elevated serum potassium. Cardiac disturbances are often the only manifestations of hyperkalaemia and regular measurement of serum potassium is necessary to keep the level within a safe range. Cardiac arrest can occur with high levels of potassium, so it is important that children and their families understand the need for good dietary compliance. Advice should be based on blood biochemistry, and monitoring of results will allow the dietitian to modify the diet for each individual child. This avoids an unnecessarily strict diet but at the same time protects against the risk

Table 12.12 Potassium in foods

	High-potassium foods	**Low-potassium alternatives**
Fruit	Bananas, oranges, grapefruit, dried fruit, tinned fruit in fruit juice	Apples, pears, tinned fruit in syrup
Vegetables	Potato Tomatoes, baked beans, mushrooms, spinach	Potato soaked overnight and boiled, rice, pasta Carrots, cabbage, swede, cauliflower
Cakes and biscuits	Fruit cake, chocolate cake Chocolate biscuits	Plain sponge cake, doughnuts Plain biscuits, custard creams
Beverages	Fruit juice Coffee, cocoa, hot chocolate	Squash, lemonade Tea
Sweets	Chocolate, toffee, fudge	Boiled sweets, jelly sweets
Snacks	Potato crisps, Hula Hoops, nuts	Corn snacks (e.g. Wotsits)
Dairy products	Milk, yoghurt	Milk substitutes

of hyperkalaemia. Children on intermittent haemodialysis will need tighter dietary control than children on daily dialysis. High-potassium foods must be avoided but it may be possible to allow treats during haemodialysis sessions. Table 12.12 shows foods with a high potassium content, and gives some low-potassium alternatives.

Sodium

In end-stage renal failure children may be advised to follow a no added salt diet, particularly if they have high blood pressure or if fluid is restricted. This also applies to children with poorly controlled nephrotic syndrome who require a low-salt diet alongside a fluid restriction to control oedema. Such a diet avoids very salty foods and contains no added salt in cooking or at the table. It is important to remember that diets need to be palatable and dietary restrictions to achieve a low salt intake should not render the diet too unappetizing.

Vitamins

As previously discussed, children with kidney failure generally have poor appetites. Inadequate food intakes and restricted diets can result in inadequate micronutrient intakes, and vitamins can also be lost during dialysis. A multivitamin supplement is advisable to ensure children meet their recommended nutrient intakes (Department of Health 1991). In addition, vitamin D supplements are necessary to replace 1,25-dihydroxycholecalciferol normally produced by the kidneys.

PHENYLKETONURIA

Phenylketonuria is a recessively inherited condition. The incidence is around 1 in 10 000 live births in the UK. All infants in the UK are screened for phenylketonuria using the Guthrie test between day 6 and 14. The basic defect is a deficiency of phenylalanine hydroxylase which is essential for the breakdown of phenylalanine to tyrosine. As a result, phenylalanine levels are raised in the blood. Untreated phenylketonuria can cause severe mental retardation and seizures.

> **KEY POINTS**
>
> - Phenylketonuria is a recessively inherited untreated disorder.
> - Untreated phenylketonuria can cause mental retardation, seizures and defects in pigmentation.
> - All infants are screened in the UK between the sixth and fourteenth day of life. Incidence is 1 in 10 000 live births.
> - Treatment is by a very low-phenylalanine diet, plus phenylalanine-free protein substitute to provide other essential amino acids, vitamins and minerals.
> - Treatment should start as early as possible.
> - It is recommended that diet is continued for life.

Principle of dietary treatment

Treatment for phenylketonuria is by a low-phenylalanine diet. This should be introduced as early as possible with an aim of achieving plasma phenylalanine levels between 120 and 360 µmol/l. This is done by reducing dietary phenylalanine intake.

Phenylalanine is an essential amino acid, and a small amount is required. Foods with a high phenylalanine concentration such as meat, fish, eggs, cheese, nuts, bread, biscuits and cakes are avoided. There are four main parts to the diet:

- Measured quantity of phenylalanine to give essential requirements in the form of a 50 mg exchange system.
- A phenylalanine-free protein substitute is required to supply all other amino acids to meet daily requirements.
- Low-phenylalanine foods are allowed freely.
- A comprehensive vitamin and mineral supplement is required, unless the protein supplement is fortified.

Phenylalanine is given in measured amounts from foods of a lower phenylalanine content such as cereals, potatoes and some vegetables. A 50 mg exchange system is generally used (see Box 12.3).

Box 12.3   Examples of 50 mg phenylalanine exchanges (NSPKU 1999)

Milk	30 ml
Single cream	40 ml
Vegetables	
Potatoes	
Boiled, boiled and mashed milk-free, jacket	80 g
Roast	55 g
Chips – frozen, fresh, oven, crinkle	45 g
Baked beans – ordinary, barbecue, curried	20 g
Peas – fresh, frozen and petit pois	25 g
Cereals	
Kelloggs Cornflakes	15 g
Rice Krispies	15 g
Weetabix, Weetaflakes	10 g
Fruits	
Passion fruit	35 g

Box 12.4   Examples of free foods (NSPKU 1999)

Fruit

Most types.

Vegetables

French beans, beetroot, cabbage, carrots, cauliflower, celery, courgettes, cucumber, gherkin, leek, lettuce, marrow, mushrooms, onion, pickled onion, parsnip, peppers (red, green, yellow and orange), swede, sweet potato, tomato, turnip. All clear vegetable pickles in vinegar.

Cereals

Cornflour, arrowroot, custard powder, blancmange powder, sago, tapioca.

Fats

Butter, margarine (but not margarine spreads which contain buttermilk – i.e., some low fat spreads), vegetable fats and oils (liquid and solid).

Miscellaneous

Sugar, glucose, jam, honey, marmalade, syrup, treacle, boiled sweets.

Drinks

Water, soda water, mineral water, aspartame-free fizzy drinks, fruit cordial and squash, black tea, black coffee and pure fruit juices.

Phenylalanine-free protein substitute

The diet must have sufficient protein to sustain normal growth, and a phenylalanine-free protein substitute is essential. Examples include: Analog LCP for infants; XP Maxamaid for children aged 1 to 8 years; XP Maxamum for children over 8 years and adults.

Protein substitutes taste unpleasant; they may be given as a drink or the powder may be given as a paste followed by a drink. They are best taken very cold using a covered cup and drunk through a straw. The daily amount should be split into three doses and given evenly throughout the day.

The restriction of phenylalanine in the diet also severely restricts vitamin and mineral intakes. The nutritionally complete protein substitutes provide sufficient vitamins and minerals if taken in sufficient volume. If a pure amino acid mixture is used, full vitamin and mineral supplementation will be required. Paediatric Seravit (SHS) or Forceval Junior Capsules plus a calcium supplement are suitable.

Free foods

Foods with very low phenylalanine content, such as sugar, butter, oil, and some fruits and vegetables, may be given freely. A range of prescribable bread flour, biscuits and pastas are available and are essential to increase variety. Box 12.4 shows some foods with very low phenylalanine content.

Monitoring

Blood phenylalanine measurements should be taken by capillary sampling at a set time, ideally early morning when levels will be highest. After stabilization, phenylalanine levels should be monitored weekly until 4 years of age. The frequency can reduce to fortnightly until 10 years of age and then monthly. Parents should be contacted with the results as soon as possible and the child's diet should be adjusted if necessary. Possible causes of high and low phenylalanine levels are given in Table 12.13.

Table 12.13 Possible causes of high and low phenylalanine levels

Causes of high phenylalanine levels	Causes of low phenylalanine levels
Catabolism (due to infection, surgery)	A growth spurt
Inadequate intake of energy or other amino acids	Anabolic phase: e.g., following an infection
Reduced requirement due to reduced growth rate	Inadequate intake of exchanges
Cheating	

Newly diagnosed infant

If plasma phenylalanine concentrations exceed 600 μmol/l while the infant is feeding normally, a low phenylalanine diet should be started. If the levels are 400 to 600 μmol/l, monitoring will be needed to decide if dietary restriction is indicated.

An infant presenting with plasma phenylalanine levels between 600 and 1000 μmol/l should have a phenylalanine-free protein substitute given in addition to breast or formula feeds. Infants with phenylalanine levels in excess of 1000 μmol/l should have all breast or formula feeds stopped for 24 to 72 hours. The phenylalanine-free protein substitute should be given. This will achieve a rapid fall in plasma phenylalanine levels. The breast or normal infant formula feeds should then be reintroduced alongside the protein substitute.

Breastfeeding

At diagnosis, if the infant is having only protein substitute, the mother must express regularly to maintain a supply of breast milk. Breast feeding may be reintroduced once levels reach 1000 μmol/l or below.

Phenylalanine levels are controlled by giving the phenylalanine-free formula in measured amounts before a breast-feed. The breast milk intake can be regulated by adjustments to the quantity of phenylalanine-free formula given. If the plasma phenylalanine level drops below 120 μmol/l, the total volume of phenylalanine-free formula is reduced so that the breast-feeds will increase. If the plasma phenylalanine level goes above 360 μmol/l, the volume of phenylalanine-free formula is increased to reduce the intake of breast milk.

Bottle-feeding

Once the phenylalanine levels reach 1000 μmol/l or below, normal formula can be reintroduced. An initial quantity of 50 to 70 mg of phenylalanine per kg may be reintroduced. This should be divided between the feeds and given before the phenylalanine-free formula, which may be given on demand.

The quantity of infant formula is adjusted according to phenylalanine levels. If the levels fall below 120 μmol/l, the infant formula should be increased by 50 mg. If it exceeds 360 μmol/l, it should be decreased by 25 to 50 mg.

Weaning

Solids are introduced at the usual time of 4 to 6 months. Initially, low-protein solids such as puréed fruit, or Aminex low-protein rusks (Gluten Free Foods Limited) can be given. These should be introduced after a feed; once weaning is established a 50 mg exchange of food may be given before feeds.

Twelve months of age

At around 12 months of age, bottle-feeding will stop. The infant protein substitute should be replaced by an alternative protein substitute such as XP Maxamaid (SHS International). Ideally, a small amount of this should be introduced as a paste before bottle-feeding stops, and should be given off a spoon so that the child gets accustomed to the taste.

The average amount of exchanges tolerated in children is between three and five, and this is unlikely to change except during periods of rapid

CASE STUDY

The table below shows a sample menu for an 8-month-old infant with PKU

6.00 am	Phenylalanine-free protein substitute
Breakfast	1 x 50 mg exchange: e.g., 10 g Weetabix + phenylalanine-free protein substitute + low protein bread and butter
Lunch	1 x 50 mg phenylalanine exchange + puréed free vegetables Diluted fruit juice Stewed fruit
Teatime	1 x 50 mg phenylalanine exchange + puréed free vegetables Phenylalanine-free protein substitute Low-protein custard made with protein-free milk
Bedtime	Measured formula feed or breast-feed Phenylalanine-free protein substitute

growth. The exchanges should be evenly distributed throughout the day. The protein substitute should be given either as a drink or as a paste off a spoon in a dose sufficient to provide adequate protein for growth. The dose should be split into three and given with meals.

If XP Maxamaid is used, no additional vitamins or minerals will be required. If Aminogran Food Supplement is used, complete vitamin and mineral supplementation will be needed.

School children

A packed lunch is usually the best option for school age children as few school canteens can cope with the diet for phenylketonuria. The child should be encouraged to take the protein substitute with the meal at school. The school should understand the importance of the diet so that the child is not inadvertently offered inappropriate foods at school.

Illness

Loss of appetite is common during illness and will contribute to raised phenylalanine levels. Phenyla-

lanine exchanges should be continued throughout illness and the protein substitute should be given in full amounts. High carbohydrate drinks such as Lucozade, squash and glucose polymers should be encouraged.

Pregnancy

It is essential that a low-phenylalanine diet is started prior to conception as high maternal phenylalanine levels carry a significant risk to the fetus, including microcephaly, congenital heart disease, mental retardation and low birth weight. The aim of the treatment should be to maintain levels between 120 and 240 µmol/l. In practice, this means a reduction in phenylalanine intake to three to seven exchanges per day. Tolerance to protein increases after 20 weeks due to the rapid growth of the fetus and phenylalanine exchanges may increase to 30 to 35 daily.

The protein substitute should provide 1 g of protein per kg of body weight. Additional tyrosine may be needed. Blood samples should be taken twice weekly to monitor both phenylalanine and tyrosine levels.

FURTHER READING

Shaw V, Lawson M 1994 Clinical paediatric dietetics. Blackwell Science, Oxford

REFERENCES

Al-Bander H, Kaysen G A 1991 Ineffectiveness of dietary protein augmentation in the management of the nephrotic syndrome. Pediatric Nephrology 5(4): 482–486

Bardella M T, Holteni N, Prampolini L et al 1994 Need for follow-up in coeliac disease. Archives of Disease in Childhood 70:211–213

Beroley D W et al 1987 Composition of four pancreatic extracts in CF. Archives of Disease in Childhood 62:564–568

British Diabetic Association 1989 Dietary recommendations for children and adolescents with diabetes. Diabetic Medicine 6(6):537–547

British Diabetic Association 1992 Dietary recommendations for people with diabetes. An update for the 1990s. Diabetic Medicine 9(2): 189–202

British Paediatric Association 1988 Working party on cystic fibrosis in the UK 1977 to 1985. British Medical Journal 297:1599–1602

British Society for Gastroenterology 1996 Guidelines for the Management of patients with coeliac disease. BSG, London

Campbell A, Forrest J, Musgrove C 1994 High strength pancreatic enzyme supplements and large bowel stricture in cystic fibrosis. Lancet 343:109

Coleman J E, Watson A R 1992 Gastrostomy buttons: the optimal route for nutritional support in children with chronic renal failure. Journal of Renal Nutrition 2(3):21–26

Collin P, Vilska S, Heinonen P K, Hallström O, Pikkarainen P 1996 Infertility and coeliac disease. Gut 39:382–384

Department of Health 1991 Report on health and social subjects No. 41. Dietary reference values for food, energy and nutrients for the United Kingdom. HMSO, London

ESPGAN 1992 Diagnostic criteria for food allergy with predominantly gastrointestinal symptoms. Journal of Paediatric Gastroenterology 14: 108–112

Farrell P M, Mischler E H, Sondel S A 1985 Predigested formula for infants with cystic fibrosis. Journal of American Dietetic Association 87:1353–1359

Francis D 1987 Diets for sick children. Blackwell Scientific, Oxford

Holmes G K T 1997 Coeliac disease and malignancy. Journal of Paediatric Gastroenterology and Nutrition 24:S20–24

Knowles M R 1988 Diabetes and cystic fibrosis. New questions emerging from increased longevity. Journal of Pediatrics 112:415–416

MacDonald A, Holden C, Harris G 1991 Nutritional strategies in cystic fibrosis. Current issues. Journal of the Royal Society of Medicine 84 (Suppl. 18):28–35

Maki M, Hallstrom O, Huupponen T, Vesikari T, Visakorpi J K 1984 Increased prevalence of coeliac disease in diabetes. Archives of Disease in Childhood 59:739–742

Murphy J L, Wootton S A, Bund S A, Jackson A A 1991 Energy content of stools in normal healthy controls and patients with cystic fibrosis. Archives of Disease in Childhood 66:495–500

NSPKU 1999 Dietary information for the treatment of phenylketonuria. NSPKU, Watford

Pierce A, Watson J B G, McKena C 1990 The Irish experience with nocturnal supplementation in cystic fibrosis. Paediatric Pulmonology (Suppl. 5):266A

Ramsey B W, Farrell P M, Pencharz P 1992 Nutritional assessment and management in cystic fibrosis. A consensus report. American Journal of Clinical Nutrition 55:108–116

Rees L, Greene S A, Adlard P et al 1988 Growth and endocrine function in steroid sensitive nephrotic syndrome. Archives of Disease in Childhood 63(5):484–490

Sigurs N 1993 Prevalence of coeliac disease in diabetic children and adolescents in Sweden. Acta Paediatrica 82(9): 748–751

Srinivasan U, Leonard N, Jones E et al 1996 Absence of oat toxicity in adult coeliac disease. British Medical Journal 313(7068): 1300–1301

Stevens F 1987 Decreasing incidence of coeliac disease. Archives of Disease in Childhood 62:465–468

Walters J R F 1994 Bone mineral density in coeliac disease. Gut 35:150–151

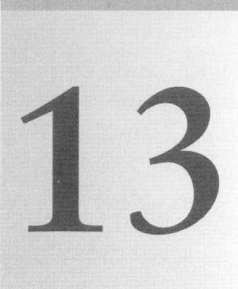

13

Nursing assessment of children's nutritional state during illness

Jane Coad   Bob Moloney

INTRODUCTION

This chapter focuses on the nursing assessment of children's nutritional needs during illness. Any nursing assessment should be viewed within the framework of children's nursing which has evolved over the last 40 years. The development of nursing models and child and family-centred care has become established as an accepted approach to the delivery of nursing care for children and their families, both in the community and in hospital. Assessing a child's nutritional status is crucial in order to plan and evaluate care. Currently, nutritional assessments are not always performed as routine practice, but rather carried out on those identified with a specific nutritional problem. However, nutritional assessment should be part of routine practice. In this chapter, a nutritional assessment tool which can be used in conjuction with any existing nursing documentation is discussed.

HISTORY AND NURSING THEORIES AND MODELS

Fifty years ago, the only acknowledged nurse theorist was Florence Nightingale, who had attempted to formulate a discreet framework of ideas in her 'Notes on nursing: what it is and what it is not' (1859). This theory focuses on nurses' manipulation of the environment, using fresh air, light, warmth, cleanliness and quiet to help the patient recover. After this, there was a dearth of nursing theory for almost a century and nursing practice came to be dominated by ideas derived from the physical sciences, essentially those associated with the medical profession.

Throughout this period, an implicit model acted as a framework for nurses and this is often referred to as the biomedical model. The beliefs underpinning this model are that patients are a collection of physiological systems which interact with each other. Health is equated with physiological homeostasis and illness with a disturbance of this balance. Also implicit in this framework is the artificial separation of body and mind, often referred to as 'Cartesian dualism' after René Descartes.

The consequences for practice were profound and included:

◆ the concentration on physical aspects of illness
◆ a focus on cure rather than care
◆ the labelling of patients as a diagnosis
◆ the relegation of psychological and emotional aspects of care to a low level of priority.

There tended to be a concentration of information, and therefore power and decision-making, in the hands of health professionals, especially doctors. Overall, the effects were to produce a health care system which could be a dehumanizing experience for patients. It was not until the 1950s that nurses began to develop alternative frameworks which could guide practice. In 1952 Hildegard Peplau published her 'Interpersonal relations theory' (Peplau 1952) in which she argues that nursing is primarily an interpersonal process and that this interaction is often therapeutic. This landmark publication was an indication of the fact that nurse education in the USA was now based in higher education and a strata of nurse academics were developing who had the time and intellectual skills necessary to be able to reflect on the fundamental nature of nursing. In doing so, they began to challenge the established biomedical framework. As an emerging profession, nursing needed its own theory base and over the next 20 years a profusion of conceptual nursing models were published. Abdellah et al (1960), Orlando (1961), Henderson (1966), Rogers (1970), King (1971), Orem (1971), Roy (1976) and Roper et al (1980) represent a few of the better known ones.

With the wisdom of hindsight, some of these frameworks seem inaccessible and removed from the realities of everyday practice. However, they contain a wealth of insights and observations which continue to influence nursing. Most of these frameworks are based on humanistic philosophies with the concept of holism as a central consideration. This period represents a unique phase in development of the nursing profession.

It is now widely accepted that no single all-encompassing theory of nursing is either possible or desirable (Castledine 1994) and many clinical areas now formulate eclectic models, combining ideas from various sources into a framework which fits their needs. In the context of these developments, a nutritional tool which reflects key values and beliefs about children's nursing has been developed.

VALUES AND BELIEFS WHICH SUPPORT CHILDREN'S NURSING

Family-centred care

In the 1950s the consequences of a disease-orientated model of nursing for children in hospital was a system of care which would now seem shocking in its lack of humanity. In particular, the separation of children from their families caused by highly restrictive visiting hours and a complete lack of residential facilities for parents emphasizes the minimal insight into the psychological needs of children. It is instructive that the impetus for change came not from a nurse but from a young social scientist, James Robertson, a colleague of John Bowlby, whose research (Robertson 1958) and tireless campaigning persuaded the Ministry of Health to set up an enquiry into the welfare of children in hospital. The result was the Platt Report (Ministry of Health 1959), which was to radically change the way children were cared for in hospital, although, sadly, the uptake was slow.

Nevertheless, the key finds of the Platt Report formed the basis of a move to a framework of care which was child-centred and family-centred and holistic in nature. These changes were fought for by an alliance of parents, nurses and medical staff, organized in the National Association for the Welfare of Children in Hospital. Today, the philosophy of family-centred care is universal in the UK, North America, Australia and New Zealand and a large part of Europe. Campbell & Glasper (1995) have identified three key elements in this philosophy:

1. It is an approach to nursing which is family-focused.
2. It accepts the family's/carer's own definition of what constitutes a family.
3. The nursing care and environment help promote the strengths and individuality of the family, in order to allow people greater scope for caring for their relatives.

Partnership in care

The concept of partnership with parents was implicit in the Platt Report and was explicitly referred to in the important Court Report (Court 1976). In the intervening years, various related ideas, such as 'involving parents in care' and 'participation in care', have been extensively debated in the nursing press (Darbyshire 1993). Casey (1988, 1993) developed this discussion and formulated a framework of care which she called 'partnership nursing'. This framework is a logical development from the philosophy of family-centred care and, indeed, most clinical areas would claim to practise some degree of partnership with parents and carers.

Negotiated care

Central to the concept of partnership is the idea that a process of negotiation takes place between nurses and parents/carer (and the child, if his or her level of understanding is appropriate), in identifying needs and formulating a plan of care. This may not be easy to implement in practice and there is evidence that such negotiation is more readily undertaken by experienced staff, whereas junior nurses and students are generally lacking in the necessary skills and confidence (Callery & Smith 1991). Partnership must be developed at an early stage in the relationship by acknowledging that the family/carer has knowledge regarding the child which nobody else has. Only when this is made explicit will families/carers feel they can engage in a genuine process of negotiation. The integration of the family's or carer's knowledge, together with the expertise of health professionals, is the key to developing quality assessment and care.

The principles outlined must, therefore, be related to any nutritional assessment. It should have social and psychological components which reflect the family's/carer's beliefs, habits, socioeconomic status and other cultural factors, such as religion and ethnicity.

NUTRITIONAL ASSESSMENT

Although assessment of a child's nutritional status is complex, it is an essential process in the planning and evaluation of care. Suskind et al (1990) suggest that 39% of pre-school children worldwide had some degree of malnutrition. Over the past 20 years a number of studies have reported a high incidence of malnutrition in hospital; this may be as high as 40% of all hospital admissions (McWhirter & Pennington 1994). Poor nutrition complicates many diseases of childhood and affects both the physical and psychological well-being of children. It can, therefore, be serious and may include:

◆ impaired gastrointestinal function
◆ growth failure
◆ pubertal delay
◆ impaired brain growth in infants
◆ development delay
◆ immune deficiency with increased susceptibility to infections
◆ altered respiratory function
◆ muscle wasting
◆ altered mood behaviour such as depression (Holden & MacDonald 1997).

However, at present it is not routine for nurses or doctors to specifically assess every child's nutritional status. Indeed, Davidson & Stables (1996) in their study found that nurses and doctors did

Table 13.1 Developmental considerations to facilitate nutritional assessment of children during illness

Baby	Birth weight is directly linked to maternal nutritional status and the required energy intake of a baby is higher than an adult.
	The infant is reliant on the parents/carers for all nutritional needs. Rhythms and daily cycles, including eating, are established very early. Questions should be centred on the parents and main carers. Examples of questions may include:
	– What type of feeding is currently used (breast/bottle)?
	– What is the normal pattern of feeding for the infant?
	– How much food is taken at each feed/meal?
	– At what stage of motor development is the infant (such as holding objects, including food pincer grip)?
	– At what stage of social development is the child (such as attempting to feed with fingers or spoon)?
	– Does the infant make any sound associated to mealtimes?
	– Has the child's normal pattern of feeding changed in the last few days?
	– Has there been any vomiting or cough during meals?
	Ask specifically about any changes such as less milk taken or gone off weaning and only wants milk.
Pre-school	The pre-school child (2–6 years) is growing rapidly, both physically and socially. During hospitalization, the food the child likes should be available in hospital and reassurances needed that the admission is not a punishment. Questions should be directed at the child, but these may need phrasing in simple terms. Examples of questions might include:
	– Do you like. . . ?
	– What do you not like? (choose foods to prompt in both cases)
	– Are you hungry now?
	– Do you use a cup (plate, spoon, chair)?
	– Do you use a spoon (plate, cup) to eat with?
	– Do you have a favourite spoon (plate, cup)?
	– Can you show me how you eat/drink?
School	The nutritional status affects the rate of puberty. Therefore, an energy-dense diet may be required.
	A child aged from 7 to 12 years is also developing social understanding (equity, fairness) and logical reasoning. They need appropriate explanation to overcome their fears about why you are asking the questions. Thus, phrasing should be open to allow them to build up a rapport with the nurse. Examples of questions might include:
	– What did you eat today?
	– What do you like?
	– What don't you like?
	– Have you any 'special' foods?
	– What meal do you like best (breakfast, dinner, tea)?
	– Ask about preferences of equipment and eating places.
Adolescent	An adolescent is able to systematically problem-solve. They may exhibit rebellious tendencies or posses idealistic values, including media images such as thinness being ideal. The nurse should encourage them to discuss their preferences and how an illness episode might affect their diet. They may also have formed strong opinions regarding their nutritional needs or practices and this must be fully respected in the assessment. Examples of questions might include:
	– Do you want to fill out the care plan, showing your own food preferences?
	– When do you normally like your meal times?

NB: Cultural special dietary requirements must always be considered for all age groups.

not consider this to be important. In 1992, the Department of Health launched 'The Health of the Nation' document; one highlighted aspect of this was nutritional needs, especially related to the education and training of health professionals. Despite this, McDowell & Green (1997) and Taylor & Baker (1997) both highlight that although health professionals have come some way in assessing children's nutritional needs, there remain large gaps in both education and practice related to nutritional needs.

Norton (1996) highlighted the fact that many nursing assessments of the child's nutritional needs were not specific enough and lacked essential information. This was particularly evident in the lack of literature found relating to the developmental and cultural conditions in the individual child's nutritional assessment.

Definition of nutritional assessment

Dudek (1993) defines nutritional assessment as 'the process of collecting and interpreting data in order to evaluate an individual's nutritional status and identify nutritional needs'. A nursing nutritional assessment is not a singular, one-off event. It is a continuous process which involves both the collection and interpretation of data and is subsequently followed by planning, implementation and evaluation (Table 13.1). Thus, the care plan can be revised as to its effectiveness.

It is essential that nurses have a good knowledge of nutrition and development as it is well known that illness affects feeding and development. The needs of the individual child should always be considered. Food and nutrition are an important component of family life and provide the basis for much social interaction. During illness, food continues to be important, arguably more so than normally. Nurses therefore need to be aware of the importance of the individual's need, and to be aware of dietary practices and cultural needs when assessing nutritional status.

McDowell & Green (1997) found that qualified nurses carried out poor dietary assessments. Vital pieces of information were missing in comparison with other health professionals, such as doctors, student nurses and medical students.

Box 13.1 Useful practical information in nutritional assessment

- Preferred choice of foods, including snacks and times of mealtimes. Ask for a normal diet history, such as what the child has for breakfast, dinner and tea, and preparation of food, such as liquid or solid foods. Include particularly favoured food including temperature and texture.

- Use of equipment such as the type of chair, utensils and cutlery.

- Feeding skills, e.g. finger foods, length of feeding.

- Record any changes such as reluctance with breast or bottle, regression of feeding patterns or behaviour changes.

- Dietary restrictions or known allergies of the child or family.

- Recent changes in body weight, such as weight loss or weight gain.

- Parental/carer observations of feeding, including any concerns such as tiredness, breathlessness during feeding or taking a much longer time over feeding.

- Awareness of any existing presence of an underlying condition, such as vomiting and diarrhoea.

- Ability to feed self, chew or swallow food and any oral or motor dysfunction.

- Any additional dietary support, such as enteral feeding.

- Dietary intake, including socioeconomic information, habits, cultural or religious preferences, food preferences and typical food patterns, such as number of meals, snacks, size or content.

- Vitamin or mineral supplements or medications being taken which may affect dietary intake, such as corticosteroids.

- Reasons for dietary and appetite changes, including teething, dental or gum problems and changes in taste, smell or ability to chew or swallow food.

It is now recognized that nutritional needs are best met by a multidisciplinary team, including dietitians, nurses, doctors and therapists (Holden & MacDonald 1997). The nurse has a key role to play in helping to identify potential or actual nutritional problems and in monitoring outcome. Nutritional assessment requires nutritional skills, knowledge, adequate time and comprehensive documentation. When nutritional assessment is implemented effectively as part of the nursing process, it enables good continuity of care.

Nutritional assessment is a complex process involving nurses gathering subjective data – such as discussing the child's eating patterns (Box 13.1) – and objective data – which should include a physical assessment and review of the child's nutritional assessment, the height, length and weight of the child (Box 13.2). This information should be gathered in conjunction with the history.

Klein et al (1997) identify the need to:

◆ identify patients who have, or are at risk of, developing protein or energy malnutrition or specific nutrient deficiencies
◆ quantify a patient's risk of developing malnutrition-related complications
◆ monitor adequacy of nutritional therapy.

A major goal of undertaking a nutritional history is to assist in identifying underlying problems or changes, such as inadequate intake or change in body weight of the baby or child. The nurse needs to develop a level of trust with the family to ensure that the nursing assessment obtained is accurate.

PROFESSIONAL ROLE AND RESPONSIBILITIES

The nurse should be aware of his or her professional responsibility when undertaking nutritional assessments. Specifically related to the Code of Professional Conduct (UKCC 1992) there are several points that are worth remembering in relation to the assessment of nutritional needs. These include:

◆ **Rule 4** 'Acknowledge any limitations' –
This incorporates the professional boundaries

Box 13.2 Useful practical information for anthropometric measurements and observations

◆ Physical observations, skin and hair condition, thinness, etc.

◆ Weight – a simple measurement which is a good indicator of current and chronic nutritional status. Should be undertaken at regular intervals and all equipment regularly serviced for accuracy. In parent-held child health records compare with weight.

◆ Height/length – a simple growth parameter used in conjunction with weight. It is essential that shoes are removed and, if the child is under 2 years, they are lying down.

◆ The height and weight can be plotted on the percentile chart.

◆ Head circumference in children up to 2 years.

◆ Note skin condition and visually assess child's overall appearance, e.g. if wasted or overweight.

◆ Clinical signs of changed nutritional status such as hair, eye, tongue, gum and lip changes.

◆ If problems are identified, the physical assessment might include some more in-depth assessments, including mid-arm circumferences and triceps skinfold thickness. These measurements are performed by staff trained in undertaking these measurements; for example, dietitians, nutritional care sisters and doctors.

which nurses work in. Therefore, if the nurse does not feel sufficiently confident to assess the child's nutrition he or she should state this to a senior nurse or consult dietetic or specialist help.

◆ **Rule 5** 'Work in a collaborative and co-operative manner with health professionals' – If nurses are to ensure that the nutritional assessment is thorough, they must liaise with all members of the multidisciplinary team.

It is worth noting that documentation by nurses is written evidence of nursing practice. The nurse assessing the child and family must therefore be

Box 13.3 The 'Kenrick' model of nutritional assessment. (Reproduced with kind permission of Sarah Kenrick.)

Physical

◆ What chair does the child sit in for meals?

◆ What texture of food does the child eat?

◆ Does the child dribble or spit food during the meals?

◆ Does the child cough during a meal? If so, how often?

◆ Does the child suffer from chest infections? How frequently?

◆ Does the child have access to speech therapy, physiotherapy and occupational therapy?

◆ How much food is eaten at each mealtime?

◆ Does the child have access to a dietitian?

◆ When was the child last weighed?

◆ Does the child have a feeding programme based on desensitization, jaw control or lip closure?

◆ Does the child become bubbly during a meal?

◆ Does the child vomit during or after meals?

◆ What type of fluid does the child take?

◆ What type of plate, spoon and cup are used?

◆ Is the child prone to urinary tract infections or constipation?

Psychological

◆ What is the child's usual mealtime routine?

◆ Who is the primary carer at mealtimes?

Observe the child being fed

◆ What cues are used? Are they consistent?

◆ Does the child exhibit choice?

◆ Is the child's appetite better at certain times of the day?

◆ Does the child experience obvious fears when being fed?

◆ Does the child exhibit any self-help skills?

Social

◆ What type of environment is the child usually fed in?

◆ Does the child concentrate on eating or is the child easily distracted?

◆ Is the child disruptive in a group setting?

◆ Does the child have specific ethnic or religious needs?

aware of his or her own personal knowledge and skills relating to nutritional assessment. Lindseth (1997) found that it was essential that student nurses acquired detailed knowledge while on their pre-registration courses and subsequently continued to build on this in their continuing post-registration education in order to acquire the skills required in nutritional assessment. It is essential both that such assessment skills are developed early in the curriculum, and that they are continually reassessed.

There is little literature specifically examining nutritional assessment tools for nurses. A useful model has been devised for use with children with special needs, based on Maslow's hierarchy of needs (Kenrick 1998). This is shown in Box 13.3. This splits the activities of eating and drinking into three sections: physical, psychological and social. As a result of the assessment tool Kenrick (1998) found that the nutritional status of children improved in 90% of cases.

PROPOSED NUTRITIONAL ASSESSMENT TOOL

A practical nutritional assessment tool has been developed by the authors and is summarized in Appendix 13.1. This tool was piloted by two qualified nurses who were looking after a caseload of 10 children. Five of the children had a variety of chronic illnesses and were being nursed at home and five were admitted to hospital with an acute illness. The nurses found it useful and easy to complete. The open framework allowed nurses, parents and children to complete the documentation in a flexible individualized format.

It was found that although evaluation took longer, issues and problems were identified at a much earlier stage instead of emerging at a later date. New and useful information was identified that would not have been obtained with existing documentation. One of the nurses who piloted it stated, 'Actually, the tool made me realize how little I did know – I'd like to keep using it so I could develop these skills further now that I've started this process'. The tool was attached to existing care plans, and was useful in facilitating further care planning and subsequent review. The nutritional assessment tool can be used as a flexible framework to guide or help nurses assess the nutritional needs of children during illness, whether this is an acute or long-term problem.

SUMMARY

This chapter has presented a specific focus on the nursing assessment of children's nutritional needs during illness. We have highlighted the need for partnership, and we have stressed that reviewing a child's nutritional status is crucial in order to plan and subsequently evaluate care required and given. We have also argued that nurses do not always perform nutritional assessments as part of routine practice. We therefore emphasize the need to develop and evaluate nutritional assessment tools to assist and support appropriate nutrition of paediatric patients. A case study reviewing a child with failure to thrive is presented to demonstrate the use of the nutritional assessment tool which we have developed (see Appendices 13.1 and 13.2). It is hoped that, as a result of this presentation, the tool will be further evaluated and subsequent tools will be developed.

 FURTHER READING

Campbell S, Glasper A E 1995 (eds) Whaley and Wongs children nursing (UK edn). Mosby, London

This is a very general but comprehensive textbook for nurses who care for children. It provides *essential information about the philosophies and frameworks that underpin children's care. It therefore expands on many of the issues the writers were only able to touch upon in this chapter.*

Holden C, MacDonald A 1994 Nutritional care. The nurse's role. Paediatric Nursing 9(4):29–34

This is a very useful article to read as it is concise and relevant to nurses in the care of children's nutritional needs. We also found it very easy to obtain and it helped provide background discussion to this chapter.

REFERENCES

Abdellah F G et al 1960 Patient centred approaches to nursing. Macmillan, New York

Callery P, Smith L 1991 A study of role negotiation between nurses and the parents of hospitalised children. Journal of Advanced Nursing 16(7):772–781

Campbell S, Glasper A E (eds) 1995 Whaley and Wongs children nursing (UK edn). Mosby, London

Castledine G 1994 Nursing can never have a unified theory. British Journal of Nursing 3(4):180–181

Casey A 1988 A partnership with child and family. Senior Nurse 8(4):8–9

Casey A 1993 Development and use of the partnership model of nursing care. In: Glasper A E, Tucker A (eds) Advances in child health nursing. Scutari, Harrow, ch. 14

Court S D M 1976 Fit for the future: report of the Committee on Child Health Services. HMSO, London

Darbyshire P 1993 Parents, nurses and paediatric nursing: a critical review. Journal of Advanced Nursing 18:1670–1680

Davidson C, Stables I 1996 Audit of nutrition screening in patients with acute illness. Nursing Times 92(8):35–37

Dudek S 1993 Nutrition handbook for nursing practice, 2nd edn. Lippincott, London

Henderson V 1966 The nature of nursing: a definition and its implication for practice, research and education. Macmillan, New York

Holden C E, MacDonald A 1997 Nutritional care: the nurse's role. Paediatric Nursing 9(4):29–34

Kenrick S 1998 The 'seeAbility' model of assessment feeding. Conference paper

King I 1971 Towards a theory of nursing: general concepts of human behaviour. John Wiley, New York

Klein S, Kinney J, Jeejeebhoy K 1997 Nutrition support in clinical practice: a review of published data and recommendations for future research directions. Journal of Parenteral and Enteral Nutrition 21(3):133–156

Lindseth G 1997 Factors affecting graduating nurses' knowledge: implications for continuing education. Journal of Continuing Education in Nursing 28(6):245–251

McDowell S, Green M R 1997 Knowledge of nutrition and its application within a children's hospital. Conference paper, Proceedings of the Nutrition Society, Blackpool, UK 56(2)

McWhirter J P, Pennington C R 1994 Incidence and recognition of malnutrition in hospital. British Medical Journal 308:945–948

Ministry of Health 1959 The welfare of children in hospital (the Platt Report). HMSO, London

Nightingale F 1859 Notes on nursing: what it is and what it is not. Appleton, London

Norton B 1996 Nutritional assessment. Nursing Times 92(26) Supplement

Orem D 1971 Nursing: concepts of practice. McGraw-Hill, Toronto

Orlando I J 1961 The dynamic nurse–patient relationship. GB Putnam, New York.

Peplau H E 1952 Interpersonal relations in nursing. GB Putnam, New York

Robertson J 1958 Young children in hospital. Tavistock Publications, London

Rogers M 1970 An introduction to the theoretical basis of nursing. FA Davis, Philadelphia

Roper N, Logan W, Tierney A 1980 The elements of nursing. Nursing Outlook, March 18:42–45

Roy Sr C 1976 Adaptation: a conceptual framework for nursing. Nursing Outlook March 18:42–45

Suskind R, Lewinter-Suskind L (eds) 1990 The malnourished child. Nestlé Nutrition Workshop Series, 19. Vevy/Raven Press, New York

Taylor R M, Baker A 1997 Nutrition knowledge in paediatric intensive care. Journal of Child Health Care 1(4)

UKCC 1992 Code of professional conduct for the nurse, midwife and health visitor. UKCC, London

Appendix 13.1 Nutritional Assessment Tool

GUIDELINES

Use the model in conjunction with the parent/carer. The parents/carers know and understand their child best and are often the primary feeders. Use Boxes 13.1 and 13.2 from this chapter to obtain data as suggested. Appendix 13.2 shows a completed assessement.

1. Complete **Section A** first, including the biographical data about the child and the reason for admission or referral. In **Section A** there is a section for physical observations. This can be completed at the initial assessment and added to after the assessment has taken place.
2. Complete **Section B**. The nurse assessing the child should include the child's past and current feeding patterns.
3. Complete **Section C**. The nurse should measure the child as instructed and plot the centile chart as attached. Use the parent-held record to help facilitate completion of this section.
4. The plan of care can be negotiated once the assessment has taken place. The nutritional assessment tool, once completed, can slot into the existing framework or care plans used in the care setting. Evaluation and review should continue in line with the care planned.
5. Observations are crucial in using the assessment tool so, if a problem is identified in the initial assessment, observation of the parent/carer feeding the child should take place. The nurse may also feed the child in order to obtain further information and a different perspective of the child's needs and abilities.

Section A

Name: . . . .

Date of Birth/Age: . . . .

Reason for Referral/Admission: . . . .

. . . .

Physical Observations: . . . .

. . . .

Section B Feeding History

	Past	Current	Plan of care
Feeding patterns: e.g., mealtimes, appetite, types of food, nutrient intake, restrictions, snacks			
Feeding environment: e.g., lap, baby chair, high chair, feed self, table, chair			
Food preferences: e.g., likes/dislikes			
Feeding skills: e.g., bottle, breastfed, cup, utensils, feed self, chewing, swallowing			
Dietary support: e.g., enteral feeds			
Ability to eat and retain food: e.g., difficulties in feeding, diarrhoea, vomiting, poor appetite, refusals			
Supplements: e.g., vitamins, medications			
Parent/carer observations: e.g., behaviour, concerns, sleep patterns			

Section C Measurements

	Past	Current	Outcomes
Height/length centile			
Weight centile			
Weight patterns (see parent-held records)			

Appendix 13.2 Completed Nutritional Assessment Tool

Kelly is 6 months old and has been admitted to hospital 'failing to thrive'. She is the first child and is cared for by both parents at home.

Section A

Name: Kelly Smith ....

Date of Birth/Age: 6 months ....

Reason for Referral/Admission: Kelly has been admitted because she is failing to thrive. She has no pre-existing conditions but Mum feels despite feeding hungrily that she is not gaining weight. ....

Physical Observations: Kelly is thin. Examination was normal. She feeds ravenously but does not vomit. Mum says stools are normal. ....

Section B Feeding history

	Past	Current	Plan of care
Feeding patterns: e.g., mealtimes, appetite, types of food, nutrient intake, restrictions, snacks	Always feed well. Mum says Kelly takes 4 oz of Cow and Gate five times a day.	Takes 4 oz Cow and Gate four times daily. Takes two bottles of juice and baby rice twice a day. Also $\frac{1}{2}$ rusk and tried her with some jar foods.	Encourage 6 oz bottles (150 ml) four times daily. Stop juice. Refer to dietitian.
Feeding environment: e.g., lap, baby chair, high chair, feed self, table, chair	Sits on mum's or dad's lap while feeding.	Currently still on lap for bottles, but mum has put Kelly in a chair for diet. Plastic spoons used only by mum.	Continue. Let Kelly start to feel the spoon.
Food preferences e.g., likes/dislikes	Enjoys milk.	Appears to like milk but mum feels Kelly spits food out.	Encourage a variety of solids.
Feeding skills: e.g., bottle, breastfed, cup, utensils, feed self, chewing, swallowing	Nil	Mum has not really let Kelly hold spoon or bottle yet.	Observe feeding behaviour and encourage Kelly to hold equipment.
Dietary support: e.g., enteral feeds	Nil	Nil	Dietitian referral has been sent.
Ability to eat and retain food: e.g., difficulties in feeding, diarrhoea, vomiting, poor appetite, food refusal	Mum says that Kelly has always had loose stools and this is normal for her.	Bowels opened at least four times a day. No change. Spits food but no vomiting.	Observe stool frequency and record accurate description. Note any spitting of food.
Supplements: e.g., vitamins, medications	Nil	Nil	Nil
Parent/carer observation: e.g., behaviour, concerns, sleep patterns	Has slept through the night since Kelly was 4 months.	Kelly has recently started to wake up crying and Mum cannot settle her.	Observe behaviour and record. Offer bottle to settle until larger volume of bottles is established.

Section C Measurements

	Past	Current	Outcomes
Height/length centile	50th centile – see chart plotted from parent-held records.	50th centile – see chart plotted from parent-held records.	Continue to plot centile chart twice weekly while in hospital.
Weight centile	50th centile – see chart plotted from parent-held records.	Less than 3rd centile – see chart plotted from parent-held records.	Continue to plot centile chart twice weekly while in hospital. Record also on hospital weight chart.
Weight patterns (see parent-held records)	Gained weight normally until 4 months.	Since 4 months has had poor weight gain which mum is very worried about.	

14

A team approach to nutritional support

Elaine Sexton   Chris Holden   Gill Abel

INTRODUCTION

There has been an upsurge in teamwork and multidisciplinary team working between dietitians, nurses, doctors, social workers and therapists working together in an aim to provide coordinated services.

Vanclay (1998) suggests that a team can be defined as a group of individuals who share goals and work together to deliver services for which they are mutually accountable. Team members are independent, although members have differentiated roles and work cooperatively.

Effective teamwork is based upon clear characteristics and is described as having.

- shared goals and objectives which take account of individuals' values and aspirations
- well-defined, complementary roles
- roles which are understood and respected by team members
- clear procedures and agreed protocols
- regular and effective communication
- support for, and recognition of, each member's contribution
- commitment by all team members
- regular audit and reflection on practice.

TEAM APPROACHES TO CHILD HEALTH

The philosophy of children's nursing is to provide family-centred care in hospital and at home or wherever the child needs care (Figure 14.1). Multidisciplinary teams should aim to work in

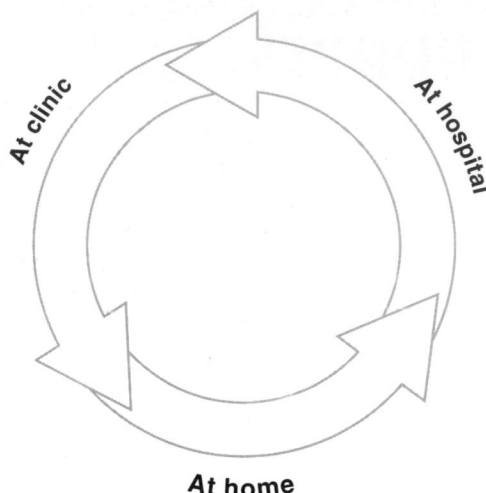

At clinic

At hospital

At home

Figure 14.1 The continuum of care–hospital–home. (After Stower 1992.)

partnership with the child and family/carer to promote the child's health and well-being (Casey 1998). Good communication skills are essential to ensure effective support for families/carers.

Child health care is constantly changing. Recent advances in high technological care has led to an increasing number of children surviving major illnesses, many of whom have complex nursing and nutritional needs (Gow 1996).

Provision of cost-effective services to children may be impeded by failures of liaison and coordination between agencies. The House of Commons Committee Report on Health Services for Children and Young People (House of Commons Health Committee 1997a,b) emphasizes problems caused by fragmentation of responsibility for services between different groups of health care providers. Team approaches to nutritional support do not appear to be a priority. Team and health care providers must establish roles and responsibilities and develop protocols to ensure nutritional aspects of a child's care are met. Multidisciplinary and cross-boundary working between agencies is vital to ensure the nutritional needs of children are met (Nutricia Clinical Care and Pharmacia 1994).

MULTIDISCIPLINARY APPROACH TO COMPLEX PROBLEMS

As clinical nutritional care becomes increasingly complex, the skills required to deal with the details of assessment, prescription, administration and

---

Box 14.1   Teamwork: Key points

Benefits of professionals working together

◆ Easier access by children, families or clients to the most appropriate professional.

◆ Collective sharing of responsibility.

◆ Better clinical risk management.

◆ Facilitation of multi-professional skills.

◆ Avoidance of isolation.

◆ Efficient sharing of education and resources.

◆ Encouragement of professional openness and sharing of information which can only enhance communication and ensure greater cohesiveness and effectiveness within an organization.

Barriers to effective teamwork

◆ Interpersonal differences.

◆ Uncertainty and fear of change.

◆ Intra- and interprofessional rivalries and misunderstanding.

◆ Perceived or real difference in power, status and income.

◆ Difference in conceptual approaches and models of health.

◆ Different management structures and lines of accountability.

◆ Differing and competing organisational priorities.

◆ Lack of training in teamwork.

◆ Encouragement of personal rather than team liability (Vanclay 1998).

monitoring of treatment will increasingly fall outside the expertise of a single practitioner, and therefore requires a team approach. However, it should be recognized that the more disciplines represented in any such team, the greater the need for excellent communication with other colleagues responsible for the child's primary problem (Smallman et al 1986). Essential communication skills within hospitals and the community can sometimes prove difficult.

Problems can be reduced by better understanding of professional roles, flexibility and patient-centred care to minimize friction. Taylor & Goodinson-McLaren (1992) argue that 'nutritional support personnel must always work through, not around, the nursing team caring for a particular patient'. Castledine (1996) realistically suggests that it takes time to establish trusting and collaborative relationships. Team members need to value and respect each other's contribution. Vanclay (1998) examines both the benefits and barriers to effective team working. These are summarized in Box 14.1.

The key principles underlying the need for professional collaboration are detailed in Figure 14.2.

The necessity of introducing a multidisciplinary nutritional care team (NCT) in a children's hospital is well-established (Puntis 1997; Puntis & Booth 1990). However, where these teams do not exist, there is a strong need for effective communication between all those directly involved with the patient's management (Silk 1983).

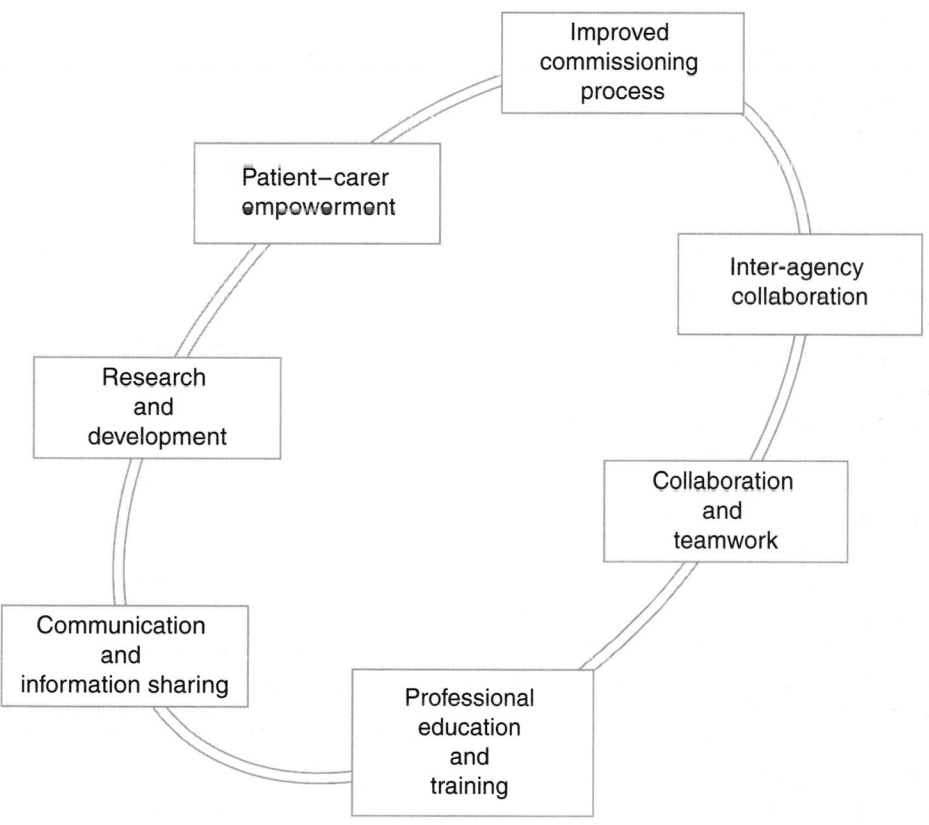

Figure 14.2 Key principles of professional collaboration

ROLES WITHIN NUTRITIONAL CARE TEAM (NCT)

The aims of a team will vary according to hospital, district and trust policies (Taylor & Goodinson-McLaren 1992). Box 14.2 outlines the role and responsibility of team members providing nutritional support in a hospital setting.

Role of individual team members

Consultant

Silk (1994) emphasizes that the clinician on the team must ensure good relationships are maintained with non-team clinicians. The team's existence and approach to patient care should have the support of colleagues. The consultant ideally should have training in clinical nutrition and nutrition support practices. Consultant duties, in addition to coordinating and overseeing the activities of the nutritional care team, should also include important teaching commitments, involving not only his or her own colleagues, but also junior medical staff.

Dietitian

The dietitian has an important role to play and will be responsible for the following:

- active promotion of nutritional support through education and training programmes for medical and paramedical staff
- assessment of the nutritional intake of children
- assessment of the nutritional status of children
- calculation of the nutritional requirements of children requiring enteral and parenteral nutrition
- formulation of an appropriate enteral feed
- monitoring nutritional status and feed tolerance and acceptability
- assessment of the effectiveness of nutritional therapy and any complications
- education, research, audit and training
- training and counselling of parents/carers and children.

Box 14.2 Roles within the nutritional care team

Role of NCT

- Provide a comprehensive and coordinated approach to nutritional support.
- Reduce the prevalence of malnutrition.
- Develop protocols and guidelines for nutritional support in hospital and at home.
- Review and rationalize use of nutritional products used in enteral and parenteral feeding.
- Act as an expert resource throughout a children's hospital.

Role of the consultant gastroenterologist

- Provide clinical expertise and team leadership.
- Liaise with consultant colleagues regarding patient referrals.
- Development of nutritional services with other team members.

Role of the paediatric surgeon

- Provide access for enteral nutrition and parenteral nutrition (placement of enteral feeding tubes and central venous catheters).
- Joint assessment and management of complex patients as required.

Role of the nutrition pharmacist

- Formulate parenteral nutrition according to the child's individual requirements using computer-assisted prescription, in consultation with doctors and dietitian.
- Monitor the progress of infants and children, ensuring parenteral feeds are properly balanced.
- Act as a resource, accessing information and advice on parenteral nutrition products, drugs and dosages.

Role of the dietitian

- Assess child's nutritional intake and requirements.
- Formulate plans for nutritional support in consultation with other team members.

Role of the dietitian (contd)

◆ Monitor and evaluate nutritional support.

◆ Advise on specialist feeds.

Role of the speech and language therapist

◆ Assess oral motor function, including the swallowing process.

◆ Monitor the development of oral motor skills.

◆ Advise on the use of food textures and utensils to promote appropriate oral motor development.

◆ Formulate oral motor programmes for children who are tube-fed, and support nurses and families/carers in carrying out these programmes.

Role of the children's nutritional nurse specialist (CNNS)

◆ Perform baseline anthropometry so that nutritional goals can be set.

◆ Prepare child and family for home enteral nutrition and home parenteral nutrition.

◆ Formulate a teaching plan and, together with ward nurses, teach child, parents/carer how to give nutritional support safely

◆ Liaise and educate with primary health care team to provide the family with continuing support.

◆ Joint home and school visits with community nurses.

◆ Organise a continuing supply of equipment.

◆ Provide support for families/carer following discharge. Reduce the need for ward outpatient attendance.

The pharmacist

The key aspects of the pharmacist's contribution to the team are as follows:

◆ formulate parenteral nutrition regimens
◆ ensure nutrition solutions are stable and contain only compatible additives
◆ advise on potential problems arising from concurrent drugs and intravenous therapy

◆ be responsible for the education and training of colleagues in the pharmaceutical aspects of parenteral nutrition.

The nurse – children's nutritional nurse specialist (CNNS)

Clinical practice is a key component of this role within the team. In addition, the CNNS is responsible for:

◆ assisting and training of ward nurses in the care of patients receiving nutritional support
◆ training, counselling and support of families/carers and children receiving parenteral or enteral nutrition in hospital or the community, and at the same time respecting their customs, values and spiritual beliefs
◆ formulating nursing policies and guidelines to achieve improved care and select and review design of equipment for nutritional support
◆ liaising with the primary health care team in the community
◆ undertaking home visits
◆ providing clear explanation of care required, in simple terms to reassure families/carers.

Successful interdisciplinary working demands professionals are valued equally and have a clear understanding of each other's technical skills (Wood 1996).

Although the formation and make-up of the team may raise funding issues, there is a large body of research emphasising that nutritional care teams have been shown to be cost-effective. This is achieved by the reduction of costly complications, minimizing waste, avoiding unnecessary treatments and simplifying treatments used (Sizer 1996, Puntis 1997, Puntis & Booth 1990).

AIMS OF A NUTRITIONAL CARE TEAM

The team at work

The team aims to promote effective liaison between the hospital and community staff, ensuring a smooth transition from hospital to home. Box 14.3 identifies the aims of a nutritional care team. Collaborative team functions must be identified and multidisciplinary care planning is essential.

Assessment and planning

Nurses have a key role to play in collaboration with health care professionals in educating the patient and family/carer, in order to ensure a successful outcome (Jackson 1994).

The Audit Commission (1991), with specific reference to discharge planning, found that assessment of need was patchy, started too late and was poorly documented or the discharge documenta-tion remained blank. This led to delayed discharge, the patient not receiving appropriate services and potential for readmission to hospital. The discharge planning process begins with assessment and this should start before or on admission (King 1994). McBridge (1995) found that the majority (57%) of discussions about discharge took place just before going home. The family's resources, individual needs and methods of coping with care require careful assessment (Corkey 1989; Jackson 1994).

DISCHARGE PLANNING FOR CHILDREN REQUIRING NUTRITIONAL SUPPORT

Good communication and liaison between the patient, family and the health professionals involved has been identified by many authors as the key to effective discharge planning (Ahula 1994; Jackson 1994; Lowenstein & Hoff 1994). These studies illustrated that discharges were poorly planned; this included the timing, the service and the equipment arranged. Abel (1997) emphasises:

◆ Communication was unsatisfactory, community nurses felt patients were inappropriately referred and some patients were completely missed.

◆ Ward nurses often fail to recognize the social, material and physical difficulties which patients face on returning home. Patients often suffer because of poor communication and assessment.

Discharge planning is a process in which the child's and family's needs are identified, negotiated and evaluated in order to prepare them for the transfer of care from hospital to home. It involves arranging and coordinating continuing care, whether the care is provided by the child, their family, health care professionals, social services, education, voluntary bodies or a combination of these options (Jackson 1994). There is a wealth of information examining discharge planning practices in adult nursing, but few studies have

Box 14.3 The aims of a nutritional care team

◆ Provide an effective advisory service at district/hospital/trust level.

◆ Identify patients requiring nutritional support.

◆ Implement and evaluate nutritional support, using support techniques.

◆ Provide a specialist service for placement and site maintenance of different types of enteral tubes or parenteral catheters.

◆ Set high standards of nutritional practice.

◆ Develop policies that are research-based, in accordance with national guidelines.

◆ Improve the quality of nutritional support by reviewing treatment/equipment usage and cost.

◆ Develop programmes for patient education in conjunction with ward staff/families/ carers.

◆ Provide in-service educational updates on clinical nutrition to staff.

◆ Undertake research locally and at national level.

explored the discharge of children requiring nutritional support from hospital and the role of the children's nurse.

Abel (1997) identified that nurses have limited knowledge of what the child and family face at home, following discharge from hospital. There is also a lack of community services available for children, and a poor understanding of those services which are available. Nurses appear to be constrained by the environment in which they practise, perceiving lack of time to be a major factor which prevents good discharge planning. The nurses need to refocus and work in closer partnership with the child and their family, and the multidisciplinary team working in the hospital and community.

Holden (1994) emphasizes that caring for children at home is likely to decrease the need for expensive hospitalization. Professional awareness of the home carer is required. There is also a need for investment in resources for continuing care of children and families at home, both locally and nationally. This is further supported by the Government White Paper (Department of Health 1997), which aims to minimize hospital stay and facilitate families' return to their homes and support them in the community.

Discharge planning is a complex and diverse process which multidisciplinary teams have to learn to manage. Nurses need to make their role explicit to others in order to help them understand the complexity of this task. Abel (1997) highlights that ward-based children's nurses concentrate on the 'high tech' and physical needs of the child and, although they recognize that discharge planning is important, it remains a low priority (Abel 1997).

Holden et al (1997) developed discharge planning grids to highlight specific roles within the team when discharging families home with enteral or parenteral feeding. Team members must be aware of their individual role, but also have an appreciation of the whole episode of the child's care (see Tables 14.1 and 14.2).

The development of protocols for discharging patients home with enteral and parenteral nutrition is essential. Each team member should identify their role, and discharge planning grids have been developed to be used in patients' notes to facilitate written communication.

Grids have been helpful in facilitating effective links and improved communication. Emphasis is placed upon the process of assessment, planning, carrying out the care and facilitating discharge planning into the community setting. The reader can see individual team roles at a glance. Even though the idea of the grid is simple, it helps to identify stages clearly and sets out the process to be seen as a whole.

KNOWLEDGE AND UNDERSTANDING OF COMMUNITY SERVICES

Community nurses usually have experience of hospital nursing, whereas ward-based nurses tend to have limited experience of community nursing.

This may explain the problems often seen in discharge planning because ward nurses have limited knowledge of continuing care at home. Nurses need to be aware of the community resources and services available and consider their appropriateness and acceptability to patients and their family. This is particularly important for children's nurses to consider, as there is a wide variation both regionally and nationally in children's community nursing service provision.

When nurses are planning discharge, home care should be considered as an alternative to hospital care. A number of studies have recommended compiling a directory of local agencies and community services to facilitate discharge planning.

Gilan (1995) commented on discharge planning and stated that 'at present the amount of time and skill involved is often under-estimated'. It is easy to criticize nurses for not always getting it right, but managers, medical staff and all the professionals involved need to collaborate effectively. There is also a need for investment in resources for continuing care of children at home, both locally and nationally. 'The Children's Charter' (Department of Health 1996b) and 'Child Health in the Community' (Department of Health 1996a) provide the framework for inter-agency collaboration. Various Department of Health documents recommend provision of a needs-led service (Box 14.4).

Table 14.1 Discharge planning grid for enteral feeding

Step	Medical staff	Dietitian	Nutritional care sister	General practitioner	Nursing staff
1. Assessment	Decision to enterally feed a child at home is discussed with dietetic/nursing staff/nutritional care sister	Decision to enterally feed Discussion with medical staff Discussion with nutritional care sister, ward and community team	Referral Assessment Discussion with medical team and dietitian re aims and duration of therapy Nutritional assessment Tolerance of enteral regimen reviewed with dietetic feeding colleagues		Discuss enteral feeding regimen with nutritional care sister and dietetic colleagues Tube intubation if able Record strict intake output chart Loose stools – send specimen to microbiology. Test for reducing substances Weight daily. Accurate height is essential Observe for any problems with vomiting
2. Discussion	Discussion with parents – likely duration of feeding Discussion with dietetic colleagues	Discussion with parents re home tube feeding Assessment of the nutritional requirements of baby/child Feeding regimen discussed with family and ward staff/nutritional care sister Choice of feed determined Assessment of feed tolerance Discussion with nursing team Feeding regimen for home discussed Oral feeding difficulties? Refer, if appropriate, to Speech Therapy, Physiotherapy, Psychology	Community Care Patient/parent details Community nursing staff contacted Health authority details obtained Discuss with business team funding issues/community managers Health visitor operational details discussed		Discussion with parents re feeding regimen
3. Liaison and training		Organization of training for parents in specialized feed unit Explanation of feed and regimen to parents/carers Contact general practitioner re feed required Discussion with parents re collection of	Discuss with parents reasons for home enteral feeding Contact primary health care team Training required insertion nasogastric/gastrostomy/jejunostomy tube Contact local hospital	Discussion with dietitians re feed	Discuss community contacts with parents Obtain written list re equipment for parents from nutrition care

		prescriptions from chemist	re tube intubation as necessary Community nursing staff paediatric trained health visitor (children under 5) Special needs health visitor Special schools/school nurse/ nursery assistant/school head Respite facilities Speech therapy Physiotherapy } Referral Psychology } if required Psychological preparation parent/child tube intubation Play therapist informed pre-post procedural preparation Interpreter contacted as necessary Training/plan care. Discuss with primary nurse/discussion about monitoring feed tolerance	
4. Administration	Letter to general practitioner Clinic appointment Follow-up assessment with dietetic colleagues/nursing staff	Contact community team, local hospital, if appropriate	Equipment supply 7 days Loan pump. Ensure medical physics has checked safety. Pump loan 7 days only On return/send back to medical physics ECR Administration Fax equipment requirements to home care company	
5. Evaluation Follow-up/ Contacts	Assessment of growth Monitor feed regimen tolerance/complications Review baby/child in clinic Routine monitoring essential Telephone contact maintained Home visits	Protocols Teaching programmes Give parents written information: tube care, procedures, emergency numbers, community contacts Appointment Telephone family next day Assessment family need/problems Liaise with community nurses Home visit, if required Further training changing route, e.g. nasogastric/gastrostomy/jejunostomy	Prescribe feed on FP10 Ongoing health special care needs	Discussion re parent competency – nutritional care – final assessment Check parents have appointment Equipment Pump Feeds Community team contact must be contacted Emergency telephone numbers given

Table 14.2 Discharge planning grid for home parenteral nutrition

	1. Assessment	2. Discussion	3. Liaison and training		4. Administration	5. Emergency procedure	6.	7. Follow-up contacts
Parents/ carers	Training ongoing	Preparation of home environment	Ensure registration with family practitioner	CASE CONFERENCE				Final discussion Ongoing 24-hour care
Medical team	Assess patient suitability (HPN)	Preliminary letters to general practitioner ◆ respite care facility ◆ shared care with hospital	Determine prescription requirements					Final discussion and assessment (1)
Nutritional care sisters (NCS)	Initial discussion Home visit Assessment of family and home	Contact company liaison nurses and community nursing staff	Commence training with family (2)			Discuss emergency procedure with family	Discuss discharge plan with pharmacy	Final discussion/ assessment provide necessary documentation for family (3) ◆ home visit arranged first night of discharge ◆ at least 3-monthly visits ◆ weekly telephone contact
Ward nursing staff	Named nurse identified to help facilitate plan of care	Assess parental progress (with NCS)						Final discussion and assessment
Dietitian	Calculate nutritional requirements for enteral/parenteral feedings	Advise suitable enteral feed, volume, rate and route, if able	Monitor response of nutritional support Review feed tolerance Monitor growth					Ongoing contact with family re growth and nutritional requirements
Registrar/ SHO	Assess central venous access. Liaise with surgeons	Assess parental progress (with NCS)						Final discussion and assessment
Business manager	Arrange funding with local authority	Confirmation of funding letter to be sent to – consultant – head of pharmacy – NCS						
Social worker	Preliminary assessment Home visit (4)		Discuss with family assistance they require, e.g. respite, laundry service, domestic help					Final discussion and assessment. Home visit

Role			**CASE CONFERENCE**		
Special pharmacist	Supply PN to ward	Informed by business manager Funding identified by health authority	**C**	Prescription identified from medical staff sent to commercial company (5)	Obtain consultant/senior registrar signature when formulation stable
Commercial secretary	Home visit by liaison nurse	Discuss service with the family	**A** **S** **E**	Stock list identified with NCS. Sister services organized (6)	Commercial liaison nurse to provide 24 hour on call emergency advice for parents
		Discuss training needs of community staff with NCS. Provide training. Inform GP of service provided	**C**		
General Practitioner		Discuss with consultant re treatment plans	**O** **N** **F** **E**		Final discussion and assessment. Assist in providing medical care following discharge of child
Paediatric community nurse/district nurse		Identify their training needs to be able to support family. Identify local support agencies available to family	**R** **E**		Final discussion – provide ongoing care to family
Health visitor		Ongoing care of family and child	**N** **C** **E**		Final discussion

Medical team
(1) Team to provide:
– prescription
– discharge summary
– line history
– follow-up plan
– check immunizations

Nutritional care sisters (NCS)
(2) Training:
– using home parenteral nutrition booklet
– monitor parents' progress using objectives set and evaluate care

(3) Parent held:
– folder
– emergency telephone numbers
– telephone number for support group HALF P.I.N.N.T.

Social worker
(4) Home visit – assess:
– psychological
– financial
– environmental issues, e.g. telephone access

Special pharmacist
(5) Ensure stability of PN:
– stability testing of home parenteral nutrition's solutions may take up to 2 weeks. Therefore, the prescription should be planned well in advance

Commercial company (6)
– refuse collection organized
– water
– electricity company contacted
– proforma sent to regional health authority informing them child going home with electrically powered equipment

LOCAL AND NATIONAL AUDIT

Auditing the indications, outcome and costs of nutritional support at home is important. It should identify the following:

◆ information regarding the adequacy of support in the hospital and community settings
◆ resources required
◆ trends and duration of treatment patterns.

An example of a local research/audit project has been undertaken by Papadopoulou et al (1995). The audit review looked at the growth of children receiving home enteral nutrition (HEN). The nutritional response to HEN was evaluated in a prospective study of 44 consecutive children (median age, 48 months) who received HEN for more than 1 month (median duration, 6 months). Three groups of children were studied and divided into groups according to their nutritional status: 17 children were stunted, 14 were wasted and 13 were adequately nourished but unlikely to maintain oral intake during anticipated nutritional stress. In the stunted group (median duration of HEN, 15 months) there was a significant correlation between improvements in height-for-age, z-scores and duration of feeds. In the wasted group (median duration of HEN, 4 months) all anthropometric indices improved significantly ($p<0.05$). HEN was also successful in maintaining nutritional status in the third group. The authors concluded that supplementary HEN is an effective method of nutritional support for a variety of indications, provided concurrent advice from a nutritional care team is available.

National audit

National audit is helpful in providing information regarding conditions which are infrequently managed at local level: for example, children requiring support for intestinal failure or metabolic disease. It provides information regarding the projection of resources required for the future. Moreover, patients should receive standardized care throughout the country and a structured national organization in theory should help to facilitate this initiative.

Box 14.4 Summary of reports on children's services

◆ 1959 Platt Report
◆ 1976 Court Report
◆ 1989 Children Act
◆ 1991 Welfare of Sick Children in Hospital
◆ 1992 A Positive Approach to Nutrition as a Treatment – British Association of Parenteral and Enteral Nutrition (BAPEN)
◆ 1993 Audit Commission – Children First
◆ 1993 Bridging the Gap
◆ 1994 Enteral and Parenteral Nutrition in the Community (BAPEN Report)
◆ 1996 Child Health in the Community
◆ 1996 Current Perspectives of Parenteral Nutrition in Adults
◆ 1997 House of Commons Report

Box 14.4 provides a summary of relevant reports which have been published.

NATIONAL INITIATIVES – THE WAY FORWARD

The British Association for Parenteral and Enteral Nutrition (BAPEN), which was formed in 1992, emphasizes the need for national standards (Box 14.5). A series of educational booklets have been produced by BAPEN to support and emphasize the need for multidisciplinary team-working to improve the nutritional treatment of all patients. Details of these are given in Box 14.6.

Sizer (1996) emphasizes the need for teams to adopt agreed standards of practice. Published information regarding the implementation of standards, procedures and protocols for nutritional support has been identified. Emphasis is based upon audit and action planning.

Box 14.5   Outline of the BAPEN policy standards for the organization and provision of nutritional support of patients in hospital

Organization and administration

◆ There is a management policy that all patients receive adequate and appropriate nutritional support, as laid down by a quality assurance programme.

◆ There is an inter-departmental, multidisciplinary nutrition steering committee, a catering liaison group and a nutritional support team. Agreed and explicit arrangements are laid down for the organization and funding for those patients continuing on artificial nutrition at home or elsewhere in the community.

Policies, protocols and procedures

◆ There is a published policy for the provision of artificial nutritional support. This policy covers screening of nutritional status and criteria for referral to the nutritional care team.

◆ Protocols and procedures are available related to feeding preparations and delivery systems, the use of oral supplements, enteral tube feeding and intravenous feeding.

◆ There are policies and procedures for the discharge of patients on nutritional support into the community.

Staff education and training

◆ There is a continuing education programme in general nutrition and techniques of nutritional support for all staff involved in the clinical care of patients.

Patients' rights

◆ Children who fulfil the criteria for referral have access to the nutritional care team, receive full explanations of the rationale for therapy and its management and are in agreement with the treatment plan.

Quality assurance and audit

◆ There is a monitoring and recording system which allows audit of catering services and nutritional support in the hospital and community.

Box 14.6   Booklets on nutrition

◆ King's Fund Report 1992 A positive approach to nutrition as treatment (ISBN 1 857170164)

◆ BAPEN 1994 Organisation of nutritional support in hospitals (ISBN 1 899467009)

◆ BAPEN 2000 Home parenteral nutrition (ISBN 1 899467 157)

◆ BAPEN 1994 Enteral and parenteral nutrition in the community (ISBN 1 9946705X)

SUMMARY

Clinical care is increasingly delivered by a multiprofessional nutritional care team. Education and training are seen as a key focus for teams (Burnam 1999). The British Association for Parenteral and Enteral Nutrition has an education and training committee. Courses are available to support interdisciplinary teamworking. Information can be obtained from the British Association for Parenteral and Enteral Nutrition.

Educational material is available to demonstrate the importance of good teamwork (Southall & Schwartz 2000).

CASE STUDY

The case study below demonstrates in detail the multidisciplinary role in discharging a patient with complex needs receiving home parenteral feeding.

Diagnosis and brief history

George is the eldest of three children. Both parents were employed but his mother gave up her job to care for George. They live in Wales, 200 miles away from the Regional Centre. They have shared care at a district general hospital, where they have a close-knit extended family who help with supporting George's siblings.

George, aged 12, presented with disseminated B-cell lymphoma. He relapsed three months after completing chemotherapy. He had a matched unrelated donor bone marrow transplant. His leukaemia relapsed in bone marrow, central nervous system, liver and subcutaneously. He developed gut graft versus host disease. He commenced on enteral nutrition, which resulted in persistent abdominal pain. At this point he was referred to a consultant surgeon and a consultant gastroenterologist for advice on how to manage his symptoms.

He underwent a ressection of part of his gut and the formation of an ileostomy and mucous fistula. Although his abdominal pain settled, he continued to need parenteral nutrition due to malabsorption problems. He developed a hyperosmolar diabetic crisis, requiring insulin and blood sugar monitoring.

Consider the case scenario presented in the case study (with reference to Table 14.2) and refer to Chapter 11 'Enteral and parenteral nutrition' before answering the following questions.

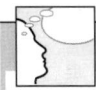

Questions

Answers are given in Appendix 2.

1. Who do you think might be in the team?

2. What would you consider to be the key issues for the team?

3. What do you think are the key issues for the family and child?

Dedication

Chapter 14 is dedicated to a child and his family who taught the team many valuable lessons.

FURTHER READING

Forsyth D R 1990 Group dynamics books. Cole Publishing, Pacific Grove, CA

This book is intended to serve as an introduction to group processes.

Miller P (ed.) 1999 Home paediatric parenteral nutrition. British Association of Parenteral and Enteral Nutrition, Maidenhead

An overview of key issues related to caring for home paediatric parenteral nutrition patients.

REFERENCES

Abel G 1997 Discharge planning; is it a priority for children's nurses? An investigation of ward-based children's nurses' knowledge, attitudes and perceptions of children discharged from hospital. BSc Dissertation, Leeds Metropolitan University

Ahula S 1994 Discharge to the community of older patients from hospital. Nursing Times 91 (28):29–30

Audit Commission 1991 The virtue of patients: making best use of the ward nursing resources. HMSO, London

Burnam P 1999 On course for better teamwork. Nursing Times 95(48) suppl.

Casey A 1998 A partnership with child and family. Senior Nurse 8(4):8–9

Castledine G 1996 Encourage team collaboration in health care. British Journal of Nursing 5:1402

Corkey 1989 In: Jackson M F 1994 Discharge planning issues and challenges for gerontological nursing: a critique of the literature. Journal of Advanced Nursing 19:492–502

Court Report 1976 Fit for the future. HMSO, London

Department of Health NHS Executive 1989a Discharge of patients from hospital: Department of Health Circular HC/89/5

Department of Health NHS Executive 1989b The Children's Act 1989: an introductory guide for the NHS:3–6

Department of Health NHS Executive 1990 The NHS and Community Care Act. HMSO, London

Department of Health NHS Executive 1991a The Welfare of Children and Young People in Hospital. HMSO, London

Department of Health NHS Executive 1991b The Patient's Charter. HMSO, London

Department of Health NHS Executive 1992 The Health of the Nation. HMSO, London

Department of Health NHS Executive 1993 New health – new opportunities. HMSO, London

Department of Health NHS Executive 1995 The Patient's Charter: Service for Children and Young People. HMSO, London

Department of Health NHS Executive 1996a Child health in the community: a guide to good practice. HMSO, London

Department of Health NHS Executive 1996b The Children's Charter. HMSO, London

Department of Health NHS Executive 1997 White Paper: The New NHS. Department of Health

Elia M (ed) 1994 Enteral and parenteral nutrition in the community. British Association for Parenteral and Enteral Nutrition, Maidenhead

Gilan J 1995 Editor's notes Nursing Times 12(91):28

Gow M A 1996 Paediatric community nursing: doctor's views. Professional Nurse 11(6):365–367

Holden C E 1994 Enteral and parenteral nutrition: feeding at home – impact on family life and the implications for home care. MSc Dissertation, Wolverhampton University

Holden C E, Brooks G, Wills J, Paul L, Sexton E 1997 Home parenteral nutrition: present management, future options. British Journal of Community Health Nursing 1(6):347–350

House of Commons Health Committee 1997a The Specific Health Needs of Children and Young People: Summary of Conclusions and Recommendations. HMSO, London

House of Commons Health Committee 1997b Health Service for Children and Young People in the Community: Home and School: Summary of Conclusions and Recommendations. HMSO, London

Jackson M F 1994 Discharge planning issues and challenges for gerontological nursing: a critique of the literature. Journal of Advanced Nursing 19:492–502

King C 1994 Documentation and discharge planning for elderly patients. Nursing Times 90(20):31–33

King's Fund Report, chaired by Professor J E Lennard-Jones 1992 A positive approach to nutrition as treatment. King's Fund, London

Lowenstein A J, Hoff P S 1994 Discharge planning: a study of nursing staff involvement. Journal of Nursing Administration 24(4):45–50

McBridge R C 1995 An audit of current discharge planning arrangements and their effectiveness on elderly care wards and community nursing services together with aspects of client satisfaction. Journal of Nursing Management 3:19–24

Miller P (ed.) 2000 Paediatric parenteral nutrition. British Association for Parenteral and Enteral Nutrition, Maidenhead

Nutricia Clinical Care and Pharmacia 1994 The management of clinical nutrition in NHS hospitals. MBA Project, Lancaster University

Papadopoulou A, Holden C E, Paul L, Sexton E, Booth I W 1995 The nutritional response to home enteral nutrition in childhood. Acta Paediatrica 84:528–531

Platt Committee Report 1959 The Welfare of Children in Hospital. HMSO, London

Puntis J W L 1997 Establishing a clinical support team. In: Ryan S W (ed.) Clinical paediatrics, international practice and research. Baillière Tindall, London, pp 177–188

Puntis J W L, Booth I W 1990 The place of a nutritional care team in paediatric practice. Intensive Therapy and Clinical Monitoring 11:132–136

Silk D B A 1983 The nutritional team. Nutritional support in hospital practice. Blackwell Scientific, Oxford

Silk D B A 1994 Organisation of nutritional support in hospitals. British Association for Parenteral and Enteral Nutrition, Maidenhead

Sizer T 1996 Standards and guidelines for nutritional support of patients in hospitals. British Association for Parenteral and Enteral Nutrition, Maidenhead

Smallman S, Handy D, Puntis J S W L, Booth I W 1986 The nutritional team in a children's hospital. Nutritional Health 5(3–4): 137–144

Southall A, Schwartz A (eds) 2000 Feeding problems in children. A practical guide. Raddiffe Medical Press, Abingdon

Standing Committee on Postgraduate Medical and Dental Education (SCOPME) 1997 Multi-professional working and learning: sharing the educational challenge. SCOPME, London

Standing Medical and Nursing Advisory Committees 1996 In the patients' interest: professional working across organisational boundaries. Department of Health NHS Executive, London

Stower S 1992 Partnership caring. Journal of Clinical Nursing 1(2): 67–72

Taylor S, Goodinson-McLaren S 1992 Nutritional support: a team approach. Clinical Skills' Series: Professional Nurse 10:10

Vanclay L 1998 Team working in primary care. Nursing Standard 12(30):37–38

Wood S 1996 Malnutrition in hospitals. The nurse's role in prevention. Nursing Times: British Association for Parenteral and Enteral Nutrition 1(1):67–68

Appendix 1 Useful Addresses

Association of Breastfeeding Mothers
26 Homeshaw Close
London SE26 4TH

Breastfeeding Network
PO Box 11126
Paisley PA2 8YB

British Association for Parenteral and Enteral
Nutrition (BAPEN)
PO Box 922
Maidenhead
Berkshire SL6 4SH

British Association of Counselling
1 Regent Place
Rugby
Warwickshire CV21 2PJ

British Dietetic Association
7th Floor, Elizabeth House
22 Suffolk Street
Queensway
Birmingham B1 1LS

British Nutrition Foundation
High Holborn House
52/54 High Holborn
London WC1V 6RQ

Caf Directory of Specific Conditions and Rare
Syndromes
Contact a Family
170 Tottenham Court Road
London W1P 0HA

Childline
Freepost 1111
Tel: 0800 1111

The Christian Lewis Trust
Child Care Centre
62 Walter Road

Swansea SA1 4PT
Tel: 0800 303031 (Childhood Cancer
Helpline)

CLIC
12–13 King Square
Bristol BS2 8JH

Children Living with Inherited Metabolic Disease
(CLIMB)
The Quadrangle
Crewe Hall
Weston Road
Crewe
Cheshire CW1 60R

Cook UK Ltd
Monroe House
Letchworth
Hertfordshire SG6 1LN

Cystic Fibrosis Trust
Alexander House
5 Blyth Road
Bromley
Kent BR1 3RS

Eating Disorders Association
First Floor, Wensum House
103 Prince of Wales Road
Norwich NR1 1DW

Edward's Trust
Edward House
St Mary's Row
Birmingham B4 6NY

Fresenius Ltd
6–8 Christleton Court
Manor Road
Runcorn
Cheshire WA7 1ST

HALF PINNT (Patients Receiving Intravenous
and Nasogastric Nutrition Therapy)
PO Box 3126
Christchurch
Dorset BH23 2XS

Health Education Authority
Trevelyan House
30 Great Peter Street
London SW1P 2HW

Kendall
154 Fareham Road
Gosport
Hampshire P013 0AS

Kidscape
152 Buckingham Palace Road
London SW1W 9TR

La Leche League
Breastfeeding Help and Information
BM 3424
London WC1 6XX

The Malcolm Sargent Cancer Fund for
Children
14 Abingdon Road
London W8 6AF

Medical Devices Agency
Hannibal House
Elephant and Castle
London SE1 6TQ

Medicina
Oak House
Lower Road
Cookham
Berkshire SL6 9HJ

Merck Biomaterial
Lenton House

Lenton Street
Alton
Hampshire GU34 1HG

National Childbirth Trust
Breastfeeding Promotion Group
Alexandra House
Oldham Terrace
Acton
London W3 6NH

NSPCC
Child Protection Helpline
67 Saffron Hill
London EC1N 8RS
Tel: 0800 800500

Paragon Model Makers
5 Host Street
Bristol BS1 5BU

Prader-Willi Syndrome Association UK
30 Follet Drive
Abbots Langley
Hertfordshire WD5 0LP

Royal College of Paediatrics and
Child Health
50 Hallam Street
London W1N 6FE

Simms Portex Ltd
Hythe
Kent CT21 6JL

UNICEF UK Baby Friendly Initiative
PO Box 29050
London WC2H 9TA

Vygon UK Ltd
Bridge Road
Cirencester
Gloucester GL7 1PT

Appendix 2 Answers to Questions

CHAPTER I

1. The young age of this mother, her low income and the short gap between pregnancies all increase her risk of nutritional deficiencies. Teenage mothers are probably more likely to smoke, take alcohol and use drugs, all of which have consequences for fetal growth. General advice regarding a nutrient-rich balanced diet should be given, taking into account her financial situation. She should be investigated for iron deficiency, and given iron supplements if indicated. Intake of vitamins A and C, folic acid, calcium and zinc are also more likely to be low, and supplementation may be required.

2. It is clearly important to establish the precise details of the vitamin preparation in question and the amount of vitamin A involved. High intakes (more than 3300 µg/day) may be associated with craniofacial, cardiac, thymic and central nervous system birth defects. The multivitamin preparation should be discontinued and liver, or products containing liver should be avoided throughout the rest of the pregnancy. A detailed fetal anomaly ultrasound scan in a fetal assessment unit could be arranged to give further reassurance if appropriate.

3. Lacto-ovo-vegetarians avoid all meat, meat products, poultry and fish; however, milk, milk products and eggs are included in the diet. Potential nutritional deficiencies include overall energy intake and vitamin D, both of which have implications for fetal growth and bone mineralization. A dietary assessment should be performed to identify any deficiency. As with all women planning pregnancy, an adequate intake of folic acid should be ensured.

CHAPTER 3

1. Aim: feed on demand
Daily requirements:
Fluid: 150 to 200 ml/kg/day
Energy: 115 kcal/kg/day
Offer: 700 ml/day

Provides: 175 ml/kg/day and 117 kcal/kg/day

Feeding plan:
Offer 100 ml every 3 hours, 7 times daily

2. The following factors are important for successful breastfeeding:

◆ good antenatal advice
◆ good postnatal advice and support
◆ early mother and baby contact
◆ frequent breastfeeding
◆ maternal diet
◆ discourage complementary feeds.

3. Energy requirements are 95 kcal/kg/day, so the baby's requirements are 713 kcal/daily. The following feeding plan would be appropriate.

	Total kcal/daily
Early morning	
I rusk mixed with breast or formula feed	70
180 ml breast or formula feed	121
Midday	
120 g puréed meat, potatoes and vegetables	84
180 ml breast or formula feed	121
Afternoon	
Water	
Evening meal	
60 g puréed meat, vegetables and pasta	42
60 g baby yoghurt	42
180 ml breast or formula feed	121
Bedtime	
180ml breast or formula feed	121
Total	**722**

CHAPTER 4

The energy requirements of a 2-year-old girl are 1165 kcal/daily.

	Energy kcals/day
Breakfast	
I Weetabix	70
100 ml whole milk	70
I banana	64
100 ml natural orange juice	36
Mid-morning	
100 ml whole milk	70
$\frac{1}{2}$ slice wholemeal bread	32
Margarine	28
Midday meal	
2 slices wholemeal bread	129
Margarine	111
Tuna	57
Tomato/cucumber	15
Low fat yoghurt	135
Sugar-free squash	
Mid-afternoon	
100 ml milk	70
Evening meal	
60 g jacket potato	46
30 g chicken	44
Carrots	12
Gravy	62
I apple	47
150 ml whole milk	105
Total	**1201**

CHAPTER 6

1. The following advice would be appropriate:

   - A haem iron source (e.g. red meat, mince dishes, grilled sausages), should be given at least once daily. Approximately 20 to 40% of haem iron is readily absorbed by the body.
   - Non-meat iron sources such as fortified breakfast cereals, eggs, baked beans, lentils and dark green vegetables (e.g., broccoli) should be given. From to 5 to 20% of iron is available from these sources, and they should be given with foods containing vitamin C, such as natural fruit juice or fresh fruit to aid absorption.
   - Useful snacks which contain iron include: cereals and milk, baked beans on toast, meat paste or egg sandwiches, scones or fruit cake.
   - There may be advantages in continuing the use of an iron-fortified infant formula or follow-on formula until 18 months to 2 years of age for faddy toddlers. Realistically, however, this is not a long-term measure; therefore, it is important to establish good eating patterns during early childhood.

2. The following advice would be appropriate:

   - At least 300 ml of cow's milk daily. This will provide 100% of a toddler's and over 50% of older children's calcium requirement.
   - One portion of yoghurt, fromage frais or cheese daily. A 150 g yoghurt or 30 g of cheese provides approximately 200 mg calcium.
   - Children who dislike milk can try milk-based puddings such as custard and instant desserts made with milk.
   - Canned fish (e.g. sardines), green leafy vegetables, calcium-enriched bread, and pulses including baked beans will provide a small source of dietary calcium.
   - Children on a vegan or milk-free diet should be given 600 ml of calcium-fortified soya milk daily. If children are unable to take this, they are likely to need a calcium supplement and their diets should be assessed by a dietitian.

3. The following advice would be appropriate:

   - At least three portions of fruit and vegetables daily should be encouraged:
     - give brightly coloured vegetables such as peas and sweetcorn
     - add extra vegetables to casseroles or soups
     - offer stir-fried vegetables
     - offer banana sandwiches
     - dried fruit such as raisins may be popular
     - offer canned fruit in its own juice as an alternative to fresh fruit.
   - Offer natural fruit juice (diluted for younger children) at mealtimes.
   - Give Mother and Children's drops to children between 1 and 5 years.

4. The majority of vitamin D is obtained by the action of sunlight on skin. Therefore:

- ◆ Encourage the use of Mother and Children's drops for all children aged 1 to 5 years and for children with little exposure to sunlight. One dose provides 7.0 μg of vitamin D.
- ◆ Encourage vitamin D fortified breakfast cereals.
- ◆ Encourage the use of fortified margarine.

CHAPTER 7

1. Exclusive breastfeeding at least until 4 months of age should be recommended. If breastfeeding is not possible, there is some evidence to suggest that routine use of a protein hydrolysate formula in children from atopic family backgrounds may reduce the risk of developing atopic symptoms; cow's milk protein should not then be introduced into the diet until after 6 months of age. Since sensitization to cow's milk protein can occur in utero, there is an argument for mother following a milk protein free diet during pregnancy, although the benefit of this is not proven. In this instance, careful dietary assessment would be required in order to ensure that overall nutrient intakes are satisfactory; a calcium supplement is likely to be necessary.

2. This really amounts to a 'near miss cot death'. Assuming that no other cause has been found for the apnoea, gastro-oesophageal reflux remains a likely explanation. Although some would suggest this scenario is an indication for fundoplication, surgery carries its own risks and cannot be a guarantee of preventing cot death in future (it is not absolutely certain that reflux was the underlying trigger for the event). For these reasons, many paediatricians would advocate a trial of medical anti-reflux treatment. The fact that apnoea could recur even with medical treatment must be explained to parents and the pros and cons of surgery must be discussed with a paediatric surgeon. Parents should be offered teaching in basic resuscitation and given the opportunity to have an apnoea alarm at home. For further reassurance, hospital outpatient follow up must be arranged, together with home visits by the health visitor or paediatric outreach nurse. Some areas have specialist health visitors who become involved when there has been a 'near miss cot death' and will teach resuscitation to parents as well as maintaining regular family contact.

3. Persistent vomiting is a recognized presentation of factitious illness. The normal investigations and previous history of cot death are worrying features which point to the possibility of this diagnosis. Nursing staff must take over the role of feeding the child from the mother so that objective evidence of feed intake and vomiting can be collected for each full 24-hour period. The child should be under continuous nursing observation (not easy in practice) and the mother should not be allowed to make up the feeds without supervision. Concerns must be discussed with social work colleagues and the GP so that the family background and medical history can be explored in detail.

4. The most likely explanations for treatment failure are inadequate laxative dosage or poor compliance with medication. Families with a high level of stress may benefit from input by a member of the child mental health team, including advice on managing toileting behaviour. Continued failure to respond requires exclusion of recognized medical and surgical causes for constipation, although investigation will usually be negative in a child who is otherwise well.

CHAPTER 9

1. The following recommendations would be appropriate:

- ◆ Plot Anna's height and weight on a centile chart.
- ◆ How does this compare to her previous position on the centile chart?
- ◆ What percentile points do her parents' heights represent? Anna's height and weight would be expected to be about 2 percentiles lower than predicted from parental height.
- ◆ Anna has had to cope with a lot of changes in the last year.
- ◆ Her visual problems will have exacerbated any feelings of insecurity associated with moving house. This may have affected her eating.

- A new school at the age of 4 years, where she does not know any of the other children, might feel like a large, bewildering and frightening place.
- She will need to feel safe and secure at school before she is likely to start eating normally.
- At school, one person should be involved with Anna's feeding so that she can gain confidence. A lot of reassurance and praise will be needed.
- At home and at school, eating should be made 'easy' for a few weeks. She should not be expected to work hard at improving the texture and type of food that she eats. She may benefit from using dietary supplements for a temporary period.
- Anna's nutritional requirements will be higher than expected as she needs to catch up to her previous growth profile.
- When Anna's growth has returned to normal, work on helping her make progress with her eating abilities can gradually be resumed. This may take many months.

2. The following recommendations would be appropriate:

- Plot Claire's height and weight on a centile chart.
- What types of exercise might Claire enjoy? Consider swimming or learning to ride an adapted bicycle. Increasing her exercise will help reduce her weight and may also help with constipation.
- If Claire becomes more overweight, this will further limit her mobility. This should be discussed with Claire and her parents as an incentive to lose weight.
- Agree some targets for Claire and her family: e.g., eating is for mealtimes only. Claire can have as many sugar-free drinks as she wants between meals, and Claire can have some sweets each Saturday after tea.
- Increasing Claire's fluid intake will help with her constipation.
- Encourage Claire to eat generous helpings of vegetables and fruit at mealtimes, both for her constipation and to help her feel satisfied at the end of a meal.

- Make sure that everyone working with Claire is following the same regimen so that she knows exactly what to expect.
- Weigh Claire when she has been following her new targets for about a month to assess her progress and set revised targets if necessary. Ask her family about any changes in bowel habits.

CHAPTER 10

1. You would require the following data:

- parental heights
- ages of parents at puberty.

2. The initial investigation would be to establish bone age.
3. The likely diagnosis is constitutional delay of growth and puberty.

CHAPTER 11

Case study: Gemma

1. There are a number of reasons for enteral feeding of Gemma:

- she only eats small amounts of feed
- she is failing to thrive
- it is a recognized treatment for severe gastro-oesophageal reflux
- improving nutrition may help her to fight infection.

2. Nasogastric feeding would be the first option to try. If long-term feeding is required:

Route	Feed	Feed administration
Nasogastric or gastrostomy	Standard paediatric feed appropriate for a child <20 kg 1–1.5 kcal/ml For example, Nutrini or Nutrini Extra Feed thickener may be used	Continuous feeding to minimize reflux Overnight feeding to cause minimal disruption to day-to-day activities
Jejunostomy	Protein hydrolysate Iso-osmolar: e.g., Pepdite 2+	Continuously

- gastrostomy feeding may be necessary
- jejunostomy feeding may be an option if Gemma is at risk of aspiration or if vomiting is affecting her nutritional status.

3. The table on p. 286 summarises the feed and administration appropriate to different feeding routes.

4. The table below summarizes the main issues and points for consideration when establishing home enteral feeding.

Case study: Katie

1. Katie is less than 12 months of age and has normal gut function. She is thriving on the 10th centile. An appropriate feed would, therefore, be a normal infant formula or follow-on formula. If Katie requires fluid restriction or if weight gain is inadequate, it may be necessary to start calorie supplements.

2. Katie should ideally be offered bottle-feeds orally without allowing her to get breathless. The volume of feed not completed by bottle should be given as a bolus via nasogastric tube.

Issues	Points to consider
Child care	Liaise with mother to arrange appointments for training to fit in with school and child care arrangements
Financial implications	*Travel* If mum is receiving any benefits (e.g., family credit) check she will be able to claim for travelling expenses to attend *Benefits* Liaise with mum to ensure that she is aware of her current financial benefit entitlement
Home issues	Ideally a home visit should be undertaken to ensure housing is suitable. It should consider: – general cleanliness of house – whether handwashing facilities are satisfactory – whether there is a clean area for feed preparation and storage Safety: – home enteral feeding pump is able to be plugged safely into electrical point next to child's bed – suitable stand is available for the pump – pump is tamper-proof and, if possible, away from any other child who may be sharing the bedroom
Community support for mother	Ideally, a paediatric community nurse (PCN) should visit to support the family Tube changes (if applicable) to be done at home with PCN Home delivery of equipment and feed to be arranged
Family support	Discuss network of family and friends (they may be able to help) Patient support group may be helpful
Schooling	The school should be given adequate information about Gemma's condition and understand the need for enteral feeding Gemma may need to have feeding during school hours if adequate nutrition cannot be delivered overnight. Facilities for storing feed may need to be investigated, and normal school activities need to be maintained as far as possible Gemma has missed a lot of school and will continue to have outpatient appointments

Issues	Points to consider
Child care	Liaise with mother: – to arrange appointments – to minimize disruptions to her working – to organize training for child minder – to arrange training for father, if he is going to be involved with her care
Financial implications	*Employment* Mum is likely to have to take some time off for training appointments Discuss with mother writing to employers to facilitate time for this without loss of earnings *Benefits* Benefits are available and should be discussed with family
Home issues	Ideally, a home visit should be undertaken to ensure housing is suitable. It should consider: – general cleanliness of house – whether handwashing facilities are satisfactory – whether there is a clean area for feed preparation and storage Safety: – home enteral feeding pump is able to be plugged safely into electrical point next to child's cot – suitable stand is available for the pump
Community support for mother	Ideally, a paediatric community nurse (PCN) and health visitor to visit and support mum: – tube changes to be done at home with PCN if possible or alternatively, arrangements to be made at hospital – home delivery of equipment and feed to be arranged – if PCN not available, liaise with local paediatric unit for support – discuss network of family and friends (they may be able to help) – discuss HALF PINNT Support Group

3. The above table summarizes the main issues and points for consideration when establishing home enteral feeding:

Case study: Mohammed

1. Mohammed's height cannot be accurately obtained. Therefore, we would use the following indices:

- mid-arm circumference is a composite measure of muscle and fat stores
- skinfold measurements
- upper arm length and lower leg length (provides upper and lower body measures of long bone growth).

2. Nasogastric feeding should be tried initially, but gastrostomy feeding may be required as long-term feeding will be necessary now that it is unsafe to feed Mohammed orally. The feeding regime should be established to fit in with the needs of Mohammed's family. Bolus feeding only may be preferred to fit in with family mealtimes; alternatively, some of the feed may be given overnight by continuous infusion to reduce the time commitment for parents at night.

3. Mohammed attends a special school. All information should be passed on to the school's multidisciplinary team, which may include the school nurse, a community dietitian, a physiotherapist, a speech therapist and a paediatrician who will be involved in Mohammed's continuing care.

4. It is important that an interpreter is used to facilitate communication with mum. Demonstrations of setting up feeding system with mother

will be extremely important. Training sessions should be kept short to minimize stress. A pictorial teaching programme (helpful videos etc.) should be used.

CHAPTER 14

1. Figure A2.1 shows some of the key workers who might be in the team.

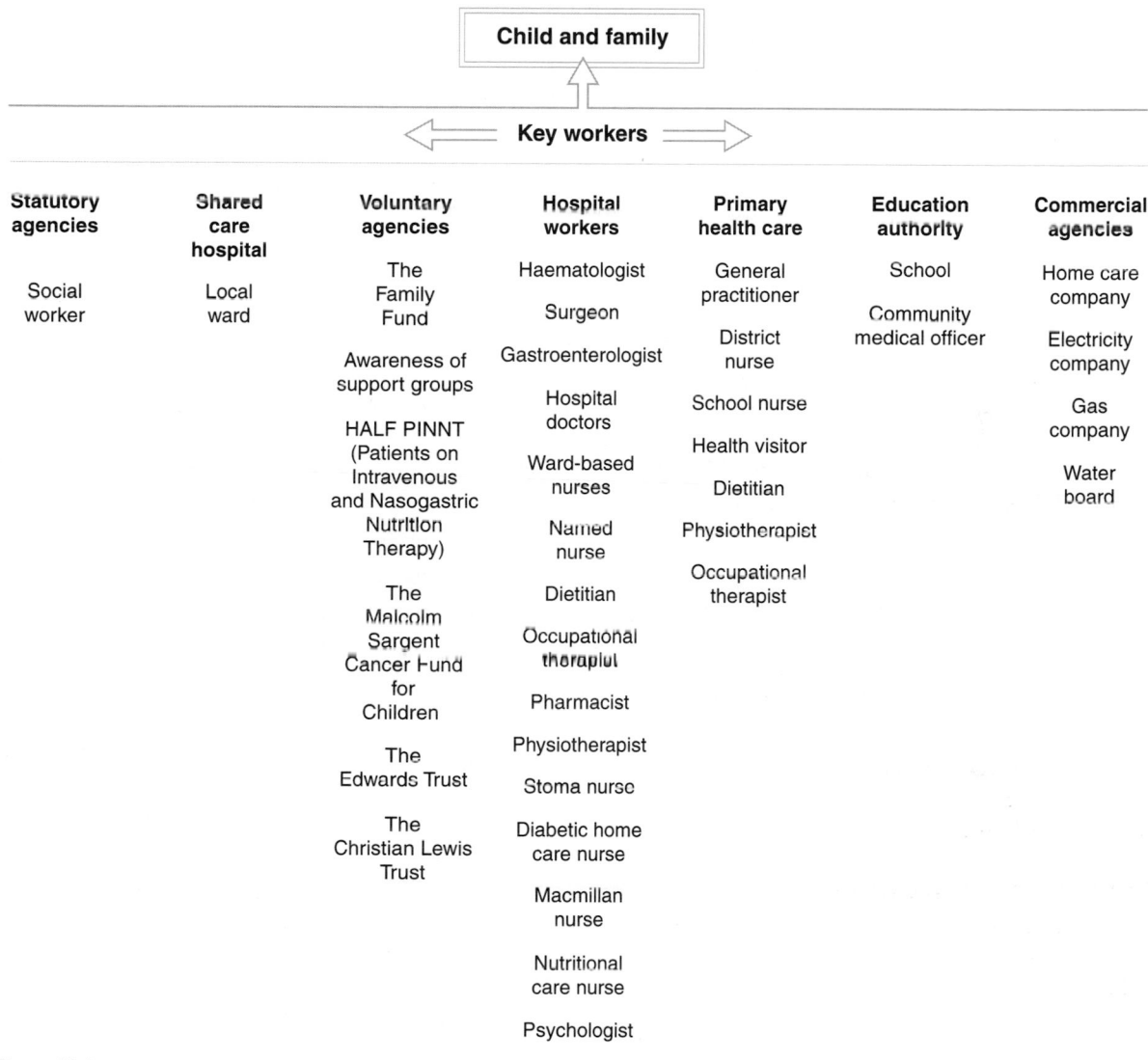

Statutory agencies	Shared care hospital	Voluntary agencies	Hospital workers	Primary health care	Education authority	Commercial agencies
Social worker	Local ward	The Family Fund	Haematologist	General practitioner	School	Home care company
		Awareness of support groups	Surgeon	District nurse	Community medical officer	Electricity company
		HALF PINNT (Patients on Intravenous and Nasogastric Nutrition Therapy)	Gastroenterologist	School nurse		Gas company
			Hospital doctors	Health visitor		Water board
			Ward-based nurses	Dietitian		
		The Malcolm Sargent Cancer Fund for Children	Named nurse	Physiotherapist		
			Dietitian	Occupational therapist		
		The Edwards Trust	Occupational therapist			
		The Christian Lewis Trust	Pharmacist			
			Physiotherapist			
			Stoma nurse			
			Diabetic home care nurse			
			Macmillan nurse			
			Nutritional care nurse			
			Psychologist			

Figure A2.1

2. The key issues would include the following

Communication:

- key worker to co-ordinate discharge planning
- key worker collates information and discusses this with the family and child
- individual and team roles to be identified
- case conference to identify needs of the child and family; discussion must take place re the responsibilities of the primary and secondary health care teams
- liaison with the child and family re their individual needs
- realistic goals to be set.

Key workers' role:

- provide easier access to the most appropriate professional
- provide realistic feedback to the family and child
- facilitate multidisciplinary discharge planning
- streamline overlapping team roles.

Professional openness:

- support for and recognition of each other member's contribution
- avoid professional rivalry.

Professional respect:

- understanding of roles and responsibilities
- recognition of families' ongoing needs for information and regular feedback

- clear, written procedures and protocols
- commitment of all team members.

3. Key issues for the family and child would include the following:

- the family and child need to know who the key worker is. Often families feel the burden of coordinating services falls upon them
- families have individual needs that must be recognised
- psychological, social and financial issues require sensitivity
- the need to understand their child's illness and how it will impact upon their lives
- support should be given as and when required in the hospital and community setting.

Key issues for the child could include:

- understanding their illness and treatment
- coping strategies required to support:
  - changing emotions
  - loss of control
  - anger
  - loss of independence
  - reliance on others
  - feeling different
  - vulnerability
  - depression
  - longing for normality at home, school, with friends and family.

Glossary

anal fissure   A small tear in the anal mucosa. It is a cause of bleeding and pain in constipation.

anorexia   Loss of appetite.

apnoea   Cessation of breathing.

appropriate for gestational age   Weight between 10th and 90th centiles for gestational age.

areola   Darker pigmented area of skin which surrounds the nipple and underneath which lie the lactiferous sinuses.

aspiration   A condition in which food or fluid is drawn into the trachea instead of the oesophagus, causing choking.

assessment tool   A tool devised to assist the collection and collation of data.

audit   A formal examination of accounts to ensure clinicians, patients and managers know of the best available evidence of clinical and cost-effectiveness.

baby-led feeding   Allowing the baby to determine the frequency and duration of the feeds.

Barker hypothesis   A hypothesis developed by Professor David Barker and colleagues at the MRC Clinical Epidemiology Unit, University of Southampton, based on epidemiological data. This group has argued convincingly that nutritional influences operating through the mother during fetal development and in early infancy determine risk of chronic disease in adult life.

cerebral palsy   A disorder of the nervous system which results in impaired movement and coordination, varying from mild involvement of a limb to severe incapacity affecting the whole body.

colostrum   Thick, yellowish, immunoglobulin-rich, vitamin-rich, high-protein milk produced during the first few days after delivery and before the production of mature breast milk.

communication   Announcement, communion, contact conversation, correspondence, despatch information, intelligence, interaction, message report.

dehydration   Lack of bodily fluids as a result of excessive loss through severe vomiting, sweating, etc., or from lack of fluid intake.

developmental age   The stage of normal development reached by an individual, regardless of his or her chronological age.

discharge planning   Coordinating all services to ensure a smooth transition from hospital to home.

dysphagia   Difficulty in swallowing.

enteral nutrition   A method of supplying nutrients to the gastro-intestinal tract. It is the term often used to describe nasogastric, nasojejunal, gastrostomy and jejunostomy feeding, although it can include food and drink taken orally.

family centred care   An approach in nursing which regards the unit of carers as being the family and where nursing care and environment help promote the strengths and individuality of the family in order to enable them greater scope for caring for their relatives.

fit   A convulsion or seizure.

foremilk   Milk produced during the early stage of a breast-feed. This high-volume milk contains more milk sugars and more protein than the hindmilk that follows it.

frenulum   The string-like membrane that attaches the tongue to the floor of the mouth. A short frenulum may cause tongue-tie, which can cause difficulty with suckling.

gastric   Pertaining to the stomach.

gastro-oesophageal reflux   The involuntary return of gastric (stomach) contents to the lower end of the oesophagus.

gastrostomy   A surgical procedure in which an artificial hole is made in the abdominal wall, through which a feeding tube can be passed.

glucose and electrolyte solution (GES)   Oral rehydration solution.

haem   An iron-containing porphyrin. This is combined with the protein globin to form haemoglobin.

hindmilk   The higher fat content, calorie-rich milk that follows the foremilk.

hypersensitivity   Increased or excessive sensitivity.

infant   A child under 12 months of age.

inter-disciplinary   The working together of two or more academic disciplines.

intrauterine growth retardation   A pathophysiological process resulting in restriction of fetal growth.

intussusception   A 'telescoping' of the bowel in a young child. This may be mistaken for gastroenteritis but is a surgical emergency.

jejunostomy   An incision into the jejunum to make an opening through which feed can be administered.

lacto-ovo-vegetarian diet   No meat, fish or poultry are consumed. Milk, eggs and other dairy products are acceptable.

lacto-vegetarian diet   No animal foods except milk and milk products are acceptable.

large for gestational age   Weight above 90th centile for gestational age.

LCPs   Long chain polyunsaturated fatty acids.

let-down reflex   The release and flow of milk that occurs as the baby starts to suckle.

low birth weight   Weight below 2500 g.

malabsorption   Faulty absorption of foodstuffs from the intestines, such as fats, vitamins and minerals.

modular feed   A feed that is formulated from separate ingredients. This allows a choice of protein, fat and carbohydrate to meet the nutritional goals and to comply with the dietary restrictions of individual patients.

Munchausen's syndrome by proxy   Fabricated illness in a child (usually fabricated by the mother). It is also known as factitious illness.

nasogastric feeding   Feeding by insertion of a tube placed in the nose and extended into the stomach.

neural tube defect   Congenital abnormalities of the brain and spinal cord comprising anencephaly, encephalocele and spina bifida.

nursing   Refers to a mother breastfeeding or suckling her child.

nursing model   A conceptual framework used in nursing to help give structure to nursing care.

nursing nutritional assessment   A holistic review by the nurse of the child's nutritional state. It includes the comprehensive information collated from all of the health care professionals involved and the child and family. Nutritional 'norms' are realized and problems identified.

nutritional needs   The identification of nutritional problems and needs, from which care and treatment are planned.

objective nutritional data   The objective data includes the physical assessment of nutritional status such as height, length and weight of the child and should be performed in conjunction with the history-taking.

occult gastro-oesophageal reflux   Gastro-oesophageal reflux disease without vomiting.

odynophagia   Pain on swallowing.

osteoporosis   A skeletal disease characterized by low bone mass and micro-architectural deterioration.

oxytocin   The hormone produced by the posterior pituitary gland which causes the let-down reflex.

parenteral nutrition The delivery of nutrients directly into the blood via an intravenous catheter.

Partnership of Care Involves parents in the care of their child in partnership with the nurse. Casey (1988, 1993) developed this discussion and formulated a framework of care which she called 'Partnership Nursing'. This framework is a logical development from the philosophy of family centred care.

peak bone mass The maximum bone mass achieved by mid-life.

pH monitoring 24-hour continuous recording by acid-sensitive probe with tip in lower oesophagus to give quantitative assessment of the severity of gastro-oesophageal reflux.

placebo An inactive 'medicine' or preparation used in the control limb of a study.

preterm infant An infant born after a gestation period of less than 37 completed weeks.

primary health care team A team of medical professionals who are involved in local health care, including the general practitioner, practice nurse and health visitor.

programming A long-lasting effect on body structure, physiology or metabolism resulting from transitory influence operating at a key stage of development.

projectile vomiting Very forceful vomits which fly out of the mouth and land some distance away. It is typical of pyloric stenosis.

prolactin A hormone produced by the anterior pituitary gland, which stimulates the breast tissue to make more breast milk.

reflux The return of food from the stomach into the mouth, short of vomiting.

rickets A disease of the immature skeleton characterized by inadequate mineralization of the bone matrix.

sham feeding A procedure carried out on babies who have not received an anastomosis (join-up operation) on their oesophagus, but have received a cervical aesophagostomy and gastrostomy. Food is given by mouth, but exits at the neck through an aesophagostomy (a surgically created opening of the upper oesophagus at the neck). Simultaneously, food is given straight into the stomach via the gastrostomy.

small for gestational age Weight below 10th centile for gestational age.

subjective nutritional data The collection of both nutritional status and nutrition intake. In order to assess this thoroughly, each child's nutritional history should be performed to assist in identifying underlying problems or changes such as inadequate intake or change in body weight. The questions should consist of questions that act as clues to the overall assessment.

team A group of individuals who share goals and work together to deliver services for which they are mutually accountable.

vegan No dairy products, eggs, meat and thus no animal foods are eaten. Vegans accept the need for vitamin B_{12} and D supplements in their diets.

very low birth weight Weight below 1500 g.

REFERENCES

Casey A 1998 A partnership with child and family. Senior Nurse 8(4):8–9

Casey A 1993 Development and use of the partnership model of nursing care. In: Glasper AE, Tucker A (eds) Advances in child health nursing. Scutari, Harrow, ch. 14

Index